A Course in Large Sample Theory

CHAPMAN & HALL TEXTS IN STATISTICAL SCIENCE SERIES

OTHER TITLES IN THE SERIES INCLUDE:

Computer-Aided Multivariate Analysis
Third edition
A. Afifi and V. Clark

Practical Statistics for Medical Research
D.G. Altman

Interpreting Data
A. J. B. Anderson

Statistical Methods for SPC and TQM
D. Bissell

Statistics in Research and Development
Second edition
R. Caulcutt

The Analysis of Time Series – An introduction
Fifth edition
C. Chatfield

Problem Solving – A statistician's guide
Second edition
C. Chatfield

Introduction to Multivariate Analysis
C. Chatfield and A. J. Collins

Modelling Binary Data
D. Collett

Modelling Survival Data in Medical Research
D. Collett

Applied Statistics
D. R. Cox and E. J. Snell

Statistical Analysis of Reliability Data
M. J. Crowder, A. C. Kimber, T. J. Sweeting and R. L. Smith

An Introduction to Generalized Linear Models
A. J. Dobson

Introduction to Optimization Methods and their Applications in Statistics
B. S. Everitt

Multivariate Statistics – A practical approach
B. Flury and H. Riedwyl

Readings in Decision Analysis
S. French

Practical Longitudinal Data Analysis
D. Hand and M. Crowder

Multivariate Analysis of Variance and Repeated Measures
D. J. Hand and C. C. Taylor

The Theory of Linear Models
B. Jørgensen

Modeling and Analysis of Stochastic Systems
V. G. Kulkarni

Statistics for Accountants
S. Letchford

Statistical Theory
Fourth edition
B. Lindgren

Randomization and Monte Carlo Methods in Biology
B. F. J. Manly

Statistical Methods in Agriculture and Experimental Biology
Second edition
R. Mead, R. N. Curnow and A. M. Hasted

Statistics in Engineering
A. V. Metcalfe

Elements of Simulation
B. J. T. Morgan

Probability – Methods and measurement
A. O'Hagan

Essential Statistics
Second edition
D. G. Rees

Large Sample Methods in Statistics
P. K. Sen and J. M. Singer

Decision analysis – A Bayesian Approach
J. Q. Smith

Applied Nonparametric Statistical Methods
Second edition
P. Sprent

Elementary Applications of Probability Theory
Second edition
H. C. Tuckwell

Statistical Process Control – Theory and practice
Third edition
G. B. Wetherill and D. W. Brown

Applied Bayesian Forecasting and Time Series Analysis
A. Pole, M. West and J. Harrison

Full information on the complete range of Chapman & Hall statistics books is available from the publishers.

A Course in Large Sample Theory

Thomas S. Ferguson
Professor of Statistics
University of California
Los Angeles
USA

CHAPMAN & HALL
London · Weinheim · New York · Tokyo · Melbourne · Madras

Published by Chapman & Hall, 2–6 Boundary Row, London SE1 8HN, UK

Chapman & Hall, 2–6 Boundary Row, London SE1 8HN, UK

Chapman & Hall GmbH, Pappelallee 3, 69469 Weinheim, Germany

Chapman & Hall USA, 115 Fifth Avenue, New York, NY 10003, USA

Chapman & Hall Japan, ITP-Japan, Kyowa Building, 3F, 2-2-1 Hirakawacho, Chiyoda-ku, Tokyo 102, Japan

Chapman & Hall Australia, 102 Dodds Street, South Melbourne, Victoria 3205, Australia

Chapman & Hall India, R. Seshadri, 32 Second Main Road, CIT East, Madras 600 035, India

First edition 1996

Typeset in the USA by Brookhaven Typesetting Systems, Brookhaven, New York
Printed in Great Britain by St Edmundsbury Press, Bury St Edmunds

ISBN 0 412 04371 8

A catalogue record for this book is available from the British Library

∞ Printed on permanent acid-free text paper, manufactured in accordance with ANSI/NISO Z39.48-1992 and ANSI/NISO Z39.48-1984 (Permanence of Paper).

Contents

Preface

The subject area of mathematical statistics is so vast that in undergraduate courses there is only time enough to present an overview of the material. In particular, proofs of theorems are often omitted, occasionally with a reference to specialized material, with the understanding that proofs will be given in later, presumably graduate, courses. Some undergraduate texts contain an outline of the proof of the central limit theorem, but other theorems useful in the large sample analysis of statistical problems are usually stated and used without proof. Typical examples concern topics such as the asymptotic normality of the maximum likelihood estimate, the asymptotic distribution of Pearson's chi-square statistic, the asymptotic distribution of the likelihood ratio test, and the asymptotic normality of the rank-sum test statistic.

But then in graduate courses, it often happens that proofs of theorems are assumed to be given in earlier, possibly undergraduate, courses, or proofs are given as they arise in specialized settings. Thus the student never learns in a general methodical way one of the most useful areas for research in statistics – large sample theory, or as it is also called, asymptotic theory. There is a need for a separate course in large sample theory at the beginning graduate level. It is hoped that this book will help in filling this need.

A course in large sample theory has been given at UCLA as the second quarter of our basic graduate course in theoretical statistics for about twenty years. The students who have learned large sample theory by the route given in this text can be said to form a large sample. Although this course is given in the Mathematics Department, the clients have been a mix of graduate students from various disciplines. Roughly 40% of the students have been from Mathematics, possibly 30% from Biostatistics, and the rest from Biomathematics, Engineering, Economics, Business, and other fields. The students generally find the course challenging and interesting, and have often contributed to the improvement of the course through questions, suggestions and, of course, complaints.

Because of the mix of students, the mathematical background required for the course has necessarily been restricted. In particular, it could not be assumed that the students have a background in measure-theoretic analysis or probability. However, for an understanding of this book, an undergraduate course in analysis is needed as well as a good undergraduate course in mathematical statistics.

Statistics is a multivariate discipline. Nearly, every useful univariate problem has important multivariate extensions and applications. For this reason, nearly all theorems are stated in a multivariate setting. Often the statement of a multivariate theorem is identical to the univariate version, but when it is not, the reader may find it useful to consider the theorem carefully in one dimension first, and then look at the examples and exercises that treat problems in higher dimensions.

The material is constructed in consideration of the student who wants to learn techniques of large sample theory on his/her own without the benefit of a classroom environment. There are many exercises, and solutions to all exercises may be found in the appendix. For use by instructors, other exercises, without solutions, can be found on the web page for the course, at http://www.stat.ucla.edu/courses/graduate/M276B/.

Each section treats a specific topic and the basic idea or central result of the section is stated as a theorem. There are 24 sections and so there are 24 theorems. The sections are grouped into four parts. In the first part, basic notions of limits in probability theory are treated, including laws of large numbers and the central limit theorem. In the second part, certain basic tools in statistical asymptotic theory, such as Slutsky's Theorem and Cramér's Theorem, are discussed and illustrated, and finally used to derive the asymptotic distribution and power of Pearson's chi-square. In the third part, certain special topics are treated by the methods of the first two parts, such as some time series statistics, some rank statistics, and distributions of quantiles and extreme order statistics. The last part contains a treatment of standard statistical techniques including maximum likelihood estimation, the likelihood ratio test, asymptotic normality of Bayes estimates, and minimum chi-square estimation. Parts 3 and 4 may be read independently. There is easily enough material in the book for a semester course. In a quarter course, some material in parts 3 and 4 will have to be omitted or skimmed.

I would like to acknowledge a great debt this book owes to Lucien Le Cam not only for specific details as one may note in references to him in the text here and there, but also for a general philosophic outlook on the subject. Since the time I learned the subject from him many years ago, he has developed a much more general and mathematical approach to the subject that may be found in his book, Le Cam (1986) mentioned in the references.

Rudimentary versions of this book in the form of notes have been in existence for some 20 years, and have undergone several changes in computer systems and word processors. I am indebted to my wife, Beatriz, for cheerfully typing some of these conversions. Finally, I am indebted to my students, too numerous to mention individually. Each class was distinctive and each class taught me something new so that the next year's class was taught somewhat differently than the last. If future students find this book helpful, they also can thank these students for their contribution to making it understandable.

Thomas S. Ferguson, April 1996

1

Basic Probability Theory

1

Modes of Convergence

We begin by studying the relationships among four distinct modes of convergence of a sequence of random vectors to a limit. All convergences are defined for d-dimensional random vectors. For a random vector $\mathbf{X} = (X_1, \ldots, X_d) \in \mathbb{R}^d$, the distribution function of $\mathbf{X}$, defined for $\mathbf{x} = (x_1, \ldots, x_d) \in \mathbb{R}^d$, is denoted by $F_{\mathbf{X}}(\mathbf{x}) = P(\mathbf{X} \le \mathbf{x}) = P(X_1 \le x_1, \ldots, X_d \le x_d)$. The Euclidean norm of $\mathbf{x} = (x_1, \ldots, x_d) \in \mathbb{R}^d$ is denoted by $|\mathbf{x}| = (x_1^2 + \cdots + x_d^2)^{1/2}$. Let $\mathbf{X}, \mathbf{X}_1, \mathbf{X}_2, \ldots$ be random vectors with values in $\mathbb{R}^d$.

Definition 1. $\mathbf{X}_n$ converges *in law* to $\mathbf{X}$, $\mathbf{X}_n \xrightarrow{\mathscr{L}} \mathbf{X}$, if $F_{\mathbf{X}_n}(\mathbf{x}) \longrightarrow F_{\mathbf{X}}(\mathbf{x})$ as $n \to \infty$, for all points $\mathbf{x}$ at which $F_{\mathbf{X}}(\mathbf{x})$ is continuous.

Convergence in law is the mode of convergence most used in the following chapters. It is the mode found in the Central Limit Theorem and is sometimes called convergence *in distribution*, or *weak* convergence.

Example 1. We say that a random vector $\mathbf{X} \in \mathbb{R}^d$ is degenerate at a point $\mathbf{c} \in \mathbb{R}^d$ if $P(\mathbf{X} = \mathbf{c}) = 1$. Let $X_n \in \mathbb{R}^1$ be degenerate at the point $1/n$, for $n = 1, 2, \ldots$ and let $X \in \mathbb{R}^1$ be degenerate at 0. Since $1/n$ converges to zero as n tends to infinity, it may be expected that $X_n \xrightarrow{\mathscr{L}} X$. This may be seen by checking Definition 1. The distribution function of X_n is $F_{X_n}(x) = I_{[1/n,\infty)}(x)$, and that of X is $F_X(x) = I_{[0,\infty]}(x)$, where $I_A(x)$ denotes the indicator function of the set A (i.e., $I_A(x)$ denotes 1 if $x \in A$, and 0 otherwise). Then $F_{X_n}(x) \longrightarrow F_X(x)$ for all x except $x = 0$, and for $x = 0$ we have $F_{X_n}(0) = 0 \nrightarrow F_X(0) = 1$. But because $F_X(x)$ is not continuous at $x = 0$, we nevertheless have $X_n \xrightarrow{\mathscr{L}} X$ from Definition 1. This shows the need, in the definition of convergence in law, to exclude points x at which $F_X(x)$ is not continuous.

Definition 2. $\mathbf{X}_n$ converges *in probability* to $\mathbf{X}$, $\mathbf{X}_n \xrightarrow{\text{P}} \mathbf{X}$, if for every $\varepsilon > 0$, $P\{|\mathbf{X}_n - \mathbf{X}| > \varepsilon\} \longrightarrow 0$ as $n \longrightarrow \infty$.

Definition 3. For a real number $r > 0$, $\mathbf{X}_n$ converges *in the rth mean* to $\mathbf{X}$, $\mathbf{X}_n \xrightarrow{r} \mathbf{X}$, if $E|\mathbf{X}_n - \mathbf{X}|^r \longrightarrow 0$ as $n \longrightarrow \infty$.

Definition 4. $\mathbf{X}_n$ converges *almost surely* to $\mathbf{X}$, $\mathbf{X}_n \xrightarrow{\text{a.s.}} \mathbf{X}$, if

$$P\{\lim_{n\to\infty} \mathbf{X}_n = \mathbf{X}\} = 1.$$

Almost sure convergence is sometimes called convergence *with probability* 1 (w.p. 1) or *strong* convergence. In statistics, convergence in the rth mean is most useful for $r = 2$, when it is called convergence *in quadratic mean*, and is written $\mathbf{X}_n \xrightarrow{\text{qm}} \mathbf{X}$. The basic relationships are as follows.

Theorem 1.

a) $\mathbf{X}_n \xrightarrow{\text{a.s}} \mathbf{X} \Rightarrow \mathbf{X}_n \xrightarrow{\text{P}} \mathbf{X}$.
b) $\mathbf{X}_n \xrightarrow{r} \mathbf{X}$ *for some* $r > 0 \Rightarrow \mathbf{X}_n \xrightarrow{\text{P}} \mathbf{X}$.
c) $\mathbf{X}_n \xrightarrow{\text{P}} \mathbf{X} \Rightarrow \mathbf{X}_n \xrightarrow{\mathscr{L}} \mathbf{X}$.

Theorem 1 states the only universally valid implications between the various modes of convergence, as the following examples show.

Example 2. To check convergence in law, nothing needs to be known about the joint distribution of $\mathbf{X}_n$ and $\mathbf{X}$, whereas this distribution must be defined to check convergence in probability. For example, if $\mathbf{X}_1, \mathbf{X}_2, \ldots$ are independent and identically distributed (i.i.d.) normal random variables, with mean 0 and variance 1, then $X_n \xrightarrow{\mathscr{L}} X_1$, yet $X_n \overset{\text{P}}{\nrightarrow} X_1$.

Example 3. Let Z be a random variable with a uniform distribution on the interval $(0, 1)$, $Z \in \mathscr{U}(0, 1)$, and let $X_1 = 1$, $X_2 = I_{[0,\,1/2)}(Z)$, $X_3 = i\mathrm{I}_{[1/2,\,1)}(Z)$, $X_4 = I_{[0,\,1/4)}(Z)$, $X_5 = I_{[1/4,\,1/2)}(Z), \ldots$. In general, if $n = 2^k + m$, where $0 \le m < 2^k$ and $k \ge 0$, then $X_n = I_{[m2^{-k},\,(m+1)2^{-k})}(Z)$. Then X_n does not converge for any $Z \in [0, 1)$, so $X_n \overset{\text{a.s.}}{\nrightarrow} 0$. Yet $X_n \xrightarrow{r} 0$ for all $r > 0$ and $X_n \xrightarrow{\text{P}} 0$.

Example 4. Let Z be $\mathscr{U}(0,1)$ and let $X_n = 2^n I_{[0,1/n)}(Z)$. Then $E|X_n|^r = 2^{nr}/n \longrightarrow \infty$, so $X_n \overset{r}{\nrightarrow} 0$ for any $r > 0$. Yet $X_n \xrightarrow{\text{a.s.}} 0$ ($\{\lim_{n\to\infty} X_n = 0\} = \{Z > 0\}$, and $P\{Z > 0\} = 1$), and $X_n \xrightarrow{\text{P}} 0$ (if $0 < \varepsilon < 1$, $P(|X_n| > \varepsilon) = P(X_n = 2^n) = 1/n \longrightarrow 0$).

In this example, we have $0 \le X_n \xrightarrow{\text{a.s.}} X$ and $\lim_{n\to\infty} EX_n > EX$. That we cannot have $0 \le X_n \xrightarrow{\text{a.s.}} X$ and $\lim_{n\to\infty} EX_n < EX$ follows from the *Fatou–Lebesgue Lemma*. This states: If $X_n \xrightarrow{\text{a.s.}} X$ and if for all n $X_n \ge Y$ for some random variable Y with $E|Y| < \infty$, then $\liminf_{n\to\infty} EX_n \ge EX$. In particular, this implies the *Monotone Convergence Theorem*: If $0 \le X_1 \le X_2 \le \cdots$ and $X_n \xrightarrow{\text{a.s.}} X$, then $EX_n \longrightarrow EX$. In these theorems, X, EX_n, and EX may take the value $+\infty$.

The Fatou–Lebesgue Lemma also implies the basic *Lebesgue Dominated Convergence Theorem*: If $X_n \xrightarrow{\text{a.s.}} X$ and if $|X_n| \le Y$ for some random variable Y with $E|Y| < \infty$, then $EX_n \longrightarrow EX$.

The following lemma contains an equivalent definition of almost sure convergence. It clarifies the distinction between convergence in probability and convergence almost surely. For convergence in probability, one needs for every $\varepsilon > 0$ that the probability that $\mathbf{X}_n$ is within ε of $\mathbf{X}$ tends to one. For convergence almost surely, one needs for every $\varepsilon > 0$ that the probability that $\mathbf{X}_k$ stays within ε of $\mathbf{X}$ for all $k \ge n$ tends to one as n tends to infinity.

Lemma 1. $\mathbf{X}_n \xrightarrow{\text{a.s.}} \mathbf{X}$ *if and only if for every* $\varepsilon > 0$,

$$P\{|\mathbf{X}_k - \mathbf{X}| < \varepsilon, \text{ for all } k \ge n\} \longrightarrow 1 \qquad \text{as } n \longrightarrow \infty. \tag{1}$$

Proof. Let $A_{n,\varepsilon} = \{|\mathbf{X}_k - \mathbf{X}| < \varepsilon \text{ for all } k \ge n\}$. Then $P\{\lim_{n\to\infty} \mathbf{X}_n = \mathbf{X}\} = P$ {for every $\varepsilon > 0$, there exists an n such that $|\mathbf{X}_k - \mathbf{X}| < \varepsilon$ for all $k \ge n\} = P\{\bigcap_{\varepsilon>0} \bigcup_n A_{n,\varepsilon}\}$. Thus, $\mathbf{X}_n \xrightarrow{\text{a.s.}} \mathbf{X}$ is equivalent to

$$P\left\{\bigcap_{\varepsilon>0} \bigcup_n A_{n,\varepsilon}\right\} = 1. \tag{2}$$

Because the sets $\bigcup_n A_{n,\varepsilon}$ decrease to $\bigcap_{\varepsilon>0} \bigcup_n A_{n,\varepsilon}$ as $\varepsilon \to 0$, (2) is equivalent to $P\{\bigcup_n A_{n,\varepsilon}\} = 1$ for all $\varepsilon > 0$. Then, because $A_{n,\varepsilon}$ increases to $\bigcup_n A_{n,\varepsilon}$ as $n \longrightarrow \infty$, this in turn is equivalent to

$$P\{A_{n,\varepsilon}\} \longrightarrow 1 \text{ as } n \longrightarrow \infty, \qquad \text{for all } \varepsilon > 0, \tag{3}$$

which is exactly (1). ∎

Proof of Theorem 1.

(a) $\mathbf{X}_n \xrightarrow{\text{a.s.}} \mathbf{X} \Rightarrow \mathbf{X}_n \xrightarrow{\text{P}} \mathbf{X}$: Let $\varepsilon > 0$. Then

$$P\{|\mathbf{X}_n - \mathbf{X}| \leq \varepsilon\} \geq P\{|\mathbf{X}_k - \mathbf{X}| \leq \varepsilon, \text{ for all } k \geq n\} \longrightarrow 1 \text{ as } n \to \infty,$$

from Lemma 1.

(b) $\mathbf{X}_n \xrightarrow{r} \mathbf{X} \Rightarrow \mathbf{X}_n \xrightarrow{\text{P}} \mathbf{X}$: We let $I(\mathbf{X} \in A)$ denote the indicator random variable that is equal to 1 if $\mathbf{X} \in A$ and to 0 otherwise. Note that

$$E|\mathbf{X}_n - \mathbf{X}|^r \geq E\big[|\mathbf{X}_n - \mathbf{X}|^r I\{|\mathbf{X}_n - \mathbf{X}| \geq \varepsilon\}\big] \geq \varepsilon^r P\{|\mathbf{X}_n - \mathbf{X}| \geq \varepsilon\}.$$

(This is *Chebyshev's Inequality*.) The result follows by letting $n \longrightarrow \infty$.

(c) $\mathbf{X}_n \xrightarrow{P} \mathbf{X} \Rightarrow \mathbf{X}_n \xrightarrow{\mathscr{L}} \mathbf{X}$: Let $\varepsilon > 0$ and let $\mathbf{1} \in \mathbb{R}^d$ represent the vector with 1 in every component. If $\mathbf{X}_n \leq \mathbf{x}_0$, then either $\mathbf{X} \leq \mathbf{x}_0 + \varepsilon\mathbf{1}$ or $|\mathbf{X} - \mathbf{X}_n| > \varepsilon$. In other words, $\{\mathbf{X}_n \leq \mathbf{x}_0\} \subset \{\mathbf{X} \leq \mathbf{x}_0 + \varepsilon\mathbf{1}\} \cup \{|\mathbf{X} - \mathbf{X}_n| > \varepsilon\}$. Hence,

$$F_{\mathbf{X}_n}(\mathbf{x}_0) \leq F_{\mathbf{X}}(\mathbf{x}_0 + \varepsilon\mathbf{1}) + P\{|\mathbf{X} - \mathbf{X}_n| > \varepsilon\}.$$

Similarly,

$$F_{\mathbf{X}}(\mathbf{X}_0 - \varepsilon\mathbf{1}) \leq F_{\mathbf{X}_n}(\mathbf{x}_0) + P\{|\mathbf{X} - \mathbf{X}_n| > \varepsilon\}.$$

Hence, since $P\{|\mathbf{X} - \mathbf{X}_n| > \varepsilon\} \longrightarrow 0$ as $n \longrightarrow \infty$,

$$F_{\mathbf{X}}(\mathbf{x}_0 - \varepsilon\mathbf{1}) \leq \liminf F_{\mathbf{X}_n}(\mathbf{x}_0) \leq \limsup \mathbf{F}_{\mathbf{X}_n}(\mathbf{x}_0) \leq F_{\mathbf{X}}(\mathbf{x}_0 + \varepsilon\mathbf{1}).$$

If $F_{\mathbf{X}}(\mathbf{x})$ is continuous at $\mathbf{x}_0$, then the left and right ends of this inequality both converge to $F_{\mathbf{X}}(\mathbf{x}_0)$ as $\varepsilon \longrightarrow 0$, implying that

$$F_{\mathbf{X}_n}(\mathbf{x}_0) \longrightarrow F_{\mathbf{X}}(\mathbf{x}_0) \text{ as } n \longrightarrow \infty. \quad \blacksquare$$

EXERCISES

1. Suppose $X_n \in \mathscr{B}e(1/n, 1/n)$ (beta) and $X \in \mathscr{B}(1, 1/2)$ (binomial). Show that $X_n \xrightarrow{\mathscr{L}} X$. What if $X_n \in \mathscr{B}e(\alpha/n, \beta/n)$?
2. Suppose X_n is uniformly distributed on the set of points $\{1/n, 2/n, \ldots, 1\}$. Show that $X_n \xrightarrow{\mathscr{L}} X$, where X is $\mathscr{U}(0, 1)$. Does $X_n \xrightarrow{\text{P}} X$?
3. (a) Show that if $0 < r' < r$ and $E|X|^r < \infty$, then $E|X|^{r'} < \infty$.
   (b) Show that if $0 < r' < r$ and $X_n \xrightarrow{r} X$ then $X_n \xrightarrow{r'} X$. You may use *Hölder's Inequality*: For nonnegative random variables X and Y with finite means, $EX^pY^{1-p} \leq (EX)^p(EY)^{1-p}$ for $0 \leq p \leq 1$.
4. Give an example of random variables X_n such that $E|X_n| \to 0$ and $E|X_n|^2 \longrightarrow 1$.

5. Let μ be a constant. Show that $X_n \xrightarrow{\text{qm}} \mu$ if and only if $EX_n \longrightarrow \mu$, and $\text{var}(X_n) \longrightarrow 0$.
6. If the limiting distribution function, $F_{\mathbf{X}}$, is continuous, then the definition of convergence in law is simply that $F_{\mathbf{X}_n}(\mathbf{x}) \longrightarrow F_{\mathbf{X}}(\mathbf{x})$ as $n \longrightarrow \infty$, for all $\mathbf{x}$. However, in this case, it automatically follows that the convergence is uniform in $\mathbf{x}$. Prove this in one dimension: If F_X is continuous and $X_n \xrightarrow{\mathscr{L}} X$ as $n \longrightarrow \infty$, then $\sup_x |F_{X_n}(x) - F_X(x)| \longrightarrow 0$ as $n \longrightarrow \infty$.
7. Using the Fatou–Lebesgue Lemma, (a) prove the Monotone Convergence Theorem, and (b) prove the Lebesgue Dominated Convergence Theorem.

2

Partial Converses to Theorem 1

Although complete converses to the statements of Theorem 1 are invalid, as we have seen, under certain additional conditions some important partial converses hold. We use the same symbol $\mathbf{c}$ to denote the point $\mathbf{c} \in \mathbb{R}^d$, as well as the degenerate random vector identically equal to $\mathbf{c}$.

Theorem 2.

(a) *If* $\mathbf{c} \in \mathbb{R}^d$, *then* $\mathbf{X}_n \xrightarrow{\mathscr{L}} \mathbf{c} \Rightarrow \mathbf{X}_n \xrightarrow{\mathrm{P}} \mathbf{c}$.
(b) *If* $\mathbf{X}_n \xrightarrow{\text{a.s.}} \mathbf{X}$ *and* $|\mathbf{X}_n|^r \le Z$ *for some* $r > 0$ *and some random variable* Z *with* $EZ < \infty$, *then* $\mathbf{X}_n \xrightarrow{r} \mathbf{X}$.
(c) [*Scheffé* (1947)]. *If* $\mathbf{X}_n \xrightarrow{\text{a.s.}} \mathbf{X}$, $\mathbf{X}_n \ge 0$, *and* $E\mathbf{X}_n \to E\mathbf{X} < \infty$, *then* $\mathbf{X}_n \xrightarrow{r} \mathbf{X}$, *where* $r = 1$.
(d) $\mathbf{X}_n \xrightarrow{\mathrm{P}} \mathbf{X}$ *if and only if every subsequence* $n_1, n_2, \ldots \varepsilon \{1, 2, \ldots\}$ *has a sub-sequence* $m_1, m_2, \ldots \varepsilon \{n_1, n_2, \ldots\}$ *such that* $\mathbf{X}_{m_j} \xrightarrow{\text{a.s.}} \mathbf{X}$ *as* $j \to \infty$.

Remarks. Part (a), together with part (c) of Theorem 1, implies that convergence in law and convergence in probability are equivalent if the limit is a constant random vector. In the following sections we use this equivalence often without explicit mention.

Part (b) gives a method of deducing convergence in the rth mean from almost sure convergence. See Exercise 3 for a strengthening of this result, and Exercise 2 for a simple sufficient condition for almost sure convergence.

Part (c) is sometimes called Scheffé's Useful Convergence Theorem because of the title of Scheffé's 1947 article. It is usually stated in terms of densities (nonnegative functions that integrate to one) as follows: If $f_n(x)$ and $g(x)$ are densities such that $f_n(x) \to g(x)$ for all x, then $\int |f_n(x) - g(x)|\, dx \to 0$. [The hypotheses $f_n(x) \ge 0$ and $\int f_n(x)\, dx \to \int g(x)\, dx$ are automatic here. The proof of this is analogous to the proof of (c) given below.]

Pointwise convergence of densities is a type of convergence in distribution that is much stronger than convergence in law. Convergence in law only requires that $P(\mathbf{X}_n \in A)$ converge to $P(\mathbf{X} \in A)$ for certain sets A of the form $\{\mathbf{x}: \mathbf{x} \le \mathbf{a}\}$. If the densities converge, then $P(\mathbf{X}_n \in A)$ converges to $P(\mathbf{X} \in A)$ for all Borel sets A, and, moreover, the convergence is uniform in A. In other words, suppose that $\mathbf{X}_n$ and $\mathbf{X}$ have densities (with respect to a measure ν) denoted by $f_n(\mathbf{x})$ and $f(\mathbf{x})$, respectively. Then, if $f_n(\mathbf{x}) \longrightarrow f(\mathbf{x})$ for all $\mathbf{x}$, we have

$$\sup_A |P(\mathbf{X}_n \in A) - P(\mathbf{X} \in A)| \longrightarrow 0.$$

The proof is an exercise. We will encounter this type of convergence later in the Bernstein–von Mises Theorem.

As an illustration of the difference between this type of convergence and convergence in law, suppose that X_n is uniformly distributed on the set $\{1/n, 2/n, \ldots, n/n\}$. Then $X_n \xrightarrow{\mathscr{L}} X \in \mathscr{U}(0,1)$, the uniform distribution on $[0,1]$, but $P(\mathbf{X}_n \in A)$ does not converge to $P(\mathbf{X} \in A)$ for all A. For example, if $A = \{x\colon x \text{ is rational}\}$, then $P(\mathbf{X}_n \in A) = 1$ does not converge to $P(\mathbf{X} \in A) = 0$.

Part (d) is a tool for dealing with convergence in probability using convergence almost surely. Generally convergence almost surely is easier to work with. Here is an example of the use of part (d). If $\mathbf{X}_n \longrightarrow \mathbf{X}$ with probability one (i.e., almost surely), and if $g(\mathbf{x})$ is a continuous function of $\mathbf{x}$, then it is immediate that $g(\mathbf{X}_n) \longrightarrow g(\mathbf{X})$ with probability one. Is the same result true if convergence almost surely is replaced by convergence in probability? Assume $\mathbf{X}_n \xrightarrow{\text{P}} \mathbf{X}$ and let $g(\mathbf{x})$ be a continuous function of $\mathbf{x}$. To show $g(\mathbf{X}_n) \xrightarrow{\text{P}} g(\mathbf{X})$, it is sufficient, according to part (d), to show that for every subsequence, $n_1, n_2, \ldots \varepsilon \{1, 2, \ldots\}$, there is a sub-subsequence, $m_1, m_2, \ldots \varepsilon \{n_1, n_2, \ldots\}$ such that $g(\mathbf{X}_{m_i}) \xrightarrow{\text{a.s.}} g(\mathbf{X})$ as $i \longrightarrow \infty$. So let $n_1, n_2, \ldots$ be an arbitrary subsequence and find, using part (d), a sub-subsequence $m_1, m_2, \ldots \varepsilon \{n_1, n_2, \ldots\}$ so that $\mathbf{X}_{m_i} \xrightarrow{\text{a.s.}} \mathbf{X}$. Then $g(\mathbf{X}_{m_i}) \xrightarrow{\text{a.s.}} g(\mathbf{X})$, since $g(\mathbf{x})$ is continuous, and the result is proved.

Proof of Theorem 2. (a) (In two dimensions)

$$\begin{aligned} P\{|\mathbf{X}_n - \mathbf{c}| \le \varepsilon\sqrt{2}\} &\ge P\left\{\mathbf{c} - \varepsilon\begin{pmatrix}1\\1\end{pmatrix} < \mathbf{X}_n \le \mathbf{c} + \varepsilon\begin{pmatrix}1\\1\end{pmatrix}\right\} \\ &= P\left\{\mathbf{X}_n \le \mathbf{c} + \varepsilon\begin{pmatrix}1\\1\end{pmatrix}\right\} - P\left\{\mathbf{X}_n \le \mathbf{c} + \varepsilon\begin{pmatrix}1\\-1\end{pmatrix}\right\} \\ &\quad - P\left\{\mathbf{X}_n \le \mathbf{c} + \varepsilon\begin{pmatrix}-1\\1\end{pmatrix}\right\} + P\left\{\mathbf{X}_n \le \mathbf{c} - \varepsilon\begin{pmatrix}1\\1\end{pmatrix}\right\} \end{aligned}$$

Here is a picture:

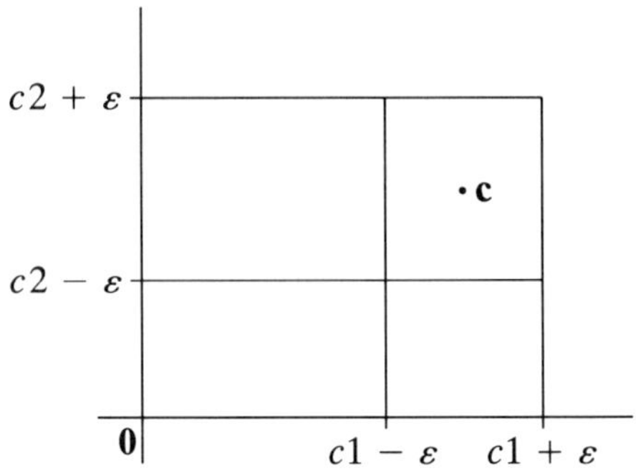

(b) This is the Lebesgue Dominated Convergence Theorem in d dimensions. Note that $\mathbf{X}_n \xrightarrow{\text{a.s.}} \mathbf{X}$ and $|\mathbf{X}_n|^r \le Z$ implies $|\mathbf{X}|^r \le Z$ a.s., so that $|\mathbf{X}_n - \mathbf{X}|^r \le (|\mathbf{X}_n| + |\mathbf{X}|)^r \le (Z^{1/r} + Z^{1/r})^r \le 2^r Z$ a.s. Now apply the Lebesgue Dominated Convergence Theorem in the form given in the previous section replacing X_n by $|\mathbf{X}_n - \mathbf{X}|^r$ and X by 0.

(c) Let x^+ denote the positive part of x: $x^+ = \max\{0, x\}$. In one dimension, for a real number x, $|x| = x + 2(-x)^+$; hence $E|X_n - X| = E(X_n - X) + 2E(X - X_n)^+$. The first term converges to zero because $EX_n \to EX$. The second term converges to zero by the Lebesgue Dominated Convergence Theorem, because $0 \le (X - X_n)^+ \le X^+$ and $EX^+ < \infty$. For dimensions greater than one, use the triangle inequality, $|\mathbf{X}_n - \mathbf{X}| \le \sum_{j=1}^{d} |X_{nj} - X_j|$, and use the above analysis on each term separately.

The proof of part (d) is based on the Borel–Cantelli Lemma. For events A_j, $j = 0, 1, \ldots,$ the event $\{A_j \text{ i.o.}\}$ (read A_j *infinitely often*), stands for the event that infinitely many A_j occur.

The Borel–Cantelli Lemma. *If* $\sum_{j=1}^{\infty} P(A_j) < \infty$, *then* $P\{A_j \text{ i.o.}\} = 0$. *Conversely, if the* A_j *are independent and* $\sum_{j=1}^{\infty} P(A_j) = \infty$, *then* $P\{A_j \text{ i.o.}\} = 1$.

Proof. (The general half) If infinitely many of the A_j occur, then for all n, at least one A_j with $j \ge n$ occurs. Hence,

$$P\{A_j \text{ i.o.}\} \le P\left\{\bigcup_{j=n}^{\infty} A_j\right\} \le \sum_{j=n}^{\infty} P(A_j) \to 0. \quad \blacksquare$$

The proof of the converse is an exercise. (See Exercise 4.)

A typical example of the use of the Borel–Cantelli Lemma occurs in coin tossing. Let $X_1, X_2, \ldots$ be a sequence of independent Bernoulli trials with probability of success on the nth trial equal to p_n. What is the probability of an infinite number of successes? Or, equivalently, what is $P\{X_n = 1 \text{ i.o.}\}$? From the Borel–Cantelli Lemma and its converse, this probability is zero or one depending on whether $\sum p_n < \infty$ or not. If $p_n = 1/n^2$, for example, then $P\{X_n = 1 \text{ i.o.}\} = 0$. If $p_n = 1/n$, then $P\{X_n = 1 \text{ i.o.}\} = 1$.

The Borel–Cantelli Lemma is useful in dealing with problems involving almost sure convergence because $\mathbf{X}_n \xrightarrow{\text{a.s.}} \mathbf{X}$ is equivalent to

$$P\{|\mathbf{X}_n - \mathbf{X}| > \varepsilon \text{ i.o.}\} = 0, \qquad \text{for all } \varepsilon > 0.$$

(d) (If) Suppose $\mathbf{X}_n$ does not converge in probability to $\mathbf{X}$. Then there exists an $\varepsilon > 0$ and a $\delta > 0$ such that $P\{|X_n - X| > \varepsilon\} > \delta$ for infinitely many n, say $\{n_j\}$. Then no subsequence of $\{n_j\}$ converges in probability, nor, consequently, almost surely.

(Only if) Let $\varepsilon_n > 0$ and $\sum_{j=1}^{\infty} \varepsilon_j < \infty$. Find n_j such that $P\{|\mathbf{X}_n - \mathbf{X}| \geq \varepsilon_j\} < \varepsilon_j$ for all $n \geq n_j$, and assume without loss of generality that $n_1 < n_2 < \ldots$. Let $A_j = \{|\mathbf{X}_{n_j} - \mathbf{X}| \geq \varepsilon_j\}$. Then, $\sum_{j=1}^{\infty} P(A_j) \leq \sum_{j=1}^{\infty} \varepsilon_j < \infty$, so by the Borel–Cantelli Lemma, $P\{A_j \text{ i.o.}\} = 0$. This says that with probability 1, $|\mathbf{X}_{n_j} - \mathbf{X}| \geq \varepsilon_j$ occurs only finitely many times. Since $\varepsilon_j \to 0$, we have for any $\varepsilon > 0$ that with probability 1, $|\mathbf{X}_{n_j} - \mathbf{X}| \geq \varepsilon$ occurs only finitely many times. Hence, $\mathbf{X}_{n_j} \xrightarrow{\text{a.s.}} \mathbf{X}$; that is $P\{|\mathbf{X}_{n_j} - \mathbf{X}| > \varepsilon \text{ i.o.}\} = 0$ for all $\varepsilon > 0$. Similarly, if n' is any subsequence, $\mathbf{X}_{n'} \xrightarrow{\text{P}} \mathbf{X}$, so we can find a sub-subsequence n'' of n' such that $\mathbf{X}_{n''} \xrightarrow{\text{a.s.}} \mathbf{X}$. ■

EXERCISES

1. Let $X_1, X_2, \ldots$ be independent identically distributed with densities $f(x) = \alpha x^{-(\alpha+1)} I_{(1,\infty)}(x)$. (a) For what values of $\alpha > 0$ and $r > 0$ is it true that $(1/n)X_n \xrightarrow{r} 0$? (b) For what values of $\alpha > 0$ is it true that $(1/n)X_n \xrightarrow{\text{a.s.}} 0$? (Use the Borel–Cantelli Lemma.)
2. Show that if $\sum E(\mathbf{X}_n - \mathbf{X})^2 < \infty$, then $\mathbf{X}_n \xrightarrow{\text{a.s.}} \mathbf{X}$ and $\mathbf{X}_n \xrightarrow{\text{qm}} \mathbf{X}$. Show that if $\sum E|\mathbf{X}_n - \mathbf{X}|^r < \infty$, then $\mathbf{X}_n \xrightarrow{\text{a.s.}} \mathbf{X}$ and $\mathbf{X}_n \xrightarrow{r} \mathbf{X}$.
3. Improve Theorem 2(b) and Theorem 2(c) by using Theorem 2(d) to show
   (a) If $\mathbf{X}_n \xrightarrow{\text{P}} \mathbf{X}$ and $|\mathbf{X}_n|^r \leq Z$ for some $r > 0$ and some random variable $\mathbf{Z}$ such that $EZ < \infty$, then $\mathbf{X}_n \xrightarrow{r} \mathbf{X}$.
   (b) If $\mathbf{X}_n \xrightarrow{\text{P}} \mathbf{X}$, $\mathbf{X}_n \geq 0$, and $E\mathbf{X}_n \to E\mathbf{X} < \infty$, then $\mathbf{X}_n \xrightarrow{r} \mathbf{X}$, where $r = 1$.

4. (a) Give an example of events $A_1, A_2, \ldots$ such that $\sum_{j=1}^{\infty} P(A_j) = \infty$ and $P(A_j \text{ i.o.}) = 0$.
   (b) Show that if $A_1, A_2, \ldots$ are independent events such that $\sum_{j=1}^{\infty} P(A_j) = \infty$, then $P(A_j \text{ i.o.}) = 1$.
   (Hint: Show that $P\{A_j \text{ finitely often}\} = P\{\cup_n \cap_{j>n} A_j^c\} = \lim_{n\to\infty} \prod_{j>n}(1 - P\{A_j\}) \le \lim_{n\to\infty} \exp\{-\sum_{j>n} P(A_j)\}$.)
5. Let $X_1, X_2, \ldots$ be independent random variables such that $P\{X_n = n^\alpha\} = 1/n$ and $P\{X_n = 0\} = 1 - 1/n$ for $n = 1, 2, \ldots,$ where α is a constant. For what values of α, $-\infty < \alpha < \infty$, is it true that
   (a) $X_n \xrightarrow{\text{P}} 0$?
   (b) $X_n \xrightarrow{\text{a.s.}} 0$?
   (c) $X_n \xrightarrow{r} 0$ for a given $r > 0$?
6. (a) Suppose $f_n(x)$ and $g(x)$ are densities such that for all x, $f_n(x) \to g(x)$ as $n \to \infty$. Show that

$$\int |f_n(x) - g(x)|\, dx \to 0 \text{ as } n \to \infty.$$

   (b) Show that if X_n has density $f_n(x)$, if X has density $g(x)$, and if $\int |f_n(x) - g(x)|\, dx \to 0$ as $n \to \infty$, then

$$\sup_A |P(X_n \in A) - P(X \in A)| \to 0 \text{ as } n \to \infty.$$

7. Prove the following strengthening of Scheffé's Theorem: If $X_n \xrightarrow{\text{a.s.}} X$ and if $E|X_n| \to E|X| < \infty$, then $E|X_n - X| \to 0$.
8. Show if $X_n \xrightarrow{\text{a.s.}} X$ and if $EX_n^2 \to EX^2$, then $X_n \xrightarrow{\text{qm}} X$.

3

Convergence in Law

In this section, we investigate the relationship between convergence in law of a sequence of random vectors and convergence of expectations of functions of the vectors. The basic result is that $\mathbf{X}_n \xrightarrow{\mathscr{L}} \mathbf{X}$ if and only if $Eg(\mathbf{X}_n) \to Eg(\mathbf{X})$ for all continuous bounded functions g. We conclude with the Continuity Theorem that relates convergence in law of a sequence of random vectors with convergence of the corresponding characteristic functions.

Let g represent a *real-valued* function defined on $\mathbb{R}^d$. We say that g vanishes outside a compact set if there is a compact set $C \subset \mathbb{R}^d$ such that $g(\mathbf{x}) = 0$ for all $\mathbf{x} \notin C$.

THEOREM 3. *The following conditions are equivalent.*

(a) $\mathbf{X}_n \xrightarrow{\mathscr{L}} \mathbf{X}$.
(b) $Eg(\mathbf{X}_n) \to Eg(\mathbf{X})$ *for all continuous functions g that vanish outside a compact set.*
(c) $Eg(\mathbf{X}_n) \to Eg(\mathbf{X})$ *for all continuous bounded functions g.*
(d) $Eg(\mathbf{X}_n) \to Eg(\mathbf{X})$ *for all bounded measurable functions g such that $P\{\mathbf{X} \in C(g)\} = 1$, where $C(g) = \{\mathbf{x}\colon g$ is continuous at $\mathbf{x}\}$ is called the continuity set of g.*

The implication (a) ⇒ (b) or (c) or (d) is known as the *Helly–Bray Theorem*. For example, it implies that $E\cos(X_n) \to E\cos(X)$ whenever $X_n \xrightarrow{\mathscr{L}} X$, because $\cos(x)$ is continuous and bounded. We now give some counterexamples to show the necessity of the boundedness and continuity conditions.

Example 1. Let $g(x) = x$, and let

$$X_n = \begin{cases} n & \text{with probability } 1/n, \\ 0, & \text{with probability } (n-1)/n. \end{cases}$$

Then $X_n \xrightarrow{\mathscr{L}} X = 0$, but $Eg(X_n) = n \cdot 1/n = 1 \nrightarrow Eg(0) = 0$. Thus in (c) and (d), one cannot remove the boundedness of g.

Example 2. Let

$$g(x) = \begin{cases} 1, & \text{if } x > 0 \\ 0, & \text{if } x = 0, \end{cases}$$

and let X_n be degenerate at $1/n$. Then $X_n \xrightarrow{\mathscr{L}} 0$, but $Eg(X_n) = 1 \nrightarrow Eg(0) = 0$. Thus in (b) and (c) one needs continuity; likewise in (d) one needs $P\{\mathbf{X} \in C(g)\} = 1$.

***Proof of Theorem* 3.** Obviously, (d) $\Rightarrow$ (c) and (c) $\Rightarrow$ (b). We will show (d) $\Rightarrow$ (a) $\Rightarrow$ (b) $\Rightarrow$ (c) $\Rightarrow$ (d).

(d) $\Rightarrow$ (a): Let $\mathbf{x}^0$ be a continuity point of $F_{\mathbf{X}}$. Then $F_{\mathbf{X}}(\mathbf{x}^0) = Eg(\mathbf{X})$, where $g(\mathbf{x})$ is the indicator function,

$$g(\mathbf{x}) = \begin{cases} 1, & \text{if } \mathbf{x} \le \mathbf{x}^0, \\ 0, & \text{otherwise}. \end{cases}$$

The continuity set of g contains all points $\mathbf{x}$ except those such that $\mathbf{x} \le \mathbf{x}^0$ with equality for at least one component. Because $\mathbf{x}^0$ is a continuity point of $F_{\mathbf{X}}$, we have $F_{\mathbf{X}}(\mathbf{x}^0 + \varepsilon\mathbf{1}) - F_{\mathbf{X}}(\mathbf{x}^0 - \varepsilon\mathbf{1}) \to 0$ as $\varepsilon \to 0$, which implies that the continuity set of g has probability 1 under the distribution of $\mathbf{X}$. Hence, $F_{\mathbf{X}_n}(\mathbf{x}^0) \to F_{\mathbf{X}}(\mathbf{x}^0)$. ■

(a) $\Rightarrow$ (b): Let g be continuous and vanishing outside a compact set, C. Then g is uniformly continuous: For every $\varepsilon > 0$, there exists a number $\delta > 0$ such that $|\mathbf{x} - \mathbf{y}| < \delta$ implies $|g(\mathbf{x}) - g(\mathbf{y})| < \varepsilon$.

Let $\varepsilon > 0$ and find such a $\delta > 0$. Slice C by finite sets of parallel hyperplanes at a distance of at most $\delta/\sqrt{d}$ apart, one set for each dimension, each hyperplane having probability zero under $F_{\mathbf{X}}$ (only countably many parallel planes can have positive mass). This cuts $\mathbb{R}^d$ into parallelepipeds of the form $(\mathbf{b}, \mathbf{c}] = \{\mathbf{x}: \mathbf{b} < \mathbf{x} \le \mathbf{c}\} = \{\mathbf{x}: b_i < x_i \le c_i, \text{ for all } i\}$. On any such parallelepiped $|g(\mathbf{x}) - g(\mathbf{c})| \le \varepsilon$. Thus, $|g(\mathbf{x}) - \tilde{g}(\mathbf{x})| \le \varepsilon$ for all $\mathbf{x}$, where $\tilde{g}(\mathbf{x}) = \sum_{\text{all } (\mathbf{b}, \mathbf{c}]} g(\mathbf{c}) I_{(\mathbf{b}, \mathbf{c}]}(\mathbf{x})$. This is essentially a finite sum since g vanishes outside a compact set, and it may be rewritten as a finite sum of the form, $\tilde{g}(\mathbf{x}) = \sum_i a_i I_{(-\infty, \mathbf{x}_i]}(\mathbf{x})$ (as in the proof of Theorem 2(a)), with $F_{\mathbf{X}}$ continuous at each $\mathbf{x}_i$. Thus, $\mathbf{X}_n \xrightarrow{\mathscr{L}} \mathbf{X}$ implies that $E\tilde{g}(\mathbf{X}_n) = \sum_i a_i F_{\mathbf{X}_n}(\mathbf{x}) \to \sum_i a_i F_{\mathbf{X}}(\mathbf{x}) = E\tilde{g}(\mathbf{X})$. Finally,

$$\begin{aligned}|Eg(\mathbf{X}_n) - Eg(\mathbf{X})| \\ &\le |Eg(\mathbf{X}_n) - E\tilde{g}(\mathbf{X}_n)| + |E\tilde{g}(\mathbf{X}_n) - E\tilde{g}(\mathbf{X})| + |E\tilde{g}(\mathbf{X}) - Eg(\mathbf{X})| \\ &\le 2\varepsilon + |E\tilde{g}(\mathbf{X}_n) - E\tilde{g}(\mathbf{X})| \to 2\varepsilon.\end{aligned}$$

Since this is true for all $\varepsilon > 0$, $Eg(\mathbf{X}_n) \to Eg(\mathbf{X})$. ■

(b) ⇒ (c): Let g be continuous, $|g(\mathbf{x})| < A$ or all $\mathbf{x}$, and $\varepsilon > 0$. Find B such that $P\{|\mathbf{X}| \ge B\} < \varepsilon/(2A)$. Find h continuous so that

$$h(\mathbf{x}) = \begin{cases} 0, & \text{if } |\mathbf{x}| \ge B + 1 \\ 1, & \text{if } |\mathbf{x}| \le B \end{cases} \qquad \text{and } 0 \le h(\mathbf{x}) \le 1 \text{ for all } \mathbf{x}.$$

Then,

$$\begin{aligned}|Eg(\mathbf{X}_n) - Eg(\mathbf{X})| \le\ & |Eg(\mathbf{X}_n) - Eg(\mathbf{X}_n)h(\mathbf{X}_n)| \\ &+ |Eg(\mathbf{X}_n)h(\mathbf{X}_n) - Eg(\mathbf{X})h(\mathbf{X})| \\ &+ |Eg(\mathbf{X})h(\mathbf{X}) - Eg(\mathbf{X})|\end{aligned}$$

The middle term $\to 0$, because $g \cdot h$ is continuous and vanishes outside a compact set. The first term is bounded by $\varepsilon/2$,

$$\begin{aligned}|Eg(\mathbf{X}_n) - Eg(\mathbf{X}_n)h(\mathbf{X}_n)| &\le E|g(\mathbf{X}_n)|\,|1 - h(\mathbf{X}_n)| \le AE(1 - h(\mathbf{X}_n)) \\ &= A(1 - Eh(\mathbf{X}_n)) \to A(1 - Eh(\mathbf{X})) \le \varepsilon/2,\end{aligned}$$

and, similarly, the last term is bounded by $\varepsilon/2$. Therefore, $|Eg(\mathbf{X}_n) - Eg(\mathbf{X})|$ is bounded by something that converges to ε. Since this is true for all $\varepsilon > 0$, $\lim_{n\to\infty} |Eg(\mathbf{X}_n) - Eg(\mathbf{X})| = 0$. ■

To prove (c) ⇒ (d), we use the following lemma.

Lemma. *Let g be bounded measurable with $P\{\mathbf{X} \in C(g)\} = 1$. Then, for every $\varepsilon > 0$ there exist bounded continuous functions f and h such that $f \le g \le h$ and $E(h(\mathbf{X}) - f(\mathbf{X})) < \varepsilon$.*

Proof. Define for $k = 1, 2, \ldots,$

$$f_k(\mathbf{x}) = \inf_{\mathbf{y}} [g(\mathbf{y}) + k|\mathbf{x} - \mathbf{y}|] \quad \text{and} \quad h_k(\mathbf{x}) = \sup_{\mathbf{y}} [g(\mathbf{y}) - k|\mathbf{x} - \mathbf{y}|].$$

Then clearly, $f_1(\mathbf{x}) \le f_2(\mathbf{x}) \le \cdots \le g(\mathbf{x}) \le \cdots \le h_2(\mathbf{x}) \le h_1(\mathbf{x})$. First note that the $f_k(\mathbf{x})$ and $h_k(\mathbf{x})$ are continuous and bounded. [Because

$$\begin{aligned} f_k(\mathbf{x}') &= \inf_{\mathbf{y}}[g(\mathbf{y}) + k|\mathbf{x}' - \mathbf{y}|] \\ &\leq \inf_{\mathbf{y}}[g(\mathbf{y}) + k|\mathbf{x} - \mathbf{y}|] + k|\mathbf{x} - \mathbf{x}'| = f_k(\mathbf{x}) + k|\mathbf{x} - \mathbf{x}'|, \end{aligned}$$

so that $|f_k(\mathbf{x}') - f_k(\mathbf{x})| \leq k|\mathbf{x} - \mathbf{x}'|$.] Let $f_0(\mathbf{x}) = \lim_{k\to\infty} f_k(\mathbf{x})$ and $h_0(\mathbf{x}) = \lim_{k\to\infty} h_k(\mathbf{x})$. Then $f_0(\mathbf{x}) \leq g(\mathbf{x}) \leq h_0(\mathbf{x})$. Second, note that if g is continuous at a point $\mathbf{x}$, then $f_0(\mathbf{x}) = g(\mathbf{x}) = h_0(\mathbf{x})$. [Let $\varepsilon > 0$ be arbitrary. We show $f_0(\mathbf{x}) \geq g(\mathbf{x}) - \varepsilon$. Find $\delta > 0$ such that $|\mathbf{y} - \mathbf{x}| < \delta$ implies $|g(\mathbf{y}) - g(\mathbf{x})| < \varepsilon$, and let B be a lower bound for the function g. Choose $k > (g(\mathbf{x}) - B)/\delta$. Then

$$\begin{aligned} f_0(\mathbf{x}) &\geq f_k(\mathbf{x}) \\ &= \min\left\{ \inf_{|\mathbf{y}-\mathbf{x}|<\delta}[g(\mathbf{y}) + k|\mathbf{x} - \mathbf{y}|], \inf_{|\mathbf{y}-\mathbf{x}|\geq\delta}[g(\mathbf{y}) + k|\mathbf{x} - \mathbf{y}|]\right\} \\ &\geq \min\{g(\mathbf{x}) - \varepsilon, B + ((g(\mathbf{x}) - B)/\delta)\delta\} = g(\mathbf{x}) - \varepsilon.] \end{aligned}$$

Third, note that $Ef_0(\mathbf{X}) = Eg(\mathbf{X}) = Eh_0(\mathbf{X})$, because $P\{\mathbf{X} \in C(g)\} = 1$. Now by the Monotone Convergence Theorem, $Ef_k(\mathbf{X}) \nearrow Ef_0(\mathbf{X})$ and $Eh_k(\mathbf{X}) \searrow Eh_0(\mathbf{X})$. So, for every $\varepsilon > 0$, there exists k such that $E(h_k(\mathbf{X}) - f_k(\mathbf{X})) < \varepsilon$. ■

Proof of (c) $\Rightarrow$ (d). Let g be bounded measurable with $P(\mathbf{X} \in C(g)) = 1$, let $\varepsilon > 0$, and find f and h as in the lemma. Then,

$$\begin{aligned} Eg(\mathbf{X}) - \varepsilon \leq Ef(\mathbf{X}) &= \lim Ef(\mathbf{X}_n) \leq \liminf Eg(\mathbf{X}_n) \\ &\leq \limsup Eg(\mathbf{X}_n) \leq \lim Eh(\mathbf{X}_n) = Eh(\mathbf{X}) \leq Eg(\mathbf{X}) + \varepsilon. \end{aligned}$$

Let $\varepsilon \to 0$, and conclude $Eg(\mathbf{X}) = \lim Eg(\mathbf{X}_n)$. ■

For $\mathbf{X} \in \mathbb{R}^d$ and $\mathbf{t} \in \mathbb{R}^d$, the characteristic function of $\mathbf{X}$ is defined as $\varphi_{\mathbf{X}}(t) = E\exp\{i\mathbf{t}^T\mathbf{X}\} = E\exp\{i(t_1X_1 + \cdots + t_dX_d)\}$, where $i = \sqrt{-1}$.

Theorem 3(e) (the Continuity Theorem)

$$\mathbf{X}_n \xrightarrow{\mathscr{L}} \mathbf{X} \Leftrightarrow \varphi_{\mathbf{X}_n}(\mathbf{t}) \to \varphi_{\mathbf{X}}(\mathbf{t}), \qquad \text{for all } \mathbf{t} \in \mathbb{R}^d.$$

Proof. ($\Rightarrow$) This follows immediately from the Helly–Bray Theorem, because $\exp\{i\mathbf{t}^T\mathbf{X} = \cos\mathbf{t}^T\mathbf{X} + i\sin\mathbf{t}^T\mathbf{X}$ is bounded and continuous.

($\Leftarrow$) Let g be continuous and vanishing outside a compact set. Then g is bounded, $|g(\mathbf{x})| \leq B$ say, and uniformly continuous. Let $\varepsilon > 0$. Find

$\delta > 0$ such that $|\mathbf{x} - \mathbf{y}| < \delta \Rightarrow |g(\mathbf{x}) - g(\mathbf{y})| < \varepsilon$. To show $Eg(\mathbf{X}_n) \to Eg(\mathbf{X})$, let $\mathbf{Y}_\sigma \in \mathscr{N}(\mathbf{0}, \sigma^2\mathbf{I})$ be independent of the $\mathbf{X}_n$ and $\mathbf{X}$. Then

$$\begin{aligned}|Eg(\mathbf{X}_n) - Eg(\mathbf{X})| \le |Eg(\mathbf{X}_n) &- Eg(\mathbf{X}_n + \mathbf{Y}_\sigma)| \\ &+ |Eg(\mathbf{X}_n + \mathbf{Y}_\sigma) - Eg(\mathbf{X} + \mathbf{Y}_\sigma)| \\ &+ |Eg(\mathbf{X} + \mathbf{Y}_\sigma) - Eg(\mathbf{X})|.\end{aligned}$$

The first term is

$$\begin{aligned}&\le E\{|g(\mathbf{X}_n) - g(\mathbf{X}_n + \mathbf{Y}_\sigma)|I(|\mathbf{Y}_\sigma| \le \delta)\} \\ &\quad + E\{|g(\mathbf{X}_n) - g(\mathbf{X}_n + \mathbf{Y}_\sigma)|I(|\mathbf{Y}_\sigma| > \delta)\} \\ &\le \varepsilon + 2BP\{|\mathbf{Y}_\sigma| > \delta\} \le 2\varepsilon\end{aligned}$$

for σ sufficiently small. Similarly, the third term $\le 2\varepsilon$. It remains to show that

$$Eg(\mathbf{X}_n + \mathbf{Y}_\sigma) \to Eg(\mathbf{X} + \mathbf{Y}_\sigma).$$

The characteristic function of $\mathscr{N}(\mathbf{0}, \alpha^2\mathbf{I})$ is

$$\varphi(\mathbf{t}) = \left[\frac{1}{\sqrt{2\pi}\,\alpha}\right]^d \int e^{i\mathbf{t}^T\mathbf{z} - \mathbf{z}^T\mathbf{z}/(2\alpha^2)}\,dz = e^{-\mathbf{t}^T\mathbf{t}\alpha^2/2}.$$

Using this with $\alpha = 1/\sigma$, and making the change of variables $\mathbf{u} = \mathbf{x} + \mathbf{y}$ for $\mathbf{y}$, we find

$$\begin{aligned}Eg(\mathbf{X}_n + \mathbf{Y}_\sigma) &= \left[\frac{1}{\sqrt{2\pi}\,\sigma}\right]^d \int\int g(\mathbf{x} + \mathbf{y})e^{-\mathbf{y}^T\mathbf{y}/(2\sigma^2)}\,d\mathbf{y}\,dF_n(\mathbf{x}) \\ &= \left[\frac{1}{\sqrt{2\pi}\,\sigma}\right]^d \int g(\mathbf{u})\int e^{-(\mathbf{u}-\mathbf{x})^T(\mathbf{u}-\mathbf{x})/(2\sigma^2)}\,dF_n(\mathbf{x})\,d\mathbf{u} \\ &= \left[\frac{1}{\sqrt{2\pi}\,\sigma}\right]^d \int g(\mathbf{u})\int\left[\frac{\sigma}{\sqrt{2\pi}}\right]^d \int e^{i\mathbf{t}^T(\mathbf{u}-\mathbf{x}) - \sigma^2\mathbf{t}^T\mathbf{t}/2}\,d\mathbf{t}\,dF_n(\mathbf{x})\,d\mathbf{u} \\ &= \left[\frac{1}{2\pi}\right]^d \int g(\mathbf{u})\int e^{i\mathbf{t}^T\mathbf{u} - \sigma^2\mathbf{t}^T\mathbf{t}/2}\varphi_{\mathbf{X}_n}(-\mathbf{t})\,d\mathbf{t}\,d\mathbf{u} \\ &\to \left[\frac{1}{2\pi}\right]^d \int g(\mathbf{u})\int e^{i\mathbf{t}^T\mathbf{u} - \sigma^2\mathbf{t}^T\mathbf{t}/2}\varphi_{\mathbf{X}}(-\mathbf{t})\,d\mathbf{t}\,d\mathbf{u},\end{aligned}$$

using the Lebesgue Dominated Convergence Theorem ($|e^{i\mathbf{t}^T\mathbf{u}}\varphi_{\mathbf{X}_n}(-\mathbf{t})| \le 1$

and g has compact support). Undoing the previous steps, we see that this last expression is equal to $Eg(\mathbf{X} + \mathbf{Y}_\sigma)$. ■

EXERCISES

1. If $X_n \xrightarrow{\mathscr{L}} X \in \mathscr{P}(\lambda)$, is it necessarily true that $Eg(X_n) \to Eg(X)$ for
   (a) $g(x) = I_{(0,10)}(x)$,
   (b) $g(x) = \exp\{-x^2\}$,
   (c) $g(x) = \text{sgn}(\cos(x))$ [where $\text{sgn}(x) = +1$ if $x > 0$, 0 if $x = 0$, and -1 if $x < 0$.]
   (d) $g(x) = x$?
   If not, give a counterexample.
2. Show that if $\mathbf{a}^T\mathbf{X}_n \xrightarrow{\mathscr{L}} \mathbf{a}^T\mathbf{X}$ for all vectors $\mathbf{a}$, then $\mathbf{X}_n \xrightarrow{\mathscr{L}} \mathbf{X}$.
3. Show that if X_n has a density $f_n(x)$, if X has density $f(x)$, and if for all x, $f_n(x) \to f(x)$ as $n \to \infty$, then for all bounded measurable functions g, $Eg(X_n) \to Eg(X)$.
4. *The Poisson Approximation to the Binomial Distribution.*
   (a) Let S_n have the binomial distribution, $\mathscr{B}(n, p_n)$, and let Z have the Poisson distribution, $\mathscr{P}(\lambda)$, and suppose that $np_n \to \lambda$ as $n \to \infty$. Using characteristic functions, show that $S_n \xrightarrow{\mathscr{L}} Z$.
   (b) Generalize as follows. Let $X_{1,n}, X_{2,n}, \ldots, X_{n,n}$ be independent Bernoulli trials with $P(X_{j,n} = 1) = p_{j,n}$. Suppose that as $n \to \infty$, $p_{1,n} + \cdots + p_{n,n} \to \lambda$, and $\max_{j \le n} p_{j,n} \to 0$. Then, $S_n \xrightarrow{\mathscr{L}} \mathscr{P}(\lambda)$.
5. *Le Cam's Inequality.* The following inequality gives a bound on the worst error that may be made using the Poisson approximation. Let $X_1, X_2, \ldots, X_n$ be independent Bernoulli trials with $P(X_i = 1) = p_i$ for $i = 1, \ldots, n$, and let $S_n = \sum_1^n X_i$. Let $\lambda = \sum_1^n p_i$, and let Z be a random variable with the Poisson distribution, $\mathscr{P}(\lambda)$. Show that for all sets A,

$$|P(S_n \in A) - P(Z \in A)| \le \sum_{i=1}^n p_i^2.$$

Note that if each $p_i = \lambda/n$, this gives Exercise 4(a). (See J. Michael Steele, "Le Cam's Inequality and Poisson Approximation," *Am. Math. Monthly* (1994), pp. 48–54, for a survey article.) [Hint: The following is a coupling argument; it couples S_n and Z by defining them on the same probability space, and making them as close as possible. For $i = 1, \ldots, n$, let U_i be independent $\mathscr{U}(0,1)$ random variables, let $X_i = I(U_i > 1 - p_i)$, and let $Y_i = 0$ if $U_i < e^{-p_i}$ and let Y_i be defined in terms of U_i in such a way that $Y_i \in \mathscr{P}(p_i)$. Show this can be done, and let $Z = \sum_1^n Y_i \in \mathscr{P}(\lambda)$. Then show (1) $|P(S_n \in A) - P(Z \in A)| \le P(S_n \ne Z)$; (2) $P(S_n \ne Z) \le \sum_1^n P(X_i \ne Y_i)$, and (3) $P(X_i \ne Y_i) \le p_i^2$.]

4

Laws of Large Numbers

The law of large numbers expresses the notion that the mean of a sample from a distribution converges to the mean of the distribution in some sense. When the convergence is in probability or, equivalently, in law, this is known as the weak law of large numbers. When the convergence is almost surely, it is the strong law of large numbers. The simplest law of large numbers, and the most useful for statistical work, is for distributions with finite second moments, and the convergence is in quadratic mean.

All three laws of large numbers are stated in a multidimensional setting. We give the proof of the weak law based on characteristic functions and the continuity theorem. For this and for the proof of the central limit theorem in the next section, we first review the properties of derivatives of vector-valued functions of a vector variable, including a Taylor-series expansion to the second order. We also review the relevant properties of characteristic functions.

These laws are related to the notion of consistency of statistical estimates and application is made to the Glivenko–Cantelli Theorem, which states that the sample distribution function is uniformly strongly consistent as an estimate of the true distribution function. Applications to estimating regression coefficients and autoregressive parameters and to finding probabilities of large deviations are left for the exercises.

Notation. If $f\colon \mathbb{R}^d \to \mathbb{R}$, the derivative of f is the row vector,

$$\dot{f}(\mathbf{x}) = \frac{d}{d\mathbf{x}} f(\mathbf{x}) = \left(\frac{\partial}{\partial x_1} f(\mathbf{x}), \ldots, \frac{\partial}{\partial x_d} f(\mathbf{x}) \right).$$

The derivative of $\mathbf{g}$: $\mathbb{R}^d \to \mathbb{R}^k$, thinking of $\mathbf{g}$ as a column vector,

$$\mathbf{g} = \begin{bmatrix} g_1 \\ \vdots \\ g_k \end{bmatrix},$$

is

$$\dot{g}(x) = \begin{bmatrix} \dot{g}_1(\mathbf{x}) \\ \vdots \\ \dot{g}_k(\mathbf{x}) \end{bmatrix} = \begin{bmatrix} \frac{\partial}{\partial x_1} g_1(\mathbf{x}) & \cdots & \frac{\partial}{\partial x_d} g_1(\mathbf{x}) \\ \vdots & & \vdots \\ \frac{\partial}{\partial x_1} g_k(\mathbf{x}) & \cdots & \frac{\partial}{\partial x_d} g_k(\mathbf{x}) \end{bmatrix}$$

(a $k \times d$ matrix). The second derivative of f: $\mathbb{R}^d \to \mathbb{R}$ is defined as

$$\ddot{f}(\mathbf{x}) = \frac{d}{d\mathbf{x}} \dot{f}(\mathbf{x})^T = \begin{bmatrix} \frac{\partial^2}{(\partial x_1)^2} f(\mathbf{x}) & \cdots & \frac{\partial^2}{\partial x_1 \, \partial x_d} f(\mathbf{x}) \\ \vdots & & \vdots \\ \frac{\partial^2}{\partial x_1 \, \partial x_d} f(\mathbf{x}) & \cdots & \frac{\partial^2}{(\partial x_d)^2} f(\mathbf{x}) \end{bmatrix}.$$

Rules

(1) If $\mathbf{f}$: $\mathbb{R}^d \to \mathbb{R}^s$, $\mathbf{g}$: $\mathbb{R}^s \to \mathbb{R}^k$, and $\mathbf{h}(\mathbf{x}) = \mathbf{g}(\mathbf{f}(\mathbf{x}))$, then $\dot{\mathbf{h}}(\mathbf{x}) = \dot{\mathbf{g}}(\mathbf{f}(\mathbf{x}))\dot{\mathbf{f}}(\mathbf{x})$.

(2) If $\mathbf{f}$: $\mathbb{R}^d \to \mathbb{R}^k$, $\mathbf{g}$: $\mathbb{R}^d \to \mathbb{R}^k$, and $h(\mathbf{x}) = \mathbf{f}(\mathbf{x})^T\mathbf{g}(\mathbf{x})$, then $\dot{h}(\mathbf{x}) = \mathbf{g}(\mathbf{x})^T\dot{\mathbf{f}}(\mathbf{x}) + \mathbf{f}(\mathbf{x})^T\dot{\mathbf{g}}(\mathbf{x})$.

(3) *The Mean-Value Theorem.* If $\mathbf{f}$: $\mathbb{R}^d \to \mathbb{R}^k$ and if $\dot{\mathbf{f}}(\mathbf{x})$ is continuous in the sphere $\{\mathbf{x}: |\mathbf{x} - \mathbf{x}_0| < r\}$, then for $|\mathbf{t}| < r$,

$$\mathbf{f}(\mathbf{x}_0 + \mathbf{t}) = \mathbf{f}(\mathbf{x}_0) + \int_0^1 \dot{\mathbf{f}}(\mathbf{x}_0 + u\mathbf{t})\, du\, \mathbf{t}.$$

Proof. Let $\mathbf{h}(u) = \mathbf{f}(\mathbf{x}_0 + u\mathbf{t})$, so that $\dot{\mathbf{h}}(u) = \dot{\mathbf{f}}(\mathbf{x}_0 + u\mathbf{t})\mathbf{t}$ from rule (1). Then, $\int_0^1 \dot{\mathbf{f}}(\mathbf{x}_0 + u\mathbf{t})\mathbf{t}\, du = \int_0^1 \dot{\mathbf{h}}(u)\, du = \mathbf{h}(1) - \mathbf{h}(0) = \mathbf{f}(\mathbf{x}_0 + \mathbf{t}) - \mathbf{f}(\mathbf{x}_0)$. ■

(4) *Taylor's Theorem.* If f: $\mathbb{R}^d \to \mathbb{R}$, and if $\ddot{f}(\mathbf{x})$ is continuous in the sphere $\{\mathbf{x}: |\mathbf{x} - \mathbf{x}_0| < r\}$, then for $|\mathbf{t}| < r$,

$$f(\mathbf{x}_0 + \mathbf{t}) = f(\mathbf{x}_0) + \dot{f}(\mathbf{x}_0)\mathbf{t} + \mathbf{t}^T \int_0^1\int_0^1 v\ddot{f}(\mathbf{x}_0 + uv\mathbf{t})\, du\, dv\, \mathbf{t}.$$

Properties of characteristic functions. $\varphi_{\mathbf{X}}(\mathbf{t}) = E\exp\{i\mathbf{t}'\mathbf{X}\}$.

(1) $\varphi_{\mathbf{X}}(\mathbf{t})$ exists for all $\mathbf{t} \in \mathbb{R}^d$ and is continuous.
(2) $\varphi_{\mathbf{X}}(0) = 1$ and $|\varphi_{\mathbf{X}}(\mathbf{t})| \leq 1$ for all $\mathbf{t} \in \mathbb{R}^d$.
(3) for a scalar $b \neq 0$, $\varphi_{\mathbf{X}/b}(\mathbf{t}) = \varphi_{\mathbf{X}}(\mathbf{t}/b)$.
(4) for a vector $\mathbf{c}$, $\varphi_{\mathbf{X}+\mathbf{c}}(\mathbf{t}) = \exp\{i\mathbf{t}^T\mathbf{c}\}\varphi_{\mathbf{X}}(\mathbf{t})$.
(5) for $\mathbf{X}$ and $\mathbf{Y}$ independent, $\varphi_{\mathbf{X}+\mathbf{Y}}(\mathbf{t}) = \varphi_{\mathbf{X}}(\mathbf{t})\varphi_{\mathbf{Y}}(\mathbf{t})$.
(6) if $E|\mathbf{X}| < \infty$, $\dot{\varphi}_{\mathbf{X}}(\mathbf{t})$ exists and is continuous and $\dot{\varphi}_{\mathbf{X}}(\mathbf{0}) = i\boldsymbol{\mu}^T$, where $\boldsymbol{\mu} = E\mathbf{X}$.
(7) if $E|\mathbf{X}|^2 < \infty$, $\ddot{\varphi}_{\mathbf{X}}(\mathbf{t})$ exists and is continuous and $\ddot{\varphi}_{\mathbf{X}}(\mathbf{0}) = -E\mathbf{X}\mathbf{X}^T$.
(8) if $\mathbf{X}$ is degenerate at $\mathbf{c}$, $\varphi_{\mathbf{X}}(\mathbf{t}) = \exp\{i\mathbf{t}^T\mathbf{c}\}$.
(9) if $\mathbf{X}$ is $\mathscr{N}(\boldsymbol{\mu}, \boldsymbol{\Sigma})$, $\varphi_{\mathbf{X}}(\mathbf{t}) = \exp\{i\mathbf{t}^T\boldsymbol{\mu} - \frac{1}{2}\mathbf{t}^T\boldsymbol{\Sigma}\mathbf{t}\}$.

Theorem 4. *Let* $\mathbf{X}, \mathbf{X}_1, \mathbf{X}_2, \ldots$ *be i.i.d. (independent, identically distributed) random vectors, and let* $\overline{\mathbf{X}}_n = (1/n)\Sigma_1^n \mathbf{X}_j$.

(a) *(Weak law) If* $E|\mathbf{X}| < \infty$, *then* $\overline{\mathbf{X}}_n \xrightarrow{\text{P}} \boldsymbol{\mu} = E\mathbf{X}$.
(b) *If* $E|\mathbf{X}|^2 < \infty$, *then* $\overline{\mathbf{X}}_n \xrightarrow{\text{qm}} \boldsymbol{\mu} = E\mathbf{X}$.
(c) *(Strong law)* $\overline{\mathbf{X}}_n \xrightarrow{\text{a.s.}} \boldsymbol{\mu} \Leftrightarrow E|\mathbf{X}| < \infty$ *and* $\boldsymbol{\mu} = E\mathbf{X}$.

Proof. (a) Let $\varphi_{\mathbf{X}}(\mathbf{t}) = E\exp\{i\mathbf{t}^T\mathbf{X}\}$. Then

$$\varphi_{\overline{\mathbf{X}}_n}(\mathbf{t}) = \varphi_{\mathbf{X}_1 + \cdots + \mathbf{X}_n}(\mathbf{t}/n) = \prod_1^n \varphi_{\mathbf{X}_j}(\mathbf{t}/n) = \varphi_{\mathbf{X}}(\mathbf{t}/n)^n$$
$$= \left(\varphi_{\mathbf{X}}(\mathbf{0}) + \left[\int_0^1 \dot{\varphi}_{\mathbf{X}}(u\mathbf{t}/n)\,du\right]\frac{\mathbf{t}}{n}\right)^n.$$

Because $\varphi_{\mathbf{X}}(\mathbf{0}) = 1$, and $\dot{\varphi}_{\mathbf{X}}(\varepsilon) \to i\boldsymbol{\mu}^T$ as $\boldsymbol{\varepsilon} \to \mathbf{0}$,

$$\varphi_{\overline{\mathbf{X}}_n}(\mathbf{t}) \to \exp\left\{\lim_{n\to\infty}\left[\int_0^1 \dot{\varphi}_{\mathbf{X}}(u\mathbf{t}/n)\,du\right]\mathbf{t}\right\} = \exp\{i\boldsymbol{\mu}^T\mathbf{t}\}.$$

Here, we use the fact that for any sequence of real numbers, a_n, for which $\lim_{n\to\infty} na_n$ exists, we have $(1 + a_n)^n \to \exp\{\lim_{n\to\infty} na_n\}$. Because $\exp\{i\boldsymbol{\mu}^T\mathbf{t}\}$ is the characteristic function of the distribution giving mass 1 to the point $\boldsymbol{\mu}$, we have from the Continuity Theorem $\overline{\mathbf{X}}_n \xrightarrow{\mathscr{L}} \boldsymbol{\mu}$ which implies from Theorem 2(a), $\overline{\mathbf{X}}_n \xrightarrow{\text{P}} \boldsymbol{\mu}$.

(b)

$$E|\overline{\mathbf{X}}_n - \boldsymbol{\mu}|^2 = E(\overline{\mathbf{X}}_n - \boldsymbol{\mu})^T(\overline{\mathbf{X}}_n - \boldsymbol{\mu}) = (1/n^2)\sum_i\sum_j E(\mathbf{X}_i - \boldsymbol{\mu})^T(\mathbf{X}_j - \boldsymbol{\mu})$$
$$= (1/n^2)\sum_i E(\mathbf{X}_i - \boldsymbol{\mu})^T(\mathbf{X}_i - \boldsymbol{\mu})$$
$$= (1/n)E(\mathbf{X} - \boldsymbol{\mu})^T(\mathbf{X} - \boldsymbol{\mu}) \to 0.$$

(Note that this proof requires only that the $\mathbf{X}_i$ be uncorrelated and have the same mean and covariance matrix; it does not require that they be independent, or that they be identically distributed.)

(c) Omitted. [See, e.g., Chung (1974), Rao (1973).] ■

The method of proof of part (b) is very general and quite useful for proving consistency in statistical estimation problems. In such problems, the underlying probability, $P_{\boldsymbol{\theta}}$, depends upon a parameter $\boldsymbol{\theta}$ in Θ in $\mathbb{R}^d$, and we are given a sequence of random vectors, $\hat{\boldsymbol{\theta}}_n$, considered as estimates of $\boldsymbol{\theta}$. We say that $\hat{\boldsymbol{\theta}}_n$ is a *consistent* sequence of estimates of $\boldsymbol{\theta}$ if for all $\boldsymbol{\theta} \in \Theta$, $\hat{\boldsymbol{\theta}}_n \xrightarrow{\text{P}} \boldsymbol{\theta}$ when $P = P_{\boldsymbol{\theta}}$ is the "true" probability distribution. This is sometimes called *weak* consistency, or consistency *in probability*. We may similarly define *strong* consistency ($\hat{\boldsymbol{\theta}}_n \xrightarrow{\text{a.s.}} \boldsymbol{\theta}$), or consistency *in quadratic mean* ($\hat{\boldsymbol{\theta}}_n \xrightarrow{\text{qm}} \boldsymbol{\theta}$), both of which imply (weak) consistency. The weak (strong) law of large numbers states the sample mean is a weakly (strongly) consistent estimate of the population mean.

Exercises 1 and 2 give extensions of the law of large numbers. In the first, the $\mathbf{X}_j$ are not identically distributed, and in the second, they are not independent.

The weak law of large numbers says that if $X_1, \ldots, X_n$ are i.i.d. random variables with finite first moment, μ, then for every $\varepsilon > 0$ we have $P(|\overline{X}_n - \mu| > \varepsilon) \to 0$ as $n \to \infty$. The argument of Theorem 2(b) only shows that $P(|\overline{X}_n - \mu| > \varepsilon) \to 0$ at rate $1/n$. Actually, the rate of convergence of $P(|\overline{X}_n - \mu| > \varepsilon)$ to zero is typically exponential at a certain rate that depends on ε and on the underlying distribution of the X's. That is, $P(|\overline{X}_n - \mu| > \varepsilon)$ behaves asymptotically like $\exp\{-n\alpha\}$ for some $\alpha > 0$, in the sense that $P(|\overline{X}_n - \mu| > \varepsilon)^{1/n} \to \exp\{-\alpha\}$ or

$$(1/n) \log P\left(|\overline{X}_n - \mu| > \varepsilon\right) \to -\alpha \text{ as } n \to \infty.$$

The study of the rate of convergence of $P(|\overline{X}_n - \mu| > \varepsilon)$ to zero is in the domain of *large deviation theory*. (See Exercises 5–8.)

Consistency of the Empirical Distribution Function. Let $X_1, \ldots, X_n$ be independent identically distributed random variables on $\mathbb{R}$ with distribution function $F(x) = P(X \leq x)$. The nonparametric maximum-likelihood estimate of F is the *sample distribution function* or *empirical distribution function* defined as

$$F_n(x) = \frac{1}{n} \sum_{i=1}^{n} I_{[X_i, \infty)}(x).$$

Thus, $F_n(x)$ is the proportion of the observations that fall less than or equal to x. For each fixed x, the strong law of large numbers implies that $F_n(x) \xrightarrow{\text{a.s.}} F(x)$, because we may consider $I_{[X_i,\infty)}(x)$ as i.i.d. random variables with mean $F(x)$. Thus, $F_n(x)$ is a strongly consistent estimate of $F(x)$ for every x.

The following corollary improves on this observation in two ways. First, the set of probability one on which convergence takes place may be chosen to be independent of x. Second, the convergence is uniform in x. This assertion, that the empirical distribution function converges uniformly almost surely to the true distribution function, is known as the *Glivenko-Cantelli Theorem.*

Corollary. $P\{sup_x|F_n(x) - F(x)| \to 0\} = 1$.

Proof. Let $\varepsilon > 0$. Find an integer $k > 1/\varepsilon$ and numbers $-\infty = x_0 < x_1 \leq x_2 \leq \cdots \leq x_{k-1} < x_k = \infty$, such that $F(x_j^-) \leq j/k \leq F(x_j)$ for $j = 1,\ldots,k-1$. [$F(x_j^-)$ may be considered notation for $P(X < x_j)$.] Note that if $x_{j-1} < x_j$, then $F(x_j^-) - F(x_{j-1}) \leq \varepsilon$. From the strong law of large numbers, $F_n(x_j) \xrightarrow{\text{a.s.}} F(x_j)$ and $F_n(x_j^-) \xrightarrow{\text{a.s.}} F(x_j^-)$ for $j = 1,\ldots,k-1$. Hence,

$$\Delta_n = \max(|F_n(x_j) - F(x_j)|, |F_n(x_j^-) - F(x_j^-)|, j = 1,\ldots,k-1) \xrightarrow{\text{a.s.}} 0.$$

Let x be arbitrary and find j such that $x_{j-1} < x \leq x_j$. Then, $F_n(x) - F(x) \leq F_n(x_j^-) - F(x_{j-1}) \leq F_n(x_j^-) - F(x_j^-) + \varepsilon$, and $F_n(x) - F(x) \geq F_n(x_{j-1}) - F(x_j^-) \geq F_n(x_{j-1}) - F(x_{j-1}) - \varepsilon$. This implies that $\sup_x|F_n(x) - F(x)| \leq \Delta_n + \epsilon \xrightarrow{\text{a.s.}} \varepsilon$. Since this holds for all $\varepsilon > 0$, the corollary follows. ∎

EXERCISES

1. (*Consistency of the least-squares estimate of a regression coefficient.*) Suppose that for given constants $z_1, z_2,\ldots$ the random variables $X_1, X_2,\ldots$ are independent with linear regression, $E(X_i) = \alpha + \beta z_i$, and constant variance, $\text{var}(X_i) = \sigma^2$. The least-squares estimates of α and β based on $X_1,\ldots,X_n$ are

$$\hat{\beta}_n = \sum_1^n X_j(z_j - \bar{z}_n) \Big/ \sum_1^n (z_j - \bar{z}_n)^2,$$

$$\hat{\alpha}_n = \bar{X}_n - \hat{\beta}_n \bar{z}_n,$$

where $\bar{z}_n = (1/n)\Sigma_1^n z_j$.
(a) Under what conditions on $z_1, z_2,\ldots$ is it true that $\hat{\beta}_n \xrightarrow{\text{qm}} \beta$?
(b) When does $\hat{\alpha}_n \xrightarrow{\text{qm}} \alpha$?

2. (*An autoregressive model.*) Suppose $\varepsilon_1, \varepsilon_2, \ldots$ are independent random variables all having the same mean μ and variance σ^2. Define X_n as the autoregressive sequence,

$$X_1 = \varepsilon_1,$$

and for $n \geq 2$,

$$X_n = \beta X_{n-1} + \varepsilon_n,$$

where $-1 \leq \beta < 1$. Show that $\overline{X}_n \xrightarrow{\text{qm}} \mu/(1-\beta)$.

3. (*Bernstein's Theorem.*) Let $X_1, X_2, \ldots$ be a sequence of random variables with $E(X_i) = 0$, $\text{var}(X_i) = \sigma_i^2$, and $\text{corr}(X_i, X_j) = \rho_{ij}$. Show that if the variances are uniformly bounded ($\sigma_i^2 \leq c$, say), and if $\rho_{ij} \to 0$ as $|i-j| \to \infty$ (i.e., for every $\varepsilon > 0$, there is an integer N such that $|i-j| > N$ implies $|\rho_{ij}| < \varepsilon$), then $\overline{X}_n \xrightarrow{\text{qm}} 0$.

4. (*Monte Carlo.*) One strategy for evaluating the integral

$$I = \int_1^\infty \frac{1}{x} \sin(2\pi x)\, dx = 0.153\ldots$$

by Monte Carlo approximation is as follows. Write integral with a change of variable, $y = 1/x$, as

$$I = \int_0^1 \frac{1}{y} \sin\left(\frac{2\pi}{y}\right) dy,$$

and approximate I by

$$\hat{I}_n = \frac{1}{n} \sum_1^n \frac{1}{Y_i} \sin\left(\frac{2\pi}{Y_i}\right),$$

where $Y_1, \ldots, Y_n$ is a sample from the uniform distribution on [0, 1]. How well does this approximation work? Does $\hat{I}_n$ converge to I?

The following four exercises deal with large deviations for sums of i.i.d. random variables. For an accessible introduction to the general theory, see the book, *Large Deviation Techniques in Decision, Simulation and Estimation* by James A. Bucklew, John Wiley & Sons, New York, 1990.

Let $X_1, \ldots, X_n$ be i.i.d. random variables with moment-generating function $M(\theta)$ finite for all θ. Let μ denote the first moment of X. To show that $P(|\overline{X}_n - \mu| > \varepsilon)$ converges to zero exponentially, it is sufficient to show that both $P(\overline{X}_n > \mu + \varepsilon)$ and $P(\overline{X}_n < \mu - \epsilon)$ tend to zero exponentially. We concentrate on the first of these two quantities, since the other is treated by symmetry. The main result is that if the large deviation rate function, $H(x)$, defined in Exercise 5, is continuous at

$\mu + \varepsilon$, then $(1/n)\log P(\overline{X}_n > \mu + \varepsilon) \to -H(\mu + \varepsilon)$. This is done in two steps in Exercises 6 and 7.

5. Let X be a random variable with moment-generating function, $M(\theta) = E\exp\{\theta X\}$ finite in a neighborhood of the origin and let μ denote the mean of X, $\mu = EX$. The quantity,

$$H(x) = \sup_{\theta}(\theta x - \log M(\theta))$$

is called the *large deviation rate function* of X.
(a) Show that $H(x)$ is a convex function of x.
(b) Show that $H(x)$ has a minimum value of zero at $x = \mu$.
(c) Evaluate $X(x)$ for the normal, Poisson, and Bernoulli distributions.

6. Show that

$$P(\overline{X}_n \geq \mu + \varepsilon) \leq \exp\{-\theta(\mu + \varepsilon) + n\log M(\theta/n)\}$$
$$\leq \exp\{-nH(\mu + \varepsilon)\}$$

for all θ and n. (Use a Chebyshev inequality type of argument.)

7. Let $f(x)$ denote the density of the common distribution of the X_i, and introduce an exponential family of distributions having density

$$f(x|\theta) = e^{\theta x}f(x)/M(\theta).$$

This reduces to the original density, $f(x)$, when $\theta = 0$. Let P_θ denote the probability measure induced by this density, and note that $P = P_0$. Let δ be an arbitrary positive number, and let $y = \mu + \varepsilon + \delta$. Find θ' such that $E_{\theta'}X = y$, or equivalently, $M'(\theta')/M(\theta') = y$.
(a) Show that $P_{\theta'}(|\overline{X}_n - y| \leq \delta) \leq \exp\{nH(y + \delta)\}P_0(|\overline{X}_n - y| \leq \delta)$.
(b) Note that $P(\overline{X}_n > \mu + \varepsilon) \geq P(|\overline{X}_n - y| < \delta) \geq \exp\{-nH(y + \delta)\}P_{\theta'}(|\overline{X}_n - y| < \delta)$, and conclude that $\liminf_{n\to\infty}(1/n)\log P(\overline{X}_n > \mu + \varepsilon) \geq -H(\mu + \varepsilon)$.

8. For the Bernoulli distribution with probability p of success, the rate function $H(x)$ is not continuous at $x = 1$. Establish the rate of convergence of $P(\overline{X}_n \geq 1)$ and $P(\overline{X}_n > 1)$ to zero directly in this case.

5

Central Limit Theorems

In this section, we present the basic Central Limit Theorem for i.i.d. variables. We do this for vector variables since the proof is essentially the same as for one-dimensional variables. The extension to independent nonidentically distributed random variables, due to Lindeberg and Feller, is stated without proof. Applications are given to some important statistical problems: to least-squares estimators of regression coefficients, to randomization tests for paired comparison experiments, and to the signed-rank test.

Theorem 5. *Let $\mathbf{X}_1, \mathbf{X}_2, \ldots$ be i.i.d. random vectors with mean $\boldsymbol{\mu}$ and finite covariance matrix, $\boldsymbol{\Sigma}$. Then $\sqrt{n}(\overline{\mathbf{X}}_n - \boldsymbol{\mu}) \xrightarrow{\mathscr{L}} \mathscr{N}(\mathbf{0}, \boldsymbol{\Sigma})$.*

Proof. Because $\sqrt{n}(\overline{\mathbf{X}}_n - \boldsymbol{\mu}) = (1/\sqrt{n})\Sigma_1^n(\mathbf{X}_j - \boldsymbol{\mu})$, we have

$$\begin{aligned} \varphi_{\sqrt{n}(\overline{\mathbf{X}}_n - \boldsymbol{\mu})}(\mathbf{t}) &= \varphi_{\Sigma_i^n(\mathbf{X}_j - \boldsymbol{\mu})}(\mathbf{t}/\sqrt{n}) \\ &= \prod_1^n \varphi_{\mathbf{X}_j - \boldsymbol{\mu}}(\mathbf{t}/\sqrt{n}) = \varphi(\mathbf{t}/\sqrt{n})^n, \end{aligned} \tag{1}$$

where $\varphi(\mathbf{t})$ is the characteristic function of $\mathbf{X}_j - \mu$. Then, because $\varphi(\mathbf{0}) = 1$, $\dot{\varphi}(\mathbf{0}) = \mathbf{0}$, and $\ddot{\varphi}(\boldsymbol{\varepsilon}) \to -\boldsymbol{\Sigma}$ as $\boldsymbol{\varepsilon} \to \mathbf{0}$, we have, applying Taylor's Theorem,

$$\begin{aligned} \varphi_{\sqrt{n}(\overline{\mathbf{X}}_n - \boldsymbol{\mu})}(\mathbf{t}) &= \left(1 + \frac{1}{n}\mathbf{t}'\int_0^1\int_0^1 v\ddot{\varphi}(uv\mathbf{t}/\sqrt{n})\,du\,dv\,\mathbf{t}\right)^n \\ &\to \exp\left\{\lim_{n\to\infty} \mathbf{t}'\int_0^1\int_0^1 v\ddot{\varphi}(uv\mathbf{t}/\sqrt{n})\,du\,dv\,\mathbf{t}\right\} \\ &= \exp\{-(1/2)\mathbf{t}'\boldsymbol{\Sigma}\mathbf{t}\}. \end{aligned} \tag{2}$$

In the convergence statement, we have used the fact that for any sequence of real numbers, a_n, for which $\lim_{n\to\infty} na_n$ exists, we have $(1 + a_n)^n \to \exp\{\lim_{n\to\infty} na_n\}$. ■

The extension of the Central Limit Theorem to the independent *non-identically* distributed case is very important for statistical work. We state the basic theorem in one dimension without proof. See Feller (1966) (Vol. 2) or Chung (1974) for a proof quite similar to the proof of Theorem 5. It is useful to state this extension in terms of a triangular array of random variables,

$$\begin{array}{l} X_{11} \\ X_{21}, X_{22} \\ X_{31}, X_{32}, X_{33} \\ \cdots, \end{array}$$

where the random variables in each row are assumed to be independent with means zero ad finite variances.

The Lindeberg–Feller Theorem. *For each* $n = 1, 2, \ldots,$ *let* X_{nj}, *for* $j = 1, 2, \ldots, n$, *be independent random variables with* $EX_{nj} = 0$ *and* $var(X_{nj}) = \sigma_{nj}^2$. *Let* $Z_n = \sum_{j=1}^n X_{nj}$, *and let* $B_n^2 = var(Z_n) = \sum_{j=1}^n \sigma_{nj}^2$. *Then,* $Z_n/B_n \xrightarrow{\mathscr{L}} \mathscr{N}(0, 1)$, *provided the Lindeberg Condition holds: For every* $\varepsilon > 0$,

$$\frac{1}{B_n^2} \sum_{j=1}^{n} E\{X_{nj}^2 I(|X_{nj}| \geq \varepsilon B_n)\} \to 0 \text{ as } n \to \infty. \tag{3}$$

Conversely, if $(1/B_n^2)\max_{j\leq n} \sigma_{nj}^2 \to 0$ *as* $n \to \infty$ *(that is, if no one term of the sum* B_n^2 *plays a significant role in the limit), and if* $Z_n/B_n \xrightarrow{\mathscr{L}} \mathscr{N}(0, 1)$, *then the Lindeberg Condition holds.*

The important special case where there is a single sequence, $X_1, X_2, \ldots,$ of independent identically distributed random variables with mean μ and $\text{var}(X_j) = \sigma^2$ can be obtained from this theorem by putting $X_{nj} = z_{nj}(X_j - \mu)$ to obtain the asymptotic normality of Z_n/B_n where $Z_n = \sum_{j=1}^n z_{nj}(X_j - \mu)$ and $B_n^2 = \sigma^2 \sum_{j=1}^n z_{nj}^2$. (See Exercise 5.)

Example 1. *Application to the asymptotic normality of the least-squares estimate of a regression coefficient.* Suppose $X_j = \alpha + \beta z_j + e_j$ for $j = 1, 2, \ldots,$ where the z_j are known numbers not all equal and the e_j are independent random variables with means zero and common variances

σ^2. In Exercise 1 of Section 4 we saw that the least-squares estimate, $\hat{\beta}_n$, of β was consistent provided $\Sigma_{j=1}(z_j - \bar{z}_n)^2 \to \infty$ as $n \to \infty$. We now show that if the conditions are strengthened to include

(a) the e_j are identically distributed, and
(b) $\max_{j \le n}(z_j - \bar{z}_n)^2/\Sigma_{j=1}^n(z_j - \bar{z}_n)^2 \to 0$ as $n \to \infty$,

then $\hat{\beta}_n$ is asymptotically normal.

Note that

$$\hat{\beta}_n = \sum_{j=1}^n X_j(z_j - \bar{z}_n) \Big/ \sum_{j=1}^n (z_j - \bar{z}_n)^2$$

$$= \beta + \sum_{j=1}^n e_j(z_j - \bar{z}_n) \Big/ \sum_{j=1}^n (z_j - \bar{z}_n)^2. \tag{4}$$

We show that the conditions of the Lindeberg–Feller Theorem are satisfied with $X_{nj} = e_j(z_j - \bar{z}_n)$. Since $EX_{nj} = 0$ and $\text{var}(X_{nj}) = \sigma^2(z_j - \bar{z}_n)^2$, we have $B_n^2 = \sigma^2\Sigma_{j=1}^n(z_j - \bar{z}_n)^2$, and

$$\frac{1}{B_n^2}\sum_{j=1}^n E\{X_{nj}^2 I(|X_{nj}| \ge \varepsilon B_n)\}$$

$$= \frac{1}{B_n^2}\sum_{j=1}^n E\{e_j^2(z_j - \bar{z}_n)^2 I(|e_j(z_j - \bar{z}_n)| \ge \varepsilon B_n)\}$$

$$\le \frac{1}{B_n^2}\sum_{j=1}^n (z_j - \bar{z}_n)^2 E\{e_j^2 I(|e_j| \ge \varepsilon\sigma/\gamma_n)\}, \tag{5}$$

where $\gamma_n^2 = \max_{j \le n}(z_j - \bar{z}_n)^2/\Sigma_{j=1}^n(z_j - \bar{z}_n)^2$. From assumption (a), the expectation term is independent of j and may be factored outside the summation sign. The terms B_n^2 cancel, and the expectation tends to zero because the variance of e_j is finite and $\gamma_n \to 0$ from assumption (b). We may conclude that

$$\sqrt{n}\, s_n(\hat{\beta}_n - \beta) \xrightarrow{\mathscr{L}} \mathscr{N}(0, \sigma^2), \tag{6}$$

where $s_n^2 = \Sigma_{j=1}^n(z_j - \bar{z}_n)^2/n$.

Example 2. *The randomization t-test for paired comparisons.* In a paired comparison experiment for comparing a treatment with a control, $2n$ experimental units are grouped into n pairs such that within each pair the units are as much alike as possible. Then for each pair, it is decided at random which member of the pair receives the treatment and which serves as control. We let (X_j, Y_j) represent the resulting measurements on the jth pair, for $j = 1, \ldots, n$, with X_j being the result of the treatment and Y_j being the result of the control.

The usual paired comparison t test for comparing treatment and control is based on the assumption that the differences, $Z_j = X_j - Y_j$, are independent and identically distributed with finite second moment. The hypothesis H_0 of no difference between treatment and control becomes the hypothesis that the distribution of the Z_j is symmetric about zero. The usual test of H_0 is based on the one-sample t statistic, $t = \sqrt{n-1}\,\overline{Z}_n/s_z = \sqrt{n-1}\,(\overline{X}_n - \overline{Y}_n)/s_z$, where s_z is the standard deviation of the sample, $s_z^2 = (1/n)\Sigma_1^n(Z_j - \overline{Z}_n)^2$. Under the hypothesis that the Z_j are i.i.d. normally distributed, t has t distribution with $n-1$ degrees of freedom.

Randomization tests (sometimes called *Permutation tests*) may also be used for this problem. This test is based solely on the fact that the assignment of treatment and control to the pairs is made independently and at random. The analysis of the test is done conditionally on the observed values of the Z_j. Because of this, the random variables Z_j, conditional on the values $|Z_j| = |z_j|$, are independent under H_0 with $P(Z_j = +|z_j|) = P(Z_j = -|z_j|) = \frac{1}{2}$. Thus under H_0, the vector $(Z_1, \ldots, Z_n)$ has 2^n equally likely possible values, $(\pm|z_1|, \ldots, \pm|z_n|)$. Any statistic based on $(Z_1, \ldots, Z_n)$ has at most 2^n values as well.

The randomization t test uses the one-sample t statistic, $t = \sqrt{n-1}\,\overline{Z}_n/s_z$. The rejection criterion is not based on the t distribution but rather on the discrete distribution generated by these 2^n equally likely values of $(Z_1, \ldots, Z_n)$. For example, testing against one-sided alternatives, one computes the t statistic for all 2^n values and rejects H_0 if the observed t falls in the upper $100\alpha\%$ of them. For small values of n, this distribution can easily be tabled by a computer by evaluating the t statistic at each of these 2^n values. For large values of n, other methods must be employed. One method is the Monte Carlo method of *approximate randomization*, where a random sample of a few hundred is drawn from the distribution and the observed t statistic is compared to the sample. The method we use here looks at the large sample distribution of the statistic under the randomization hypothesis.

First, consider the randomization test applied to the statistic $\overline{Z}_n$. We show that if the z_j satisfy the condition

$$\max_{j \le n} z_j^2 \Big/ \sum_{j=1}^{n} z_j^2 \to 0, \tag{7}$$

then $\sqrt{n}\,\overline{Z}_n/\sigma_n \xrightarrow{\mathscr{L}} \mathscr{N}(0,1)$ under H_0, where $\sigma_n^2 = (1/n)\Sigma_1^n z_j^2$. We let

$X_{nj} = Z_j$ in the notation of the Lindeberg–Feller Theorem. Then $EX_{nj} = 0$ and $\operatorname{var} X_{nj} = z_j^2$, so that $B_n^2 = \sum_1^n z_j^2$. We show $\sum_1^n Z_j/B_n \xrightarrow{\mathscr{L}} \mathscr{N}(0,1)$ by checking the Lindeberg Condition. Because $|X_{nj}|$ is degenerate at $|z_j|$,

$$\frac{1}{B_n^2}\sum_1^n E\{X_{nj}^2 I(|X_{nj}| > \varepsilon B_n)\} = \frac{1}{B_n^2}\sum_1^n z_j^2 I(|z_j| > \varepsilon B_n)$$

$$\leq \frac{1}{B_n^2}\sum_1^n z_j^2 I\Big(\max_{j\leq n}|z_j| > \varepsilon B_n\Big)$$

$$= I\Big(\max_{j\leq n} z_j^2/B_n^2 > \varepsilon^2\Big). \tag{8}$$

From condition (7), this is equal to zero for all n sufficiently large. Thus, we conclude that $\sqrt{n}\,\overline{Z}_n/\sigma_n = \sum_1^n Z_j/B_n \xrightarrow{\mathscr{L}} \mathscr{N}(0,1)$.

The randomization t test is based on the t statistic rather than $\overline{Z}_n$. However, one can show that these two randomization tests are equivalent. This is because $t = \sqrt{n-1}\,\overline{Z}_n/s_z$ is an increasing function of $v = \sqrt{n}\,\overline{Z}_n/\sigma_n$. To see this, note that t and v always have the same sign, and that

$$v^2 = n\overline{Z}_n^2/\sigma_n^2 = n\overline{Z}_n^2/\left(s_z^2 + \overline{Z}_n^2\right) = n\left(\frac{n-1}{t^2} + 1\right)^{-1}.$$

The conclusion to be drawn from this is that the randomization t test is asymptotically normal and has asymptotically the same cutoff points as the usual t test provided (7) is satisfied. This result can be considered as a nonparametric justification of the usual t test for paired comparisons when the sample size is large.

Example 3. *The signed-rank test for paired comparisons.* One may also apply the signed-rank test to this problem. This test, like the randomization t test, is based on the assumption that under H_0 the random variables Z_j, conditional on the values $|Z_j| = |z_j|$, are independent with $P(Z_j = +|z_j|) = P(Z_j = -|z_j|) = \frac{1}{2}$. The signed-rank statistic is defined as follows. Let R_j denote the rank of $|z_j|$ in the ranking of $|z_1|, \ldots, |z_n|$ from smallest to largest. (We assume that all the $|z_j|$ are different and that no $|z_j|$ is zero.) Then the signed-rank statistic, W_+, is the sum of the ranks R_j for those Z_j that are positive:

$$W_+ = \sum_1^n R_j I(Z_j > 0). \tag{9}$$

If we reorder the subscripts of the Z_j so that $0 < |z_1| < |z_2| < \cdots < |z_n|$, then we have $W_+ = \sum_1^n jI(Z_j > 0)$. Because under H_0, the $I(Z_j > 0)$ are i.i.d. Bernoulli variables equally likely to be zero as one, we find

$$EW_+ = \frac{1}{2}\sum_1^n j = \frac{n(n+1)}{4}$$

$$\operatorname{var} W_+ = \frac{1}{4}\sum_1^n j^2 = \frac{n(n+1)(2n+1)}{24}. \qquad (10)$$

To show asymptotic normality of $(W_+ - EW_+)/\sqrt{\operatorname{var} W_+}$, note that $W_+ = \sum_1^n jI(Z_j > 0)$ may be reduced to a form of the randomization test based on Z_n. In fact, if W_n denotes the sum of the ranks of the positive Z_j, minus the sum of the ranks of the negative Z_j, then (assuming no $z_j = 0$), $W_n = \sum_1^n jI(Z_j > 0) - \sum_1^n jI(Z_j < 0) = 2W_+ - \sum_1^n j$. This shows that W_+ is linearly related to W_n. But $(1/n)W_n$ is exactly of the form of Z_n of the randomization test with $|z_j| = j$. We merely have to show that the sequence $|z_j| = j$ satisfies (7). This follows because $\max_{j \le n} j^2 = n^2$, and $\sum_1^n j^2 = n(n+1)(2n+1)/6$. We may conclude that W_n and hence W_+ are asympotically normal; $(W_+ - EW_+)/\sqrt{\operatorname{var} W_+} \xrightarrow{\mathscr{L}} \mathscr{N}(0,1)$.

Improving the Approximation

The convergence in the Central Limit Theorem is not uniform in the underlying distribution. For any fixed sample size n, there are distributions for which the normal distribution approximation to the distribution function of $\sqrt{n}(\overline{X}_n - \mu)/\sigma$ is arbitrarily poor. However, there is an upper bound, due to Berry (1941) and Esseen (1942), to the error of the Central Limit Theorem approximation that shows the convergence is uniform for the class of distributions for which $E|X - \mu|^3/\sigma^3$ is bounded above by a finite bound. We state this theorem without proof in one dimension.

Berry–Esseen Theorem. *If $X_1, X_2, \ldots, X_n$ are i.i.d. with mean μ, variance $\sigma^2 > 0$, and absolute third moment $\rho = E|X - \mu|^3 < \infty$, then*

$$|F_n(x) - \Phi(x)| < c\rho/(\sqrt{n}\,\sigma^3), \qquad \text{for all } x \text{ and } n, \qquad (11)$$

where $F_n(x)$ is the distribution function of $\sqrt{n}(\overline{X}_n - \mu)/\sigma$, where $\Phi(x)$ is the distribution function of $\mathscr{N}(0,1)$, and where c is a universal constant known to be greater than 0.4097 *and less than* 0.7975. [*See van Beek* (1972).]

When we have information about the third and higher moments of the underlying distribution, we may often improve on the normal approximation by considering higher-order terms in the expansion of the characteristic function. This leads to asymptotic expansions known as *Edgeworth Expansions*. We present without proof the two next terms in the Edgeworth Expansion approximations of $F_n(x)$:

$$F_n(x) \sim \Phi(x) - \frac{\beta_1(x^2 - 1)}{6\sqrt{n}}\varphi(x) - \left[\frac{\beta_2(x^3 - 3x)}{24n} + \frac{\beta_1^2(x^5 - 10x^3 + 15x)}{72n}\right]\varphi(x). \quad (12)$$

where $\beta_1 = E(X - \mu)^3/\sigma^3$ and $\beta_2 = E(X - \mu)^4/\sigma^4 - 3$ are the coefficient of skewness and the coefficient of kurtosis, respectively, and where $\varphi(x)$ represents the density of the standard normal distribution. This approximation is to be understood in the sense that the difference of the two sides when multiplied by n tends to zero as $n \to \infty$. Assuming the fourth moment exists, it is valid under the condition that

$$\limsup_{|t| \to \infty} |E(\exp\{itX\})| < 1. \quad (13)$$

This condition is known as *Cramér's Condition*. It holds, in particular, if the underlying distribution has a nonzero absolutely continuous component. The expansion to the term involving $1/\sqrt{n}$ is valid if the third moment exists, provided only that the underlying distribution is nonlattice, and even for lattice distributions it is valid provided a correction for continuity is made. See Feller (Vol. 2, Chap. XVI.4) for details.

Let us inspect this approximation. If we stop at the first term, $F_n(x) \sim \Phi(x)$, we have the approximation given by the Central Limit Theorem. The next term is of order $1/\sqrt{n}$ and represents a correction for skewness, since this term is zero if $\beta_1 = 0$. In particular, if the underlying distribution is symmetric, the Central Limit Theorem approximation is accurate up to terms of order $1/n$. The remaining term is a correction for kurtosis (and skewness) or order $1/n$.

The Edgeworth Expansion is an asymptotic expansion, which means that continuing with further terms in the expansion with n fixed may not converge. In particular, expanding to further terms for fixed n may make the accuracy worse. There are a number of books treating the more advanced theory of Edgeworth and allied expansions. The review by Bhattacharya (1990), treats the more mathematical aspects of the theory and the book of Barndorff-Nielsen and Cox (1989) the more statistical.

Table 1. Normal and Edgeworth approximations of the normalized mean of a sample of size 5 from an exponential distribution

x	$\Phi(x)$	$E_1(x)$	$E_2(x)$	Exact
−2.0	0.023	−0.001	−0.007	0.000
−1.8	0.036	0.010	0.000	0.003
−1.6	0.055	0.029	0.017	0.015
−1.4	0.081	0.059	0.047	0.042
−1.2	0.115	0.102	0.091	0.086
−1.0	0.159	0.159	0.151	0.147
−0.8	0.212	0.227	0.223	0.221
−0.6	0.274	0.306	0.305	0.305
−0.4	0.345	0.391	0.392	0.392
−0.2	0.421	0.477	0.478	0.478
0.0	0.500	0.559	0.559	0.560
0.2	0.579	0.635	0.634	0.634
0.4	0.655	0.702	0.700	0.701
0.6	0.726	0.758	0.758	0.758
0.8	0.788	0.804	0.808	0.807
1.0	0.841	0.841	0.849	0.847
1.2	0.885	0.872	0.883	0.881
1.4	0.919	0.898	0.910	0.908
1.6	0.945	0.919	0.931	0.929
1.8	0.964	0.938	0.947	0.946
2.0	0.977	0.953	0.959	0.959

Hall (1992) is concerned with the application of Edgeworth Expansion to the bootstrap.

We conclude with a simple example to illustrate the improvement in accuracy afforded by the Edgeworth Expansion. Suppose that $n = 5$ and that $X_1, X_2, \ldots, X_n$ is a sample from the exponential distribution with density $\exp\{-x\}$ on $(0, \infty)$. For this distribution, $\mu = 1$, $\sigma^2 = 1$, $\beta_1 = 2$, and $\beta_2 = 6$. In Table 1, the exact values of $F_n(x)$ may be compared with the normal approximation, $\Phi(x)$, and the Edgeworth Expansions to terms of order $1/\sqrt{n}$ and $1/n$, denoted by $E_1(x)$ and $E_2(x)$, respectively. The exact values may be obtained from the χ^2 distribution with 10 degrees of freedom, normalized to have mean 0 and variance 1.

It may be seen that the normal approximation is only moderately good, being off by 0.060 at $x = 0$. The approximation $E_1(x)$ is much better, the maximum error having been reduced to .018, occurring at $x = -1.4$. Finally, the approximation $E_2(x)$ is remarkably good, having a maximum error of 0.005 at $x = -1.2$. The negative values of E_1 and E_2 may be replaced by zeros.

EXERCISES

1. (a) If $X_1, X_2, \ldots$ are i.i.d. in $\mathbb{R}^2$ with distribution giving probability θ_1 to $\begin{bmatrix}1\\0\end{bmatrix}$, θ_2 to $\begin{bmatrix}0\\1\end{bmatrix}$, and $(1 - \theta_1 - \theta_2)$ to $\begin{bmatrix}0\\0\end{bmatrix}$, where $\theta_1 \geq 0$, $\theta_2 \geq 0$, and $\theta_1 + \theta_2 \leq 1$, what is the asymptotic distribution of $\overline{\mathbf{X}}_n$ given by the Central Limit Theorem?

   (b) Let $X_1, X_2, \ldots, X_n$ be a sample from the Poisson distribution with density $f(x|\theta) = e^{-\theta}\theta^x/x!$ for $x = 0, 1, \ldots,$ and let Z_n be the proportion of zeros observed, $Z_n = (1/n)\Sigma_{j=1}^n I(X_j = 0)$. Find the joint asymptotic distribution of $(\overline{X}_n, Z_n)$.
2. Let $X_1, X_2, \ldots$ be independent and suppose that $X_n = \sqrt{n}$ with probability $\frac{1}{2}$ and $X_n = -\sqrt{n}$ with probability $\frac{1}{2}$, for $n = 1, 2, \ldots$. Find the asymptotic distribution of $\overline{X}_n$. (Check the Lindeberg Condition.)
3. Show that the Lindeberg–Feller Theorem implies the Central Limit Theorem in one dimension.
4. Give a counterexample to the conjecture: If $X_1, X_2, \ldots$ are independent random variables, and $EX_j = 0$ and $\operatorname{var} X_j = 1$ for all j, then $\sqrt{n}\,\overline{X}_n \xrightarrow{\mathscr{L}} \mathscr{N}(0,1)$. (Consider distributions of the form $P\{X_j = v_j\} = p_j/2$, $P\{X_j = -v_j\} = p_j/2$, and $P\{X_j = 0\} = 1 - p_j$, for some numbers v_j and p_j.)
5. (All the applications of this section may be based on the following special case of the Lindeberg–Feller Theorem.) Suppose $X_1, X_2, \ldots$ are i.i.d. random variables with mean μ and variance σ^2. Let $T_n = \Sigma_{j=1}^n z_{nj} X_j$, where the z_{nj} are given numbers. Let $\mu_n = ET_n$ and $\sigma_n^2 = \operatorname{var} T_n$. Using the Lindeberg–Feller Theorem, show that $(T_n - \mu_n)/\sigma_n \xrightarrow{\mathscr{L}} \mathscr{N}(0,1)$ provided $\max_{j \leq n} z_{nj}^2 / \Sigma_{j=1}^n z_{nj}^2 \to 0$ as $n \to \infty$.
6. *Records*. Let $Z_1, Z_2, \ldots$ be i.i.d. continuous random variables. We say a record occurs at k if $Z_k > \max_{i<k} Z_i$. Let $R_k = 1$ if a record occurs at k, and let $R_k = 0$ otherwise. Then $R_1, R_2, \ldots$ are independent Bernoulli random variables with $P(R_k = 1) = 1 - P(R_k = 0) = 1/k$ for $k = 1, 2, \ldots$. Let $S_n = \Sigma_1^n R_k$ denote the number of records in the first n observations. Find ES_n and $\operatorname{var} S_n$, and show that $(S_n - ES_n)/\sqrt{\operatorname{var} S_n} \xrightarrow{\mathscr{L}} \mathscr{N}(0,1)$. (The distribution of S_n is also the distribution of the number of cycles in a random permutation.)
7. *Kendall's τ*. Let $Z_1, Z_2, \ldots$ be i.i.d. continuous random variables, and let X_k denote the number of Z_i for $i < k$ that are out of order, that is, have values greater than Z_k, $X_k = \Sigma_1^{k-1} I(Z_i > Z_k)$. It is known that the X_k are independent random variables and that X_k is uniformly distributed on the set $\{0, 1, \ldots, k-1\}$. The statistic $T_n = \Sigma_1^n X_k$ represents the total number of discrepancies in the ordering. It is zero

if the observations are in increasing order, and it takes on its maximum value of $\Sigma_1^n(k-1) = n(n-1)/2$ when the observations are in decreasing order. It may be used as a nonparametric test of randomness against the hypothesis that there is a trend in the observations, increasing or decreasing. The statistic, $\tau_n = 1 - 4T_n/(n(n-1))$, is always between -1 and $+1$ and is called Kendall's coefficient of rank correlation. It is a measure of agreement between two rankings of n objects. Find ET_n and $\operatorname{var} T_n$, and show that $(T_n - ET_n)/\sqrt{\operatorname{var} T_n} \xrightarrow{\mathscr{L}} \mathscr{N}(0, 1)$.

8. If $X_1, X_2, \ldots, X_n$ are i.i.d. in $\mathbb{R}^1$ with distribution giving probability $\frac{1}{2}$ to -1 and $+1$, find c_n for $n = 1$ and 2 such that $\sup_x |F_n(x) - \Phi(x)| = c_n \rho/(\sqrt{n}\,\sigma^3)$. What do you conjecture for $\lim_{n\to\infty} c_n$? (Use Stirling's formula: $n! \cong (n^n/e^n)\sqrt{2\pi n}$.) What does this say about the constant c in the Berry–Esseen Theorem?
9. Show that if $X_1, X_2, \ldots, X_n$ are samples from a distribution with coefficient of skewness β_1, and coefficient of kurtosis β_2, then the coefficient of skewness β_{1n} and the coefficient of kurtosis β_{2n} of $S_n = X_1 + X_2 + \cdots + X_n$ are given by $\beta_{1n} = \beta_1/\sqrt{n}$ and $\beta_{2n} = \beta_2/n$. Conclude that Table 1 also represents the Edgeworth Expansion approximations for the mean of a sample of size 10 from the χ^2 distribution with 1 degree of freedom, or the Edgeworth Expansion approximations for a sample of size 1 from the χ^2 distribution with 10 degrees of freedom.
10. Suppose that X_1, X_2, X_3 is a sample of size 3 from the uniform distribution on $(0, 1)$. Compare the exact probability, $P(X_1 + X_2 + X_3 \leq 2)$, to its normal and Edgeworth approximations.

2

Basic Statistical Large Sample Theory

6

Slutsky Theorems

A common problem in large sample theory is the following. Given a sequence of random vectors, $\{\mathbf{X}_n\}$, and given its limit law, say $\mathbf{X}_n \xrightarrow{\mathscr{L}} \mathbf{X}$, find the limiting distribution of $f(\mathbf{X}_n)$ for a given function, $f(\mathbf{x})$. The Slutsky Theorems provide a powerful technique for attacking this problem. For example, it gives a simple method for showing that the t-statistic for a sample from a distribution with finite variance is asymptotically normal, as we shall see.

Theorem 6. (a) *If* $\mathbf{X}_n \in \mathbb{R}^d$, $\mathbf{X}_n \xrightarrow{\mathscr{L}} \mathbf{X}$, *and if* $\mathbf{f}$: $\mathbb{R}^d \to \mathbb{R}^k$ *is such that* $P\{\mathbf{X} \in C(\mathbf{f})\} = 1$, *where* $C(\mathbf{f})$ *is the continuity set of* $\mathbf{f}$, *then* $\mathbf{f}(\mathbf{X}_n) \xrightarrow{\mathscr{L}} f(\mathbf{X})$.

(b) *If* $\mathbf{X}_n \xrightarrow{\mathscr{L}} \mathbf{X}$ *and* $(\mathbf{X}_n - \mathbf{Y}_n) \xrightarrow{\mathrm{P}} \mathbf{0}$, *then* $\mathbf{Y}_n \xrightarrow{\mathscr{L}} \mathbf{X}$.

(c) *If* $\mathbf{X}_n \in \mathbb{R}^d$, $\mathbf{Y}_n \in \mathbb{R}^k$, $\mathbf{X}_n \xrightarrow{\mathscr{L}} \mathbf{X}$, *and* $\mathbf{Y}_n \xrightarrow{\mathscr{L}} \mathbf{c}$, *then*

$$\begin{pmatrix} \mathbf{X}_n \\ \mathbf{Y}_n \end{pmatrix} \xrightarrow{\mathscr{L}} \begin{pmatrix} \mathbf{X} \\ \mathbf{c} \end{pmatrix}.$$

Note: We say $\mathbf{X}_n$ and $\mathbf{Y}_n$ are *asymptotically equivalent* if $(\mathbf{X}_n - \mathbf{Y}_n) \xrightarrow{\mathrm{P}} \mathbf{0}$. Thus, part (b) states that asymptotically equivalent sequences have the same limit laws.

Example 1. Suppose $X_n \xrightarrow{\mathscr{L}} X \in \mathscr{N}(0, 1)$. Then, using $f(x) = x^2$, part (a) gives $X_n^2 \xrightarrow{\mathscr{L}} X^2$, because f is continuous. Since $X^2 \in \chi_1^2$ when $X \in \mathscr{N}(0, 1)$, we have $X_n^2 \xrightarrow{\mathscr{L}} \chi_1^2$.

Example 2. If $X_n \xrightarrow{\mathscr{L}} X \in \mathscr{N}(0,1)$, then $1/X_n \xrightarrow{\mathscr{L}} Z$, where Z has the distribution of $1/X$, even though the function $f(x) = 1/x$ is not continuous at 0, because $P(X = 0) = 0$. Z has the reciprocal normal distribution with density,

$$g(z) = \frac{1}{\sqrt{2\pi z^2}} \exp\left\{-\frac{1}{2z^2}\right\}.$$

Example 3. However, if $X_n = 1/n$ and

$$f(x) = \begin{cases} 1, & \text{if } x > 0, \\ 0, & \text{if } x \leq 0, \end{cases}$$

then $X_n \xrightarrow{\mathscr{L}} 0$, but $f(X_n) \overset{\mathscr{L}}{\nrightarrow} f(0)$.

Example 4. Part (c) cannot be improved by assuming $\mathbf{Y}_n \xrightarrow{\mathscr{L}} \mathbf{Y}$ and concluding $\begin{pmatrix} \mathbf{X}_n \\ \mathbf{Y}_n \end{pmatrix} \xrightarrow{\mathscr{L}} \begin{pmatrix} \mathbf{X} \\ \mathbf{Y} \end{pmatrix}$. For example, if X is $\mathscr{U}(0,1)$ and $X_n = X$ for all n, and $Y_n = X$ for n odd and $Y_n = 1 - X$ for n even, then $X_n \xrightarrow{\mathscr{L}} X$ and $Y_n \xrightarrow{\mathscr{L}} \mathscr{U}(0,1)$, yet $\begin{pmatrix} X_n \\ Y_n \end{pmatrix}$ does not converge in law.

Example 5. Suppose $X_n \xrightarrow{\mathscr{L}} X$ and $Y_n \xrightarrow{P} c$. Does $X_n + Y_n \xrightarrow{\mathscr{L}} X + c$? First we note from (c) that $\begin{pmatrix} X_n \\ Y_n \end{pmatrix} \xrightarrow{\mathscr{L}} \begin{pmatrix} X \\ c \end{pmatrix}$, and then from (a) with $f(x,y) = x + y$ that $X_n + Y_n \xrightarrow{\mathscr{L}} X + c$. This combination of (a) and (c) is worth stating as a corollary.

Corollary. *If* $\mathbf{X}_n \in \mathbb{R}^d$, $\mathbf{Y}_n \in \mathbb{R}^k$, $\mathbf{X}_n \xrightarrow{\mathscr{L}} \mathbf{X}$, $\mathbf{Y}_n \xrightarrow{\mathscr{L}} \mathbf{c}$, *and* $\mathbf{f}\colon \mathbb{R}^{d+k} \to \mathbb{R}^r$ *is such that* $P\left\{\begin{pmatrix} \mathbf{X} \\ \mathbf{c} \end{pmatrix} \in C(\mathbf{f})\right\} = 1$, *then* $\mathbf{f}(\mathbf{X}_n, \mathbf{Y}_n) \xrightarrow{\mathscr{L}} \mathbf{f}(\mathbf{X}, \mathbf{c})$.

This follows directly from (a) and (c).

Example 6. If $\mathbf{X}_n \xrightarrow{\mathscr{L}} \mathbf{X}$ and $\mathbf{Y}_n \xrightarrow{\mathscr{L}} \mathbf{c}$, then $\mathbf{Y}_n^T \mathbf{X}_n \xrightarrow{\mathscr{L}} \mathbf{c}^T \mathbf{X}$.

Example 7. In one dimension, if $c \neq 0$ and $X_n \xrightarrow{\mathscr{L}} X$ and $Y_n \xrightarrow{P} c$, then $X_n/Y_n \xrightarrow{\mathscr{L}} X/c$. In this last, we are using the function

$$f(x,y) = \begin{cases} x/y, & \text{if } y \neq 0, \\ 0, & \text{if } y = 0, \end{cases}$$

which is discontinuous at all points of the line $y = 0$. However, the limiting distribution of $\begin{pmatrix} X \\ c \end{pmatrix}$ gives mass 0 to this line if $c \neq 0$, so the result follows from the corollary.

Proof of Theorem 6. (a) Let $g: \mathbb{R}^k \to \mathbb{R}$ be bounded and continuous. From Theorem 3(c), it is sufficient to show that $Eg(\mathbf{f}(\mathbf{X}_n)) \to Eg(\mathbf{f}(\mathbf{X}))$. Let $h(\mathbf{x}) = g(\mathbf{f}(\mathbf{x}))$. Then, a point of continuity of $\mathbf{f}$ is also a point of continuity of h; that is, $C(\mathbf{f}) \subset C(h)$, so from Theorem 3(d), $Eg(\mathbf{f}(\mathbf{X}_n)) = Eh(\mathbf{X}_n) \to Eh(\mathbf{X}) = Eg(\mathbf{f}(\mathbf{X}))$.

(b) Let g be continuous vanishing outside a compact set. From Theorem 3(b), it is sufficient to show that $Eg(\mathbf{Y}_n) \to Eg(\mathbf{X})$. Because g is uniformly continuous, let $\varepsilon > 0$, and find $\delta > 0$ such that

$$|\mathbf{x} - \mathbf{y}| < \delta \Rightarrow |g(\mathbf{x}) - g(\mathbf{y})| < \varepsilon.$$

Also g is bounded, say $|g(\mathbf{x})| < B$. Thus,

$$\begin{aligned}
|Eg(\mathbf{Y}_n) - Eg(\mathbf{X})| &\le |Eg(\mathbf{Y}_n) - Eg(\mathbf{X}_n)| + |Eg(\mathbf{X}_n) - Eg(\mathbf{X})| \\
&= E|g(\mathbf{Y}_n) - g(\mathbf{X}_n)| I(|\mathbf{X}_n - \mathbf{Y}_n| \le \delta) \\
&\quad + E|g(\mathbf{Y}_n) - g(\mathbf{X}_n)| I(|\mathbf{X}_n - \mathbf{Y}_n| > \delta) \\
&\quad + |Eg(\mathbf{X}_n) - Eg(\mathbf{X})| \\
&\le \varepsilon + 2BP\{|\mathbf{X}_n - \mathbf{Y}_n| > \delta\} + |Eg(\mathbf{X}_n) - Eg(\mathbf{X})| \to \varepsilon.
\end{aligned}$$

(c) $P\{|\binom{\mathbf{X}_n}{\mathbf{Y}_n} - \binom{\mathbf{X}_n}{\mathbf{c}}| > \varepsilon\} = P\{|\mathbf{Y}_n - \mathbf{c}| > \varepsilon\} \to 0.$

So from (b), it is sufficient to show that $\binom{\mathbf{X}_n}{\mathbf{c}} \xrightarrow{\mathscr{L}} \binom{\mathbf{X}}{\mathbf{c}}$. But if g is continuous bounded, $Eg(\mathbf{X}_n, \mathbf{c}) \to Eg(\mathbf{X}, \mathbf{c})$ because $\mathbf{X}_n \xrightarrow{\mathscr{L}} \mathbf{X}$. ■

Asymptotic Normality of the t Statistic. If $X_1, X_2, \ldots$ is a sample from a distribution with mean μ and variance $\sigma^2 > 0$ (on the real line), then

$$\bar{X}_n \xrightarrow{\mathscr{L}} \mu \quad \text{and} \quad (1/n)\sum_1^n X_j^2 \xrightarrow{\mathscr{L}} EX^2,$$

from the Law of Large Numbers, so from the corollary,

$$s_n^2 = (1/n)\sum_1^n X_j^2 - \bar{X}_n^2 \xrightarrow{\mathscr{L}} EX^2 - \mu^2 = \sigma^2.$$

In addition,

$$\sqrt{n}\,(\bar{X}_n - \mu)/\sigma \xrightarrow{\mathscr{L}} \mathscr{N}(0,1)$$

from the Central Limit Theorem. Hence, again from the corollary,

$$\sqrt{n}\,(\bar{X}_n - \mu)/s_n \xrightarrow{\mathscr{L}} \mathscr{N}(0,1).$$

The left side is defined as zero (or anything else) if $s_n = 0$, as in Example 7. From this it follows that the t statistic is asymptotically normal,

$$t_{n-1} = \sqrt{n-1}\left(\overline{X}_n - \mu\right)/s_n \xrightarrow{\mathscr{L}} \mathscr{N}(0,1). \quad \blacksquare$$

The Slutsky Theorems for convergence in probability are quite analogous to Theorem 6, but part (c) can be strengthened:

Theorem 6′. (a) *If* $\mathbf{X}_n \in \mathbb{R}^d$, $\mathbf{X}_n \xrightarrow{\text{P}} \mathbf{X}$, *and* $\mathbf{f}\colon \mathbb{R}^d \to \mathbb{R}^k$ *is such that* $P\{\mathbf{X} \in C(\mathbf{f})\} = 1$, *then* $\mathbf{f}(\mathbf{X}_n) \xrightarrow{\text{P}} \mathbf{f}(\mathbf{X})$.

(b) *If* $\mathbf{X}_n \xrightarrow{\text{P}} \mathbf{X}$ *and* $\mathbf{X}_n - \mathbf{Y}_n \xrightarrow{\text{P}} 0$, *then* $\mathbf{Y}_n \xrightarrow{\text{P}} \mathbf{X}$.

(c) *If* $\mathbf{X}_n \xrightarrow{\text{P}} \mathbf{X}$ *and* $\mathbf{Y}_n \xrightarrow{\text{P}} \mathbf{Y}$, *then* $\begin{pmatrix}\mathbf{X}_n\\ \mathbf{Y}_n\end{pmatrix} \xrightarrow{\text{P}} \begin{pmatrix}\mathbf{X}\\ \mathbf{Y}\end{pmatrix}$.

The Slutsky Theorems for convergence almost surely, obtained by replacing $\xrightarrow{\text{P}}$ wherever it occurs in Theorem 6′ by $\xrightarrow{\text{a.s.}}$, are also valid and easy to prove.

EXERCISES

1. Prove Theorem 6′. Hint: For (a), use Theorem 2(d).
2. Show that if $\{X_n\}$ and $\{Y_n\}$ are independent, and if $X_n \xrightarrow{\mathscr{L}} X$ and $Y_n \xrightarrow{\mathscr{L}} Y$, then $\begin{pmatrix}X_n\\ Y_n\end{pmatrix} \xrightarrow{\mathscr{L}} \begin{pmatrix}X\\ Y\end{pmatrix}$, where X and Y are taken to be independent.
3. Consider the autoregressive scheme,

$$X_n = \beta X_{n-1} + \varepsilon_n, \qquad \text{for } n = 1, 2, 3, \ldots,$$

where $\varepsilon_1, \varepsilon_2, \ldots$ are i.i.d., $E\varepsilon_n = \mu$, $\operatorname{var}(\varepsilon_n) = \sigma^2$, $-1 \le \beta < 1$, and $X_0 = 0$. Show that $\overline{X}_n = (1/n)\sum_1^n X_j$ is asymptotically normal:

$$\sqrt{n}\left(\overline{X}_n - \mu/(1-\beta)\right) \xrightarrow{\mathscr{L}} \mathscr{N}\left(0, \sigma^2/(1-\beta)^2\right), \qquad \text{if } -1 < \beta < 1,$$

$$\sqrt{n}\left(\overline{X}_n - \mu/2\right) \xrightarrow{\mathscr{L}} \mathscr{N}\left(0, \sigma^2/2\right), \qquad \text{if } \beta = -1.$$

Note the discontinuity at $\beta = -1$. What happens at $\beta = +1$?
4. (a) Show that two sequences of normalized random variables are asymptotically equivalent if their correlation converges to one. (A random variable is normalized if it has mean 0 and variance 1.) Conclude that if $(X_n - EX_n)/\sqrt{\operatorname{var} X_n} \xrightarrow{\mathscr{L}} X$ and if $\operatorname{corr}(X_n, Y_n) \to 1$, then $(Y_n - EY_n)/\sqrt{\operatorname{var} Y_n} \xrightarrow{\mathscr{L}} X$.

   (b) Suppose X_n and Y_n have zero means and equal variances. Is it true that if $X_n \xrightarrow{\mathscr{L}} X$ and $\operatorname{corr}(X_n, Y_n) \to 1$, then $Y_n \xrightarrow{\mathscr{L}} X$?

5. Show that if $E(X_n - Y_n)^2/\text{var}\,X_n \to 0$, then $\text{corr}(X_n, Y_n) \to 1$. Conclude using Exercise 4,

$$\frac{X_n - EX_n}{\sqrt{\text{var}\,X_n}} \xrightarrow{\mathscr{L}} X \quad \text{and} \quad \frac{E(X_n - Y_n)^2}{\text{var}\,X_n} \to 0$$

imply

$$\frac{Y_n - EY_n}{\sqrt{\text{var}\,Y_n}} \xrightarrow{\mathscr{L}} X.$$

6. The following version of Theorem 6(b) is often useful for nonnegative random variables.
   (a) Show that if $X_n \xrightarrow{\mathscr{L}} X > 0$ and $X_n/Y_n \xrightarrow{\text{P}} 1$, then $Y_n \xrightarrow{\mathscr{L}} X$.
   (b) Extend this result to random vectors.

7

Functions of the Sample Moments

We continue investigating the implications of the Slutsky Theorems. Here we study Cramér's Theorem on the asymptotic normality of functions of the sample moments through a Taylor-series expansion to one term. In some situations, the rate of convergence to normality is exceedingly slow. Hence, we conclude this section by studying improvements to the normal approximation that take more terms of the series expansion into account.

The analysis of the asymptotic distribution of the t-statistic given in the previous section may be extended to d dimensions as follows. From the central limit theorem, we have $\sqrt{n}(\overline{\mathbf{X}}_n - \boldsymbol{\mu}) \xrightarrow{\mathscr{L}} \mathscr{N}(\mathbf{0}, \boldsymbol{\Sigma})$ where $\boldsymbol{\Sigma} = \mathrm{var}(\mathbf{X})$, and from the Law of Large Numbers, with some help from the Slutsky Theorems, we have $\mathbf{S}_n = (1/n)\sum_1^n(\mathbf{X}_j - \overline{\mathbf{X}}_n)(\mathbf{X}_j - \overline{\mathbf{X}}_n)^T \xrightarrow{\mathrm{P}} \boldsymbol{\Sigma}$. If $\boldsymbol{\Sigma}$ is non-singular, then $P\{\mathbf{S}_n$ is nonsingular$\} \to 1$ and $\mathbf{S}_n^{-1/2}\sqrt{n}(\overline{\mathbf{X}}_n - \boldsymbol{\mu}) \xrightarrow{\mathscr{L}} \boldsymbol{\Sigma}^{-1/2}\mathbf{Y}$ where $\mathbf{Y} \in \mathscr{N}(\mathbf{0}, \boldsymbol{\Sigma})$. Since $\boldsymbol{\Sigma}^{-1/2}\mathbf{Y} \in \mathscr{N}(\mathbf{0}, \boldsymbol{\Sigma}^{-1/2}\boldsymbol{\Sigma}\boldsymbol{\Sigma}^{-1/2}) = \mathscr{N}(\mathbf{0}, \mathbf{I})$, we conclude that $\mathbf{S}_n^{-1/2}\sqrt{n}(\overline{\mathbf{X}}_n - \boldsymbol{\mu}) \xrightarrow{\mathscr{L}} \mathscr{N}(\mathbf{0}, \mathbf{I})$.

This is an example of a more general theorem, due to Cramér, that states that smooth functions of the sample moments are asymptotically normal. First, it is clear from the Central Limit Theorem that the sample moments about zero, things like $(1/n)\sum_1^n X_j$, $(1/n)\sum_1^n X_j^3$, and $(1/n)\sum_1^n X_j^2 Y_j$, are jointly asymptotically normal if the expectations of the squares of all terms exist. Then, repeated application of the following theorem shows that moments centered at the sample mean and smooth differentiable functions of them are also asymptotically normal.

Theorem 7 (Cramér). *Let* $\mathbf{g}$ *be a mapping* $\mathbf{g}\colon \mathbb{R}^d \to \mathbb{R}^k$ *such that* $\dot{\mathbf{g}}(\mathbf{x})$ *is continuous in a neighborhood of* $\boldsymbol{\mu} \in \mathbb{R}^d$. *If* $\mathbf{X}_n$ *is a sequence of d-dimensional random vectors such that* $\sqrt{n}(\mathbf{X}_n - \boldsymbol{\mu}) \xrightarrow{\mathscr{L}} \mathbf{X}$, *then* $\sqrt{n}(\mathbf{g}(\mathbf{X}_n) - \mathbf{g}(\boldsymbol{\mu})) \xrightarrow{\mathscr{L}} \dot{\mathbf{g}}(\boldsymbol{\mu})\mathbf{X}$. *In particular, if* $\sqrt{n}(\mathbf{X}_n - \boldsymbol{\mu}) \xrightarrow{\mathscr{L}} \mathscr{N}(0, \boldsymbol{\Sigma})$ *where* $\boldsymbol{\Sigma}$ *is a* $d \times d$ *covariance matrix, then*

$$\sqrt{n}(\mathbf{g}(\mathbf{X}_n) - \mathbf{g}(\boldsymbol{\mu})) \xrightarrow{\mathscr{L}} \mathscr{N}\left(\mathbf{0}, \dot{\mathbf{g}}(\boldsymbol{\mu})\boldsymbol{\Sigma}\dot{\mathbf{g}}(\boldsymbol{\mu})^T\right). \tag{1}$$

Proof. First note that $\sqrt{n}(\mathbf{X}_n - \boldsymbol{\mu}) \xrightarrow{\mathscr{L}} \mathbf{X}$ implies that $\mathbf{X}_n \xrightarrow{\mathscr{L}} \boldsymbol{\mu}$. Now if $\dot{\mathbf{g}}(\mathbf{x})$ is continuous in $\{\mathbf{x}\colon |\mathbf{x} - \boldsymbol{\mu}| < \delta\}$, then for $|\mathbf{x} - \boldsymbol{\mu}| < \delta$,

$$\mathbf{g}(\mathbf{x}) = \mathbf{g}(\boldsymbol{\mu}) + \int_0^1 \dot{\mathbf{g}}(\boldsymbol{\mu} + v(\mathbf{x} - \boldsymbol{\mu}))\, dv(\mathbf{x} - \boldsymbol{\mu}), \tag{2}$$

so for $|\mathbf{X}_n - \boldsymbol{\mu}| < \delta$,

$$\sqrt{n}(\mathbf{g}(\mathbf{X}_n) - g(\boldsymbol{\mu})) = \int_0^1 \dot{\mathbf{g}}(\boldsymbol{\mu} + v(\mathbf{X}_n - \boldsymbol{\mu}))\, dv\sqrt{n}(\mathbf{X}_n - \boldsymbol{\mu}). \tag{3}$$

Since $\mathbf{X}_n \xrightarrow{\mathscr{L}} \boldsymbol{\mu}$, we have $P(|\mathbf{X}_n - \boldsymbol{\mu}| < \delta) \to 1$ and $\int_0^1 \dot{\mathbf{g}}(\boldsymbol{\mu} + v(\mathbf{X}_n - \boldsymbol{\mu}))\, dv \xrightarrow{\mathscr{L}} \dot{\mathbf{g}}(\boldsymbol{\mu})$, so $\sqrt{n}(\mathbf{g}(\mathbf{X}_n) - \mathbf{g}(\boldsymbol{\mu})) \xrightarrow{\mathscr{L}} \dot{\mathbf{g}}(\boldsymbol{\mu})\mathbf{X}$. If $\mathbf{X} \in \mathscr{N}(\mathbf{0}, \boldsymbol{\Sigma})$, then because $E\dot{\mathbf{g}}(\boldsymbol{\mu})\mathbf{X} = \mathbf{0}$ and $\mathrm{var}(\dot{\mathbf{g}}(\boldsymbol{\mu})\mathbf{X}) = \dot{\mathbf{g}}(\boldsymbol{\mu})\boldsymbol{\Sigma}\dot{\mathbf{g}}(\boldsymbol{\mu})^T$ we have $\dot{\mathbf{g}}(\boldsymbol{\mu})\mathbf{X} \in \mathscr{N}(\mathbf{0}, \dot{\mathbf{g}}(\boldsymbol{\mu})\boldsymbol{\Sigma}\dot{\mathbf{g}}(\boldsymbol{\mu})^T)$.

Example 1. For a sample from a one-dimensional distribution with mean μ and variance σ^2, $\sqrt{n}(\overline{X}_n - \mu) \xrightarrow{\mathscr{L}} \mathscr{N}(0, \sigma^2)$. What is the asymptotic distribution of $\overline{X}_n^2$?

Solution. Let $g(x) = x^2$. Then $\dot{g}(x) = 2x$, and $\dot{g}(\mu) = 2\mu$. Hence, from Theorem 7,

$$\sqrt{n}\left(\overline{X}_n^2 - \mu^2\right) \xrightarrow{\mathscr{L}} \mathscr{N}(0, 4\mu^2\sigma^2). \tag{4}$$

Note: This example and those that follow bring out several points to be aware of in large sample theory. First, the rate of convergence to normality in Theorem 7 can vary widely with variation in either g or μ.

Second, the asymptotic variance can be zero as in Example 1 when $\mu = 0$. All this example says when $\mu = 0$ is that $\sqrt{n}\,\overline{X}_n^2 \xrightarrow{\mathscr{L}} 0$, and this is not what one means by asymptotic distribution. We would like to find an asymptotic scaling sequence a_n such that $a_n\overline{X}_n^2$ has a *nondegenerate* distribution. In fact, when $\mu = 0$, $n\overline{X}_n^2 \xrightarrow{\mathscr{L}} \sigma^2\chi_1^2$, because by Slutsky $n\overline{X}_n^2 = (\sqrt{n}\,\overline{X}_n)^2 \to Y^2$ where $Y \in \mathscr{N}(0, \sigma^2)$ so that $(Y/\sigma)^2 \in \chi_1^2$.

Third, the moments of the limit need not be the limit of the moments, as the following example indicates.

Example 2. Suppose that $\sqrt{n}(X_n - \mu) \xrightarrow{\mathscr{L}} \mathscr{N}(0, \sigma^2)$. What is the asymptotic distribution of $1/X_n$? Let $g(x) = 1/x$. Then $\dot{g}(x) = -1/x^2$ and $\dot{g}(\mu) = -1/\mu^2$. Therefore, by Cramér's Theorem, when $\mu \neq 0$,

$$\sqrt{n}\left(\frac{1}{X_n} - \frac{1}{\mu}\right) \xrightarrow{\mathscr{L}} \mathscr{N}\left(0, \frac{\sigma^2}{\mu^4}\right). \tag{5}$$

However, when $X_n \in \mathscr{N}(\mu, \sigma^2/n)$, $E(1/X_n)$ does not exist, because for any distribution with density positive and continuous at the origin, $E(1/|X|) = \infty$.

Example 3. Assuming finite fourth moments, what is the asymptotic distribution of the sample variance, $s_x^2 = (1/n)\Sigma_1^n(X_j - \overline{X}_n)^2$? Since $s_x^2 = (1/n)\Sigma_1^n X_j^2 - \overline{X}_n^2$, we must first find the asymptotic joint distribution of the first two moments. Since s_x^2 does not depend on location, we may as well assume $\mu = 0$ (or equivalently, work with $X_j - \mu$). Let $m_{xx} = (1/n)\Sigma_1^n X_j^2$ and $m_x = (1/n)\Sigma_1^n X_j$. From the Central Limit Theorem,

$$\sqrt{n}\left[\begin{pmatrix} m_x \\ m_{xx} \end{pmatrix} - \begin{pmatrix} 0 \\ \sigma^2 \end{pmatrix}\right] \xrightarrow{\mathscr{L}} \mathscr{N}(\mathbf{0}, \mathbf{\Sigma}),$$

where

$$\mathbf{\Sigma} = \begin{bmatrix} \operatorname{var} X & \operatorname{cov}(X^2, X) \\ \operatorname{cov}(X^2, X) & \operatorname{var} X^2 \end{bmatrix}.$$

To find the asymptotic distribution of s_x^2, let $g(m_x, m_{xx}) = m_{xx} - m_x^2 = s_x^2$, and note that $\dot{g}(m_x, m_{xx}) = (-2m_x, 1)$ and $\dot{g}(0, \sigma^2) = (0, 1)$. Hence,

$$\begin{aligned}\sqrt{n}(s_x^2 - \sigma^2) &\xrightarrow{\mathscr{L}} \mathscr{N}\left(0, \dot{g}(0, \sigma^2)\mathbf{\Sigma}\dot{g}(0, \sigma^2)^T\right) \\ &= \mathscr{N}(0, \operatorname{var} X^2) = \mathscr{N}\left(0, EX^4 - (EX^2)^2\right) \\ &= \mathscr{N}(0, \mu_4 - \sigma^4). \end{aligned} \tag{6}$$

If the parent distribution is normal, then $\mu_4 = 3\sigma^4$, so

$$\sqrt{n}(s_x^2 - \sigma^2) \xrightarrow{\mathscr{L}} \mathscr{N}(0, 2\sigma^4).$$

Improving the Approximation. We return to the observation in Example 1 that if $\sqrt{n}\,(\overline{X}_n - \mu) \xrightarrow{\mathscr{L}} \mathscr{N}(0, \sigma^2)$ and $g(x) = x^2$, then Cramér's Theorem yields

$$\sqrt{n}\left(\overline{X}_n^2 - \mu^2\right) \xrightarrow{\mathscr{L}} \mathscr{N}(0, 4\mu^2\sigma^2). \tag{7}$$

When $\mu = 0$, this gives $\sqrt{n}\,\overline{X}_n^2 \xrightarrow{\mathscr{L}} \mathscr{N}(0,0)$, but more accuracy can be obtained using instead

$$n\overline{X}_n^2 \xrightarrow{\mathscr{L}} \sigma^2 x_1^2. \tag{8}$$

This clearly implies a danger from using (7) when μ is close to but not equal to zero. No matter how large n is, there is a μ sufficiently close to zero for which the approximation (7) is very poor. One can often obtain a definite improvement in the approximation by taking more terms in the expansion of the function g into account in the proof of Cramer's Theorem.

Suppose that $\sqrt{n}\,(X_n - \mu) \xrightarrow{\mathscr{L}} \mathscr{N}(0, \sigma^2)$, and suppose we are interested in estimating $g(\mu)$ where $g(\mu)$ has a continuous second derivative with $g''(\mu) \neq 0$. To improve upon the approximation given in Theorem 7, we expand $g(x)$ about μ to second-order terms and complete the square in $x - \mu$:

$$\begin{aligned} g(x) - g(\mu) &\sim g'(\mu)(x-\mu) + \frac{g''(\mu)}{2}(x-\mu)^2 \\ &= \frac{g''(\mu)}{2}\left[\left(x - \mu + \frac{g'(\mu)}{g''(\mu)}\right)^2 - \frac{g'(\mu)^2}{g''(\mu)^2}\right]. \end{aligned} \tag{9}$$

Replacing x by X_n, we may conclude that

$$n(g(X_n) - g(\mu)) \sim \frac{\sigma^2 g''(\mu)}{2}\left[\left(\sqrt{n}\,(X_n - \mu)/\sigma + \gamma_n\right)^2 - \gamma_n^2\right] \tag{10}$$

where

$$\gamma_n = \frac{\sqrt{n}\,g'(\mu)}{\sigma g''(\mu)}.$$

The distribution of the square of a normal random variable with mean γ and variance 1 is the noncentral chi-square distribution with 1 degree of freedom and noncentrality parameter γ^2, denoted by $\chi_1^2(\gamma^2)$. Therefore, we may rewrite (10) with the notation

$$n(g(X_n) - g(\mu)) \sim \frac{\sigma^2 g''(\mu)}{2}\left[\chi_1^2(\gamma_n^2) - \gamma_n^2\right]. \tag{11}$$

When $g(x) = x^2$, this gives in comparison to (7)

$$n(X_n^2 - \mu^2) \sim \sigma^2\left[\chi_1^2(\gamma_n^2) - \gamma_n^2\right], \tag{12}$$

where $\gamma_n = \sqrt{n}\,\mu/(2\sigma)$. When $\mu = 0$, this reduces to (8). For γ_n^2 close to zero, this provides a big improvement over (7). Even for γ_n^2 large, (12) is approximately the same as (7), because $\chi_1^2(\gamma_n^2) - \gamma_n^2$ is approximately $\mathscr{N}(0, 4\gamma_n^2)$ [see Exercise 2(b) of Section 10].

We conclude with a numerical example of the accuracy of these approximations. The function $g(x) = x^2$ is a little too simple, because the expansion (9) becomes exact. Instead we take $g(x) = \exp\{x\}$, and we suppose that $\sqrt{n}\,(X_n - \mu)$ is exactly $\mathscr{N}(0, \sigma^2)$. To keep things simple, we take $\mu = 0$ and $\sigma^2 = 1$. Let $Z = \sqrt{n}\,(\exp\{X_n\} - \exp\{\mu\})/(\sigma \exp\{\mu\}) = \sqrt{n}\,(\exp\{X_n\} - 1)$. Under the normal approximation (7), the distribution of Z is $\Phi(z)$. From the noncentral χ^2 approximation (11), the distribution of Z is (using $\gamma_n = \sqrt{n}$)

$$\begin{aligned} P(Z \le z) &\sim P\left((\mathscr{N}(0,1) + \gamma_n)^2 \le \gamma_n^2 + 2\sqrt{n}\,z\right) \\ &= \Phi\left(\sqrt{n + 2\sqrt{n}\,z} - \sqrt{n}\right) - \Phi\left(-\sqrt{n + 2\sqrt{n}\,z} - \sqrt{n}\right). \end{aligned} \tag{13}$$

The exact distribution of $\exp\{X_n\}$ is lognormal, and

$$P(Z \le z) = P\left(\exp\{\mathscr{N}(0, 1/n)\} \le 1 + z/\sqrt{n}\right) = \Phi\left(\sqrt{n}\,\log(1 + z/\sqrt{n})\right). \tag{14}$$

In Table 2, we take $n = 5$ and compare the two approximations with the exact probabilities.

If X_n is not exactly normal, for example, if it were the mean of a sample for an exponential distribution, the above approximations can be improved by considering the Edgeworth Expansion, $E_2(x)$, of Table 1 in place of $\Phi(x)$ in Table 2.

Table 2. Normal and noncentral χ^2 approximations of the distribution of $\sqrt{n}\,(g(\overline{X}_n) - g(0))/g'(0)$ for a sample of size $n = 5$ from a standard normal distribution with $g(x) = \exp\{x\}$.

z	$\Phi(z)$	(13)	(14)
−2.0	0.0228	0.0000	0.0000
−1.8	0.0359	0.0000	0.0001
−1.6	0.0548	0.0000	0.0025
−1.4	0.0808	0.0000	0.0139
−1.2	0.1151	0.0000	0.0427
−1.0	0.1587	0.0641	0.0925
−0.8	0.2119	0.1481	0.1610
−0.6	0.2743	0.2375	0.2424
−0.4	0.3446	0.3285	0.3297
−0.2	0.4207	0.4169	0.4170
0.0	0.5000	0.5000	0.5000
0.2	0.5793	0.5760	0.5760
0.4	0.6554	0.6441	0.6436
0.6	0.7257	0.7040	0.7025
0.8	0.7881	0.7558	0.7530
1.0	0.8413	0.8000	0.7958
1.2	0.8849	0.8374	0.8316
1.4	0.9192	0.8686	0.8615
1.6	0.9452	0.8944	0.8863
1.8	0.9641	0.9156	0.9067
2.0	0.9772	0.9330	0.9234

EXERCISES

1. Find the asymptotic distribution of $\log s_x^2$.
2. Show that the joint asymptotic distribution $\overline{X}_n$ and s_x^2 is

$$\sqrt{n}\left[\begin{pmatrix}\overline{X}_n \\ s_x^2\end{pmatrix} - \begin{pmatrix}\mu \\ \sigma^2\end{pmatrix}\right] \xrightarrow{\mathscr{L}} \mathscr{N}\left(\mathbf{0}, \begin{bmatrix}\sigma^2 & \mu_3 \\ \mu_3 & \mu_4 - \sigma^4\end{bmatrix}\right).$$

3. Find the asymptotic distribution of
   (a) $s_x/\overline{X}_n$ (the coefficient of variation).
   (b) $m_3 = (1/n)\Sigma_1^n(X_j - \overline{X})^3$.
4. Let $X_1, \ldots, X_n$ be a sample of size n from the beta distribution, $\mathscr{Be}(\theta, 1)$, $\theta > 0$. The method-of-moments estimate of θ is $\hat{\theta}_n = \overline{X}_n/(1 - \overline{X}_n)$. Find its asymptotic distribution.

5. *The Poisson Dispersion Test*. A standard test of the hypothesis H_0 that a distribution is Poisson, $\mathscr{P}(\lambda)$ for some λ, is to reject H_0 if the ratio of the sample variance to the sample mean, $s_x^2/\overline{X}_n$, is too large. This test is good against alternatives whose variance is greater than the mean, such as the negative binomial distribution or any other mixture of Poisson distributions.
   (a) Find the asymptotic distribution of $s_x^2/\overline{X}_n$ for general distributions.
   (b) Find the asymptotic distribution of $x_x^2/\overline{X}_n$ under H_0 and show that it is independent of λ.
6. Suppose we are interested in estimating the variance, $g(p) = p(1-p)$, of the Bernoulli distribution with probability p of success, based on a sample of size n. Let X_n denote the proportion of successes, $X_n = X/n$, where X has the binomial distribution, $\mathscr{B}(n, p)$, and consider the estimate $g(X_n) = X_n(1 - X_n)$.
   (a) Find the asymptotic distribution of $g(X_n)$. What happens when $p = \frac{1}{2}$?
   (b) What is the asymptotic expansion (11) for the distribution of $g(X_n)$?
   (c) Take $p = 0.6$ and $n = 100$. Compare the approximations to $P(g(X_n) \leq y)$ given by (a) and (b) at the points $y = 0.23$, 0.24, and 0.25.

8

The Sample Correlation Coefficient

The last example of Section 6, namely, that

$$t_{n-1} = \sqrt{n-1}\,(\bar{X}_n - \mu)/s_n \xrightarrow{\mathscr{L}} \mathscr{N}(0,1),$$

shows that the t test is *asymptotically robust* or *asymptotically distribution-free* within the class of distributions with finite second moments. In particular, the confidence interval for the mean μ of a distribution, given by

$$\bar{X}_n - \left(s_n/\sqrt{n-1}\,\right)t_{n-1;\,\alpha} \le \mu \le \bar{X}_n + \left(s_n/\sqrt{n-1}\,\right)t_{n-1;\,\alpha},$$

has approximate probability $1 - 2\alpha$ whatever be the true distribution of the X_i, provided it has a finite variance and n is sufficiently large.

The usual test or confidence interval for the variance of a distribution when sampling from a normal distribution is based on the statistic $(ns_x^2)/\sigma^2$ which has a χ^2_{n-1} distribution. Example 3 of Section 7 shows that this test is not asymptotically distribution-free. The asymptotic distribution of $(ns_x^2)/\sigma^2$ depends on the fourth moment of the true distribution. For the normal distribution, $\mu_4 = 3\sigma^4$, and so the usual test will be asymptotically valid for any true distribution with $\mu_4 = 3\sigma^4$. But we often expect sampling distributions to have somewhat thicker tails than the normal. For example, $\mu_4 = 6.111\ldots\sigma^4$ for the double exponential distribution with density $f(x) = (1/2)e^{-|x|}$.

Even worse in this regard is the sample correlation coefficient, $r = s_{xy}/s_x s_y$, when used for testing hypotheses concerning the correlation coefficient, $\rho = \sigma_{xy}/\sigma_x\sigma_y$. The asymptotic distribution of r, when sampling from distributions with finite fourth moments, may be found by the methods of Section 7.

Theorem 8. *Let $(X_1, Y_1), (X_2, Y_2), \ldots$ be a sample from a bivariate distribution with finite fourth moments, EX^4 and EY^4. Then,*

(a)

$$\sqrt{n}\left[\begin{bmatrix} s_x^2 \\ s_{xy} \\ s_y^2 \end{bmatrix} - \begin{bmatrix} \sigma_x^2 \\ \sigma_{xy} \\ \sigma_y^2 \end{bmatrix}\right] \xrightarrow{\mathscr{L}} \mathscr{N}\left(\mathbf{0}, \begin{bmatrix} C(XX,XX) & C(XX,XY) & C(XX,YY) \\ C(XX,XY) & C(XY,XY) & C(XY,YY) \\ C(XX,YY) & C(XY,YY) & C(YY,YY) \end{bmatrix}\right),$$

where

$$C(XX,XX) = \mathrm{cov}\big((X-\mu_x)^2, (X-\mu_x)^2\big) = E(X-\mu_x)^4 - \big(E(X-\mu_x)^2\big)^2,$$

$$C(XX,XY) = \mathrm{cov}\big((X-\mu_x)^2, (X-\mu_x)(Y-\mu_y)\big)$$

$$= E(X-\mu_x)^3(Y-\mu_y) - \sigma_x^2\sigma_{xy}, \text{ etc.}$$

(b)

$$\sqrt{n}\,(r-\rho) \xrightarrow{\mathscr{L}} \mathscr{N}(0, \gamma^2),$$

where

$$\gamma^2 = \frac{1}{4}\rho^2\left[\frac{C(XX,XX)}{\sigma_x^4} + 2\frac{C(XX,YY)}{\sigma_x^2\sigma_y^2} + \frac{C(YY,YY)}{\sigma_y^4}\right]$$

$$- \rho\left[\frac{C(XX,XY)}{\sigma_x^3\sigma_y} + \frac{C(XY,YY)}{\sigma_x\sigma_y^3}\right] + \frac{C(XY,XY)}{\sigma_x^2\sigma_y^2}.$$

Outline of Proof. The proof follows the steps of the last example of Section 7. Assume without loss of generality that $\mu_x = \mu_y = 0$. First, use the Central Limit Theorem to find the joint asymptotic distribution of $\mathbf{M}_n = (m_x, m_y, m_{xx}, m_{xy}, m_{yy})^T$, where $m_x = (1/n)\Sigma_1^n X_j$, $m_{xx} = (1/n)\Sigma_1^n X_j^2$ and $m_{xy} = (1/n)\Sigma_1^n X_jY_j$, etc. Then, apply Cramér's Theorem to the function, $\mathbf{g}(\mathbf{M}_n) = (m_{xx} - m_x^2, m_{xy} - m_xm_y, m_{yy} - m_y^2)^T$.

Moments of the Bivariate Normal Distribution. To find the value of γ^2 for the bivariate normal distribution, we may assume the means are 0 and the variances are 1, because γ^2 is independent of a change in location and scale in X or Y. The moments EX^3Y, et cetera, may be found by integrating, or by taking the appropriate derivatives of the characteristic function,

$$\varphi(t_1, t_2) = \exp\{-(1/2)(t_1^2 + 2\rho t_1 t_2 + t_2^2)\},$$

and setting $(t_1, t_2) = (0, 0)$. We find

$$E(X - \mu_x)^4 = 3\sigma_x^4,$$

$$E(X - \mu_x)^3(Y - \mu_y) = 3\rho\sigma_x^3\sigma_y,$$

and

$$E(X - \mu_x)^2(Y - \mu_y)^2 = (1 + 2\rho^2)\sigma_x^2\sigma_y^2.$$

Hence,

$$\begin{aligned}\gamma^2 &= (1/4)\rho^2[2 + 2(2\rho^2) + 2] - \rho[(3\rho - \rho)\cdot 2] + (1 + 2\rho^2 - \rho^2)\\ &= \rho^2[1 + \rho^2] - 4\rho^2 + 1 + \rho^2 = (1 - \rho^2)^2,\end{aligned}$$

so that for normal populations,

$$\sqrt{n}\,(r - \rho) \xrightarrow{\mathscr{L}} \mathscr{N}\big(0, (1 - \rho^2)^2\big).$$

Robustizing. The usual χ^2 test for a variance is based on the fact that for normal distributions $(ns_x^2)/\sigma^2$ has a χ_{n-1}^2 distribution. For n large, the χ_{n-1}^2 distribution is approximately $\mathscr{N}(n - 1, 2(n - 1))$. Hence, the confidence intervals for σ^2 obtained from this test are asymptotically those obtained from

$$\frac{ns_x^2/\sigma^2 - (n - 1)}{\sqrt{2(n - 1)}} \sim \frac{\sqrt{n}}{\sqrt{2}}\left[\frac{s_x^2}{\sigma^2} - 1\right] \xrightarrow{\mathscr{L}} \mathscr{N}(0, 1).$$

If the population is not normal, we should be using, as seen at the end of Section 7,

$$\frac{\sqrt{n}\,[s_x^2/\sigma^2 - 1]}{\sqrt{\mu_4/\sigma^4 - 1}} \xrightarrow{\mathscr{L}} \mathscr{N}(0, 1).$$

Because μ_4 is not known, this statistic cannot be used directly. However, it may be robustized by replacing the coefficient of kurtosis, $\beta_2 = \mu_4/\sigma^4$, by an estimate, $b_2 = m_4/s_x^4$, the sample coefficient of kurtosis. The confidence interval resulting from

$$\left|\frac{s_x^2}{\sigma^2} - 1\right| < \frac{\sqrt{b_2 - 1}}{\sqrt{n}}\mathscr{N}_{\alpha/2}$$

may be written

$$\frac{s_x^2}{1 + \frac{\sqrt{b_2 - 1}}{\sqrt{n}}\mathcal{N}_{\alpha/2}} < \sigma^2 < \frac{s_x^2}{1 - \frac{\sqrt{b_2 - 1}}{\sqrt{n}}\mathcal{N}_{\alpha/2}}.$$

The usual confidence interval based on the χ_n^2 distribution may be obtained from this, approximately for large n, by replacing b_2 by the coefficient of kurtosis for the normal distribution, namely, $\beta_2 = 3$.

One may similarly robustize tests and confidence intervals for ρ by replacing the moments in γ^2 by their sample estimates to obtain $\hat{\gamma}^2$ and using $\sqrt{n}(r - \rho)/\hat{\gamma} \xrightarrow{\mathscr{L}} \mathcal{N}(0, 1)$. However, these procedures must be used with caution; estimates of fourth and cross-second moments have large standard error.

Variance-stabilizing Transformations. For normal populations, $\sqrt{n}(r - \rho) \xrightarrow{\mathscr{L}} \mathcal{N}(0, (1 - \rho^2)^2)$. We seek a transformation, $g(r)$, such that $\sqrt{n}(g(r) - g(\rho)) \xrightarrow{\mathscr{L}} \mathcal{N}(0, 1)$. Such a transformation is called variance-stabilizing. From Cramér's Theorem $\sqrt{n}(g(r) - g(\rho)) \xrightarrow{\mathscr{L}} \mathcal{N}(0, \dot{g}(\rho)^2(1 - \rho^2)^2)$, so we must solve the differential equation

$$\dot{g}(\rho)^2(1 - \rho^2)^2 = 1 \quad \text{or} \quad \dot{g}(\rho) = 1/(1 - \rho^2).$$

The solution is known as Fisher's transformation:

$$g(\rho) = \int \frac{1}{1 - \rho^2}\, d\rho = \int \left[\frac{1/2}{1 - \rho} + \frac{1/2}{1 + \rho}\right] d\rho = \frac{1}{2}\log\frac{1 + \rho}{1 - \rho}.$$

also known as $\tanh^{-1} \rho$. Therefore,

$$\sqrt{n}\left[\frac{1}{2}\log\frac{1 + r}{1 - r} - \frac{1}{2}\log\frac{1 + \rho}{1 - \rho}\right] \xrightarrow{\mathscr{L}} \mathcal{N}(0, 1).$$

EXERCISES

1. Find the asymptotic distribution of the estimate of the regression coefficient, $\hat{\beta} = s_{xy}/s_x^2$, when sampling from a bivariate distribution. What is its asymptotic variance when sampling from a bivariate normal distribution?
2. Find an asymptotically robustized version of the confidence intervals for σ_{xy}.

3. Find variance-stabilizing transformations for $\overline{X}_n$ when sampling from (a) the Poisson distribution, $\mathscr{P}(\lambda)$, (b) the Bernoulli distribution, $\mathscr{B}(1, p)$.
4. The usual F test for the equality of variances of two independent normal populations is based on the ratio of the two sample variances, s_x^2/s_y^2. Show that this test is not asymptotically distribution-free within the class of distributions with finite fourth moments, by finding the asymptotic distribution of $\sqrt{n}\,(s_x^2/s_y^2 - \sigma_x{}^2/\sigma_y{}^2)$ within this class. Suppose both samples are of size n.

9

Pearson's Chi-Square

In this section we derive the asymptotic distribution of the Pearson χ^2 statistic as another application of the theorems of Slutsky. We first present three general lemmas relating quadratic forms in normal or asymptotically normal variables to the chi-square distribution. After describing multinomial experiments and the Pearson χ^2 statistic for testing a simple null hypothesis, we present two derivations of the asymptotic distribution of Pearson's χ^2 under the null hypothesis. The first, contained in the proof of Theorem 9, is based on the matrix theory notions of rank and projection. The second uses the fact that Pearson's χ^2 is just a version of Hotelling's T^2 and is postponed to the exercises (Exercise 3). We also mention two important variations of Pearson's χ^2, one based on transformations (Hellinger's χ^2) and the other based on the principle of modification (Neyman's χ^2 of Exercise 1).

Recall that the χ^2 distribution with d degrees of freedom, denoted by χ^2_d, is defined as the distribution of $\mathbf{X}^T\mathbf{X}$, where $\mathbf{X}$ is d-dimensional with $\mathbf{X} \in \mathscr{N}(\mathbf{0}, \mathbf{I})$ [the sum of squares of d independent $\mathscr{N}(0, 1)$'s].

Lemma 1. *If* $\mathbf{X} \in \mathscr{N}(\boldsymbol{\mu}, \boldsymbol{\Sigma})$ *with* $\boldsymbol{\Sigma}$ *nonsingular, then*

$$Z = (\mathbf{X} - \boldsymbol{\mu})^T \boldsymbol{\Sigma}^{-1} (\mathbf{X} - \boldsymbol{\mu}) \in \chi^2_d$$

Proof. Let $\mathbf{Y} = \boldsymbol{\Sigma}^{-1/2}(\mathbf{X} - \boldsymbol{\mu})$. Then $\mathbf{Y} \in \mathscr{N}(\mathbf{0}, \mathbf{I})$ and $Z = \mathbf{Y}^T\mathbf{Y}$. ■

Lemma 2. *If* $\mathbf{X}_1, \mathbf{X}_2, \ldots$ *are i.i.d. with mean* $\boldsymbol{\mu}$ *and nonsingular covariance matrix* $\boldsymbol{\Sigma}$, *then*

$$T^2 = (n-1)\left(\overline{\mathbf{X}}_n - \boldsymbol{\mu}\right)^T \mathbf{S}_n^{-1} \left(\overline{\mathbf{X}}_n - \boldsymbol{\mu}\right) \xrightarrow{\mathscr{L}} \chi^2_d,$$

where $\mathbf{S}_n$ *is the sample covariance matrix,*

$$\mathbf{S}_n = (1/n)\sum_1^n (\mathbf{X}_i - \overline{\mathbf{X}})(\mathbf{X}_i - \overline{\mathbf{X}})^T$$

Proof. By the Central Limit Theorem, $\sqrt{n}\,(\overline{\mathbf{X}}_n - \boldsymbol{\mu}) \xrightarrow{\mathscr{L}} \mathbf{Y} \in \mathscr{N}(\mathbf{0}, \boldsymbol{\Sigma})$, and by the Weak Law of Large Numbers and Slutsky's Theorem $\mathbf{S}_n \xrightarrow{\mathscr{L}} \boldsymbol{\Sigma}$. Hence by Slutsky, $T^2 \xrightarrow{\mathscr{L}} \mathbf{Y}^T\boldsymbol{\Sigma}^{-1}\mathbf{Y} \in \chi_d^2$.

Note: T^2 is known as *Hotelling's* T^2. It is known that if $\mathbf{X}_1, \mathbf{X}_2, \ldots, \mathbf{X}_n$ is a sample from $\mathscr{N}(\boldsymbol{\mu}, \boldsymbol{\Sigma})$ with $\boldsymbol{\Sigma}$ nonsingular, then $((n-d)/(n-1)d)T^2$ has an exact $F_{d,n-d}$ distribution.

The characteristic function of the χ_d^2 distribution is $\varphi(t) = (1 - 2it)^{-d/2}$.

A square matrix $\boldsymbol{\Sigma}$ is a *projection* if $\boldsymbol{\Sigma}^2 = \boldsymbol{\Sigma}$. (If $\mathbf{y} = \boldsymbol{\Sigma}\mathbf{x}$, then $\mathbf{y}$ is the projection of $\mathbf{x}$ onto the range space of $\boldsymbol{\Sigma}$. Further application of $\boldsymbol{\Sigma}$ to $\mathbf{y}$ does not change it: $\boldsymbol{\Sigma}y = \boldsymbol{\Sigma}^2x = \boldsymbol{\Sigma}\mathbf{x} = \mathbf{y}$.) If in addition $\boldsymbol{\Sigma}$ is symmetric, the projection is perpendicular onto its range. [That is, $\mathbf{y} = \boldsymbol{\Sigma}\mathbf{x}$ is perpendicular to $\mathbf{x} - \mathbf{y} = (\mathbf{I} - \boldsymbol{\Sigma})\mathbf{x}$: $(\boldsymbol{\Sigma}\mathbf{x})^T(\mathbf{I} - \boldsymbol{\Sigma})\mathbf{x} = \mathbf{x}^T\boldsymbol{\Sigma}^T(\mathbf{I} - \boldsymbol{\Sigma})\mathbf{x} = \mathbf{x}^T(\boldsymbol{\Sigma}^2 - \boldsymbol{\Sigma})\mathbf{x} = 0$.]

LEMMA 3. *Let* $\mathbf{X} \in \mathscr{N}(\mathbf{0}, \boldsymbol{\Sigma})$. *Then* $\mathbf{X}^T\mathbf{X} \in \chi_r^2$ *if and only if* $\boldsymbol{\Sigma}$ *is a projection of rank* r.

Proof. Since $\boldsymbol{\Sigma}$ is symmetric, there exists an orthogonal matrix $\mathbf{Q}$ ($\mathbf{Q}^T\mathbf{Q} = \mathbf{I}$) such that $\mathbf{D} = \mathbf{Q}\boldsymbol{\Sigma}\mathbf{Q}^T$ is a diagonal matrix. Then,

$$\begin{aligned} &\boldsymbol{\Sigma}^2 = \boldsymbol{\Sigma} \text{ and } \boldsymbol{\Sigma} \text{ has rank } r \\ &\quad\Leftrightarrow \mathbf{D}^2 = \mathbf{D} \text{ and } \mathbf{D} \text{ has rank } r \\ &\quad\Leftrightarrow r \text{ of the diagonal elements of } \mathbf{D} \text{ are 1 and the rest 0.} \end{aligned}$$

Let $\mathbf{Y} = \mathbf{Q}\mathbf{X}$. Then $\mathbf{Y} \in \mathscr{N}(\mathbf{0}, \mathbf{D})$ and $\mathbf{Y}^T\mathbf{Y} = \mathbf{X}^T\mathbf{Q}^T\mathbf{Q}\mathbf{X} = \mathbf{X}^T\mathbf{X}$. If d_j denotes the jth diagonal element of $\mathbf{D}$, the characteristic function of $\mathbf{Y}^T\mathbf{Y} = \sum_j Y_j^2$ is $\prod_j(1 - 2id_jt)^{-1/2}$, which is equal to the characteristic function of χ_r^2, $(1 - 2it)^{-r/2}$, if and only if r of the d_j are 1 and the rest are 0. ■

Note: The d_j are the eigenvalues of $\boldsymbol{\Sigma}$. For any symmetric projection, $\boldsymbol{\Sigma}$,

$$\operatorname{rank}(\boldsymbol{\Sigma}) = \operatorname{trace}(\boldsymbol{\Sigma}),$$

because both are equal to the sum of the eigenvalues.

Multinomial Experiments. Consider n independent trials, each resulting in one of c possible outcomes or cells and each trial having the same probability $p_j > 0$ of resulting in outcome j for $j = 1, \ldots, c$. Let n_j denote the number of trials that result in outcome j for $j = 1, \ldots, c$, so that $\sum n_j = n$. Pearson's χ^2 is defined to be

$$\chi^2 = \sum_{\text{cells}} \frac{(\text{obs} - \text{exp})^2}{\text{exp}} = \sum_1^c \frac{(n_j - np_j)^2}{np_j}.$$

To find the asymptotic distribution of this statistic as $n \to \infty$, we use the following vector notation. Let $\mathbf{e}_j$ denote the jth unit vector in c dimensions (1 in the jth coordinate, 0's elsewhere), and define the random vector $\mathbf{X}_i$ to be $\mathbf{e}_j$ if the ith trial resulted in outcome j. Then $\mathbf{X}_1, \ldots, \mathbf{X}_n$ are i.i.d. with mean vector $E\mathbf{X} = \mathbf{p}$ and covariance matrix $\mathbf{\Sigma} = \text{cov}(\mathbf{X})$, where

$$\mathbf{p} = \begin{bmatrix} p_1 \\ \vdots \\ p_c \end{bmatrix} \quad \text{and} \quad \mathbf{\Sigma} = \begin{bmatrix} p_1(1-p_1) & -p_1p_2 & \cdots & -p_1p_c \\ -p_1p_2 & p_2(1-p_2) & \cdots & -p_2p_c \\ \vdots & \vdots & & \vdots \\ -p_1p_c & -p_2p_c & \cdots & p_c(1-p_c) \end{bmatrix}.$$

and Pearson's χ^2 may be written

$$\chi^2 = n\sum_1^c \frac{((n_j/n) - p_j)^2}{p_j} = n(\overline{\mathbf{X}}_n - \mathbf{p})^T \mathbf{P}^{-1}(\overline{\mathbf{X}}_n - \mathbf{p})$$

where

$$\mathbf{P} = \begin{bmatrix} p_1 & 0 & \cdots & 0 \\ 0 & p_2 & \cdots & 0 \\ \vdots & \vdots & \ddots & \vdots \\ 0 & 0 & \cdots & p_c \end{bmatrix}.$$

Note that $\mathbf{\Sigma} = \mathbf{P} - \mathbf{p}\mathbf{p}^T$.

Theorem 9

$$\chi^2 \xrightarrow{\mathscr{L}} \chi^2_{c-1}.$$

Proof. From the Central Limit Theorem, $\sqrt{n}\,(\overline{\mathbf{X}}_n - \mathbf{p}) \xrightarrow{\mathscr{L}} \mathbf{Y} \in \mathscr{N}(\mathbf{0}, \mathbf{\Sigma})$. Hence, from Slutsky's Theorem

$$\chi^2 = \sqrt{n}\left(\overline{\mathbf{X}}_n - \mathbf{p}\right)^T \mathbf{P}^{-1} \sqrt{n}\left(\overline{\mathbf{X}}_n - \mathbf{p}\right) \xrightarrow{\mathscr{L}} \mathbf{Y}^T\mathbf{P}^{-1}\mathbf{Y}.$$

To show that $\mathbf{Y}^T\mathbf{P}^{-1}\mathbf{Y} \in \chi^2_{c-1}$, let $\mathbf{Z} = \mathbf{P}^{-1/2}\mathbf{Y}$, so that $\mathbf{Z}^T\mathbf{Z} = \mathbf{Y}^T\mathbf{P}^{-1}\mathbf{Y}$ and $\mathbf{Z} \in \mathscr{N}(\mathbf{0}, \mathbf{P}^{-1/2}\mathbf{\Sigma}\mathbf{P}^{-1/2})$. To show that the covariance matrix of $\mathbf{Z}$ is a projection, replace $\mathbf{\Sigma}$ by $\mathbf{P} - \mathbf{p}\mathbf{p}^T$ to find that $\mathbf{P}^{-1/2}\mathbf{\Sigma}\mathbf{P}^{-1/2} = \mathbf{I} - \mathbf{P}^{-1/2}\mathbf{p}\mathbf{p}^T\mathbf{P}^{-1/2}$. It is easy to check that this is a projection and has trace, and hence rank, $c - 1$, using the fact that trace($\mathbf{AB}$) = trace($\mathbf{BA}$). ■

Transformed χ^2. We may extend Theorem 9 by combining it with Cramér's Theorem. We consider differentiable transformations of the form $\mathbf{g}(\mathbf{x}) = (g_1(x_1), \ldots, g_c(x_c))^T$, such that the jth component of the transformation is a function only of the jth component of $\mathbf{x}$. As a consequence, the gradient $\dot{\mathbf{g}}(\mathbf{x})$ is a diagonal matrix with the derivatives $\dot{g}_1(x_1), \ldots, \dot{g}_c(x_c)$ down the diagonal. As in the proof of Cramér's Theorem, $\sqrt{n}\,(\mathbf{g}(\overline{\mathbf{X}}_n) - \mathbf{g}(\mathbf{p}))$ is asymptotically equivalent to $\sqrt{n}\,\dot{\mathbf{g}}(\mathbf{p})(\overline{\mathbf{X}}_n - \mathbf{p})$, so that in Pearson's χ^2, we may replace $\sqrt{n}\,(\overline{\mathbf{X}}_n - \mathbf{p})$ by $\sqrt{n}\,\dot{\mathbf{g}}(\mathbf{p})^{-1}(\mathbf{g}(\overline{\mathbf{X}}_n) - \mathbf{g}(\mathbf{p}))$ and obtain the transformed χ^2,

$$\begin{aligned}\chi^2_{\mathbf{g}} &= n\left(\mathbf{g}(\overline{\mathbf{X}}_n) - \mathbf{g}(\mathbf{p})\right)^T \dot{\mathbf{g}}(\mathbf{p})^{-1}\mathbf{P}^{-1}\dot{\mathbf{g}}(\mathbf{p})^{-1}\left(\mathbf{g}(\overline{\mathbf{X}}_n) - \mathbf{g}(\mathbf{p})\right)\\ &= n\sum_1^c \frac{\left(g_j(n_j/n) - g_j(p_j)\right)^2}{p_j\dot{g}_j(p_j)^2} \xrightarrow{\mathscr{L}} \chi^2_{c-1}.\end{aligned}$$

Example. Although the variance-stabilizing transformation for the binomial distribution is the arcsin function (Exercise 3 of Section 8), the transformation that makes the denominator in Pearson's χ^2 a constant is the square-root function. We are led to investigate the transformed χ^2 with $\mathbf{g}(\mathbf{x}) = (\sqrt{x_1}, \sqrt{x_2}, \ldots, \sqrt{x_c})^T$. The transformed χ^2, with $\dot{g}_j(p_j) = 0.5/\sqrt{p_j}$, becomes

$$\chi^2_H = 4n\sum_1^c\left(\sqrt{n_j/n} - \sqrt{p_j}\right)^2.$$

This is known as the *Hellinger* χ^2 because of its relation to Hellinger distance. [The Hellinger distance between two densities, $f(x)$ and $g(x)$, is $d(f, g)$ where $d(f, g)^2 = \int(\sqrt{f(x)} - \sqrt{g(x)})^2\,dx$.]

EXERCISES

1. *Modified* χ^2. Pearson's χ^2 may be modified by replacing the expected number of observations in the denominator by the observed number. The resulting χ^2 is known as *Neyman's* χ^2, χ_N^2:

$$\chi_N^2 = \sum_{\text{cells}} \frac{(\text{obs} - \text{exp})^2}{\text{obs}} = \sum_1^c \frac{(n_j - np_j)^2}{n_j}.$$

Show that $\chi_N^2 \xrightarrow{\mathscr{L}} \chi_{c-1}^2$.

2. Let $\mathbf{X} \in \mathscr{N}(\mathbf{0}, \mathbf{I})$, $\mathbf{P}$ symmetric. Show that $\mathbf{X}^T\mathbf{P}\mathbf{X} \in \chi_r^2 \Leftrightarrow \mathbf{P}$ is a projection of rank $\mathbf{r}$.
3. *Alternate Proof of Theorem* 9. Define the $(c-1)$-vector $\mathbf{Y}_i$ to be $\mathbf{X}_i$ with the last component deleted, let $\mathbf{q}$ denote $\mathbf{p}$ with the last component deleted, and let $\mathbf{\Phi}$ denote $\mathbf{\Sigma}$ with the last row and column deleted. Show the identity

$$\text{Pearson's } \chi^2 = n(\overline{\mathbf{Y}}_n - \mathbf{q})^T \mathbf{\Phi}^{-1}(\overline{\mathbf{Y}}_n - \mathbf{q}).$$

Thus, Pearson's χ^2 is just a version of Hotelling's T^2, and we may conclude Theorem 9 directly from Lemma 2. (Let $\mathbf{Q}$ denote $\mathbf{P}$ with the last row and column deleted. Show $\mathbf{\Phi} = \mathbf{Q} - \mathbf{q}\mathbf{q}^T$ and $\mathbf{\Phi}^{-1} = \mathbf{Q}^{-1} + \mathbf{1}\cdot\mathbf{1}^T/p_c$, where $\mathbf{1}$ denotes the $(c-1)$-vector of all 1's.)

4. What is the transformed χ^2 for the transformation that replaces each cell frequency by its logarithm? What is the modified transformed χ^2 for this transformation?

10

Asymptotic Power of the Pearson Chi-Square Test

It is important to be able to judge the sensitivity of the χ^2 test in distinguishing the null hypothesis from nearby alternatives. We would like to find the probabilities of rejecting the null hypothesis when some relevant alternatives are true; that is, we would like to find the power function of the test. In this section, we find an asymptotic approximation to the power function based on the noncentral χ^2 distribution. In addition to allowing us to measure the sensitivity of the test, this approximation helps solve the important problem of finding the sample size required to obtain a fixed power at a fixed alternative for a given level of significance. The Fix Tables (Table 3) for noncentral χ^2 are in a convenient form for solving this problem for levels 0.05 and 0.01.

Consider a multinomial experiment consisting of n independent trials with c possible outcomes having probabilities $p_1, \ldots, p_c$ as in Section 9. Let $p_1^0, \ldots, p_c^0$ be a given set of probabilities with $p_j^0 > 0$ for all j and with $\Sigma_1^c p_j^0 = 1$, and consider testing H_0: $p_j = p_j^0$ for $j = 1, \ldots, c$. The goodness-of-fit test based on Pearson's χ^2 rejects H_0 if

$$\chi^2 = \sum_{\text{cells}} \frac{(\text{obs} - \exp)^2}{\exp} = \sum_1^c \frac{\left(n_j - np_j^0\right)^2}{np_j^0}$$

is too large, where n_j denotes the number of trials that resulted in

Table 3. Fix Tables of Noncentral χ^2. The quantity tabled is that value of the parameter λ that satisfies the equation

$$e^{-(\lambda/2)} \sum_{k=0}^{\infty} \frac{\lambda^k}{k!\, 2^{(1/2 f + 2k - 1)} \Gamma(f/2 + k)} \int_{x_f(\alpha)}^{\infty} x^{f+2k-1} e^{-(1/2)x^2}\, dx = \beta,$$

where f = number of degrees of freedom and $\chi_f(\alpha)$ is such that

$$\frac{1}{2^{(1/2)f-1}\Gamma(f/2)} \int_{x_f(\alpha)}^{\infty} x^{f-1} e^{-(1/2)x^2}\, dx = \alpha.$$

$\alpha = 0.05$

f \ β	0.1	0.2	0.3	0.4	0.5	0.6	0.7	0.8	0.9
1	0.426	1.242	2.058	2.911	3.841	4.899	6.172	7.849	10.509
2	0.624	1.731	2.776	3.832	4.957	6.213	7.702	9.635	12.655
3	0.779	2.096	3.302	4.501	5.761	7.154	8.792	10.903	14.172
4	0.910	2.401	3.737	5.050	6.420	7.924	9.683	11.935	15.405
5	1.026	2.667	4.117	5.529	6.991	8.591	10.453	12.828	16.470
6	1.131	2.907	4.458	5.957	7.503	9.187	11.141	13.624	17.419
7	1.228	3.128	4.770	6.349	7.971	9.732	11.768	14.350	18.284
8	1.319	3.333	5.059	6.713	8.405	10.236	12.349	15.022	19.083
9	1.404	3.525	5.331	7.053	8.811	10.708	12.892	15.650	19.829
10	1.485	3.707	5.588	7.375	9.194	11.153	13.404	16.241	20.532
11	1.562	3.880	5.831	7.680	9.557	11.575	13.890	16.802	21.198
12	1.636	4.045	6.064	7.971	9.903	11.977	14.353	17.336	21.833
13	1.707	4.204	6.287	8.250	10.235	12.362	14.796	17.847	22.440
14	1.775	4.357	6.502	8.519	10.554	12.733	15.221	18.338	23.022
15	1.840	4.501	6.709	8.777	10.862	13.090	15.631	18.811	23.583
16	1.904	4.646	6.909	9.027	11.159	13.435	16.027	19.268	24.125
17	1.966	4.784	7.103	9.269	11.447	13.768	16.411	19.710	24.650
18	2.026	4.918	7.291	9.505	11.726	14.092	16.783	20.139	25.158
19	2.085	5.049	7.474	9.734	11.998	14.407	17.144	20.556	25.652
20	2.142	5.176	7.653	9.956	12.262	14.714	17.496	20.961	26.132

$\alpha = 0.01$

f \ β	0.1	0.2	0.3	0.4	0.5	0.6	0.7	0.8	0.9
1	1.674	3.007	4.208	5.394	6.635	8.004	9.611	11.680	14.879
2	2.299	3.941	5.372	6.758	8.190	9.752	11.567	13.881	17.427
3	2.763	4.624	6.218	7.745	9.311	11.008	12.970	15.458	19.248
4	3.149	5.188	6.914	8.557	10.231	12.039	14.121	16.749	20.737
5	3.488	5.682	7.523	9.265	11.033	12.936	15.120	17.871	22.033
6	3.794	6.126	8.069	9.899	11.751	13.738	16.014	18.873	23.187
7	4.075	6.534	8.569	10.480	12.408	14.473	16.831	19.788	24.238
8	4.337	6.912	9.033	11.019	13.017	15.153	17.589	20.636	25.211
9	4.583	7.267	9.469	11.524	13.588	15.790	18.297	21.429	26.122
10	4.816	7.603	9.880	12.000	14.126	16.391	18.965	22.177	26.981
11	5.038	7.922	10.271	12.453	14.638	16.961	19.599	22.887	27.797
12	5.250	8.227	10.644	12.885	15.126	17.505	20.204	23.563	28.575
13	5.453	8.520	11.002	13.299	15.594	18.027	20.784	24.211	29.319
14	5.649	8.801	11.346	13.698	16.043	18.528	21.341	24.833	30.034
15	5.838	9.072	11.678	14.082	16.476	19.011	21.878	25.433	30.722
16	6.021	9.335	11.999	14.454	16.895	19.478	22.396	26.013	31.387
17	6.198	9.590	12.310	14.814	17.301	19.930	22.898	26.574	32.031
18	6.371	9.837	12.612	15.163	17.695	20.369	23.385	27.118	32.655
19	6.539	10.078	12.906	15.502	18.078	20.796	23.859	27.647	33.262
20	6.702	10.312	13.192	15.833	18.451	21.211	24.320	28.162	33.852

outcome j. Under H_0, this statistic has approximately a χ^2_{c-1} distribution when n is large.

If some alternative $\mathbf{p} = (p_1, \ldots, p_c) \neq (p_1^0, \ldots, p_c^0) = \mathbf{p}^0$ is the true value of the parameter, then the probability of rejecting H_0, using this test with a fixed size α, tends to 1 as $n \to \infty$. To obtain an approximation to the power, we fix $\mathbf{p}$ and consider a sequence of null hypotheses, say $H_0(n)$: $\mathbf{p} = \mathbf{p}_n^0$, where $\mathbf{p}_n^0 = (p_{n1}^0, \ldots, p_{nc}^0)^T$ is a fixed sequence of values converging to $\mathbf{p}$ at rate $1/\sqrt{n}$, say $\mathbf{p}_n^0 = \mathbf{p} - (1/\sqrt{n})\boldsymbol{\delta}$ for some fixed vector $\boldsymbol{\delta} = (\delta_1, \ldots, \delta_c)^T$. Note that because both $\mathbf{p}$ and $\mathbf{p}_n^0$ are probability vectors, we have $\sum_1^c \delta_i = 0$. We show that the limiting distribution of the above χ^2 statistic is a noncentral χ^2 distribution with $c - 1$ degrees of freedom and noncentrality parameter

$$\lambda = \boldsymbol{\delta}^T \mathbf{P}^{-1} \boldsymbol{\delta} = \sum_1^c \delta_j^2 / p_j \sim \sum_1^c \delta_j^2 / p_{nj}^0.$$

The *noncentral* χ^2 *distribution with d degrees of freedom and noncentrality parameter* $\lambda = \boldsymbol{\delta}^T\boldsymbol{\delta}$, denoted by $\chi_d^2(\lambda)$, is defined as the distribution of $Z = \mathbf{X}^T\mathbf{X}$, where $\mathbf{X} \in \mathcal{N}(\boldsymbol{\delta}, \mathbf{I})$ is a d-dimensional vector. (It should be first noted that this distribution depends on $\boldsymbol{\delta}$ only through $\lambda = \boldsymbol{\delta}^T\boldsymbol{\delta}$.) We need the following generalization of the important half of Lemma 3 of Section 9.

Lemma. *Suppose* $\mathbf{X} \in \mathcal{N}(\boldsymbol{\delta}, \boldsymbol{\Sigma})$. *If* $\boldsymbol{\Sigma}$ *is a projection of rank r, and* $\boldsymbol{\Sigma\delta} = \boldsymbol{\delta}$, *then* $\mathbf{X}^T\mathbf{X} \in \chi_r^2(\boldsymbol{\delta}^T\boldsymbol{\delta})$.

Proof. Find $\mathbf{Q}$ orthogonal such that $\mathbf{D} = \mathbf{Q\Sigma Q}^T$ is diagonal. Then $\mathbf{D}$ is a projection of rank r, so that r of the diagonal elements of $\mathbf{D}$ are ones and the rest zeros. Assume that $\mathbf{Q}$ has been chosen so that the first r diagonal elements of $\mathbf{D}$ are 1's. Let $\mathbf{Y} = \mathbf{QX}$. Then $\mathbf{Y} \in \mathcal{N}(\mathbf{Q}\boldsymbol{\delta}, \mathbf{D})$ and $\mathbf{Y}^T\mathbf{Y} = \mathbf{X}^T\mathbf{X}$, and $\mathbf{DQ}\boldsymbol{\delta} = \mathbf{Q\Sigma Q}^T\mathbf{Q}\boldsymbol{\delta} = \mathbf{Q\Sigma}\boldsymbol{\delta} = \mathbf{Q}\boldsymbol{\delta}$. The Y_j are independent normal with variance 1 for $j = 1, \ldots, r$ and variance 0 for $j = r + 1, \ldots, d$. Since $\mathbf{Q}\boldsymbol{\delta} = \mathbf{DQ}\boldsymbol{\delta}$, the last $d - r$ components of $E\mathbf{Y}$ are zero; thus, $Y_{r+1}, \ldots, Y_n$ are identically zero, so that $\mathbf{Y}^T\mathbf{Y} = Y_1^2 + \cdots + Y_r^2$. Moreover, the sum of squares of the means on the first r components is then $(\mathbf{Q}\boldsymbol{\delta})^T(\mathbf{Q}\boldsymbol{\delta}) = \boldsymbol{\delta}^T\mathbf{Q}^T\mathbf{Q}\boldsymbol{\delta} = \boldsymbol{\delta}^T\boldsymbol{\delta}$. Thus, $\mathbf{Y}^T\mathbf{Y} \in \chi_r^2(\boldsymbol{\delta}^T\boldsymbol{\delta})$. ∎

The converse to this lemma can be proved, as for Lemma 3, Section 9, using characteristic functions.

THEOREM 10. *Let* $\mathbf{p}$ *be the vector of true cell probabilities, and let* $\boldsymbol{\delta} = \sqrt{n}\,(\mathbf{p} - \mathbf{p}_n^0)$. *Then*

$$\chi^2 = n \sum_1^c \frac{\left(n_j/n - p_{nj}^0\right)^2}{p_{nj}^0} \xrightarrow{\mathscr{L}} \chi^2_{c-1}(\lambda),$$

where $\lambda = \sum_1^c \delta_j^2/p_j$.

REMARK. There is a simple, easily remembered principle embodied here, namely that the noncentrality parameter may be found by replacing the observed frequencies, n_j/n, in Pearson's χ^2 by the expected values, p_j.

Proof. As in the proof of Theorem 9, let

$$\mathbf{p} = \begin{bmatrix} p_1 \\ \vdots \\ p_c \end{bmatrix}, \qquad \mathbf{P} = \begin{bmatrix} p_1 & 0 & \cdots & 0 \\ 0 & p_2 & \cdots & 0 \\ \vdots & \vdots & \ddots & \vdots \\ 0 & 0 & \cdots & p_c \end{bmatrix}, \qquad \boldsymbol{\Sigma} = \mathbf{P} - \mathbf{p}\mathbf{p}^T,$$

$$\mathbf{p}_n^0 = \begin{bmatrix} p_{n1}^0 \\ \vdots \\ p_{nc}^0 \end{bmatrix}, \qquad \mathbf{P}_n^0 = \begin{bmatrix} p_{n1}^0 & 0 & \cdots & 0 \\ 0 & p_{n2}^0 & \cdots & 0 \\ \vdots & \vdots & \ddots & \vdots \\ 0 & 0 & \cdots & p_{nc}^0 \end{bmatrix},$$

and

$$\overline{\mathbf{X}}_n = \begin{bmatrix} n_1/n \\ \vdots \\ n_c/n \end{bmatrix},$$

Then, $\sqrt{n}\,(\overline{\mathbf{X}}_n - \mathbf{p}_n^0) = \sqrt{n}\,(\overline{\mathbf{X}}_n - \mathbf{p}) + \boldsymbol{\delta} \xrightarrow{\mathscr{L}} \mathbf{Y} \in \mathscr{N}(\boldsymbol{\delta}, \boldsymbol{\Sigma})$ and $\mathbf{P}_n^0 \to \mathbf{P}$. Hence from Slutsky's Theorem,

$$\chi^2 = \sqrt{n}\left(\overline{\mathbf{X}}_n - \mathbf{p}_n^0\right)^T \mathbf{P}_n^{0-1} \sqrt{n}\left(\overline{\mathbf{X}}_n - \mathbf{p}_n^0\right) \xrightarrow{\mathscr{L}} \mathbf{Y}\mathbf{P}^{-1}\mathbf{Y}.$$

Let $\mathbf{Z} = \mathbf{P}^{-1/2}\mathbf{Y}$. Then $\mathbf{Z}^T\mathbf{Z} = \mathbf{Y}^T\mathbf{P}^{-1}\mathbf{Y}$ and

$$\mathbf{Z} \in \mathscr{N}(\mathbf{P}^{-1/2}\boldsymbol{\delta}, \mathbf{P}^{-1/2}\boldsymbol{\Sigma}\mathbf{P}^{-1/2}) = \mathscr{N}(\mathbf{P}^{-1/2}\boldsymbol{\delta}, \mathbf{I} - \mathbf{P}^{-1/2}\mathbf{p}\mathbf{p}^T\mathbf{P}^{-1/2}).$$

As in Theorem 9, $\mathbf{I} - \mathbf{P}^{-1/2}\mathbf{p}\mathbf{p}^T\mathbf{P}^{-1/2}$ is a projection of rank $c - 1$. In addition, $(\mathbf{I} - \mathbf{P}^{-1/2}\mathbf{p}\mathbf{p}^T\mathbf{P}^{-1/2})\mathbf{P}^{-1/2}\boldsymbol{\delta} = \mathbf{P}^{-1/2}\boldsymbol{\delta} - \mathbf{P}^{-1/2}\mathbf{p}\mathbf{p}^T\mathbf{P}^{-1}\boldsymbol{\delta} = \mathbf{P}^{-1/2}\boldsymbol{\delta}$, since $\mathbf{p}^T\mathbf{P}^{-1}\boldsymbol{\delta} = \sum_1^c \delta_j = 0$. Therefore, the theorem follows from the lemma. ∎

Example. A die is tossed 300 times. Let H_0 denote the hypothesis that all faces are equally likely, H_0: $p_i = \frac{1}{6}$, $i = 1, \ldots, 6$. To test H_0, the χ^2 test would reject H_0 if $\chi^2 = \sum_1^6 (n_j - 50)^2/50$ were too large, where n_j is the number of times that face j turned up. At the 5% level, we reject H_0 if $\chi^2 > 11.07$, and at the 1% level, we reject H_0 if $\chi^2 > 15.09$. What is the approximate power at the alternative $p_1 = p_2 = 0.13$, $p_3 = p_4 = 0.17$, $p_5 = p_6 = 0.20$? We compute the noncentrality parameter, $\lambda = \sum_1^c \delta_j^2/p_j$ or $\lambda^0 = \sum_1^6 \delta_j^2/p_j^0$. (They are asymptotically equivalent.) Since $\boldsymbol{\delta} = \sqrt{n}\,(\mathbf{p} - \mathbf{p}^0)$, we have $\lambda^0 = \sum_1^6 n(p_j - p_j^0)^2/p_j^0$, and

$$\frac{n(p_1 - p_1^0)^2}{p_1^0} = \frac{n(p_2 - p_2^0)^2}{p_2^0} = \frac{300(0.13 - \frac{1}{6})^2}{\frac{1}{6}} = 2.42,$$

$$\frac{n(p_3 - p_3^0)^2}{p_3^0} = \frac{n(p_4 - p_4^0)^2}{p_4^0} = 0.02,$$

$$\frac{n(p_5 - p_5^0)^2}{p_5^0} = \frac{n(p_6 - p_6^0)^2}{p_6^0} = 2.00.$$

Hence, $\lambda = 2.42 + 2.42 + 0.02 + 0.02 + 2.00 + 2.00 = 8.88$. From the Fix Tables (Table 3) of noncentral χ^2, we find power approximately 0.61 at the 5% level, and power approximately 0.38 at the 1% level.

Approximately how large a sample size is needed to obtain power 0.90 at this alternative when testing at the 5% level? We must increase n so that $\lambda = 16.470$. Solving $(n/300)\,8.88 = 16.470$, we find n approximately 556.

EXERCISES

1. In a multinomial experiment with sample size 100 and 3 cells with null hypothesis H_0: $p_1 = \frac{1}{4}$, $p_2 = \frac{1}{2}$, $p_3 = \frac{1}{4}$, what is the approximate power at the alternative $p_1 = 0.2$, $p_2 = 0.6$, $p_3 = 0.2$ when the level of significance is $\alpha = 0.05$? $\alpha = 0.01$? How large a sample size is needed to achieve power 0.9 at this alternative when $\alpha = 0.05$? $\alpha = 0.01$?

2. (a) Show $\chi_r^2(\lambda)$ has mean $r + \lambda$ and variance $2r + 4\lambda$.
   (b) Show $[\chi_r^2(\lambda) - (r + \lambda)]/\sqrt{2r + 4\lambda} \xrightarrow{\mathcal{L}} \mathcal{N}(0, 1)$ as $\max(r, \lambda) \to \infty$.
   (c) Assuming (b), compare the value of λ given in the Fix Table for $\alpha = 0.05$ and $\beta = 0.5$ and $r = 20$, with the asymptotic value.
3. Show that the transformed χ^2 has the same (first-order) power as Pearson's χ^2; that is, show

$$\chi_g^2 = n \sum_1^c \frac{\left(g_j(n_j/n) - g_j\left(p_{nj}^0\right)\right)^2}{p_{nj}^0 \dot{g}_j\left(p_{nj}^0\right)^2} \xrightarrow{\mathcal{L}} \chi_{c-1}^2(\lambda)$$

as $n \to \infty$, where $\lambda = \sum_1^c \delta_j^2/p_j$.

3

Special Topics

11

Stationary *m*-Dependent Sequences

In this section we prove a theorem that allows us to show asymptotic normality for sums of random variables for certain statistical problems with a limited amount of dependence between the variables. A sequence of random variables, $Y_1, Y_2, \ldots,$ is said to be *m-dependent* if for every integer, $s \geq 1$, the sets of random variables $\{Y_1, \ldots, Y_s\}$ and $\{Y_{m+s+1}, Y_{m+s+2}, \ldots\}$ are independent. (For $m = 0$, this is equivalent to independence of the sequence.)

A sequence of random variables $Y_1, Y_2, \ldots$ is said to be (*strict sense*) *stationary* if for any positive integers s and t, the joint distribution of the vector $(Y_t, \ldots, Y_{t+s})$ does not depend on t. In other words, a sequence is stationary if the distribution of a sequence of any s consecutive observations does not depend on the time one starts observing.

We are interested in the asymptotic distribution of $S_n = \Sigma_{i=1}^n Y_i$ for a stationary, m-dependent sequence of random variables $Y_1, Y_2, \ldots$. Such a sequence arises in time-series analysis, for example, in computing the asymptotic distribution of the autoproduct moment at lag m, which is defined for a sequence of random variables, $X_1, X_2, \ldots$ as $S_n/n = (1/n)\Sigma_{i=1}^n X_i X_{i+m}$. If the X_i are assumed to be i.i.d., then the sequence, $Y_i = X_i X_{i+m}$ forms a stationary m-dependent sequence.

Let the mean of the Y_t be denoted by $\mu = EY_t$ the variance by $\sigma_{00} = \text{var}(Y_t)$, and the covariances by $\sigma_{0i} = \text{cov}(Y_t, Y_{t+i})$. These quantities are independent of t due to the stationarity assumption. Also, $\sigma_{0i} = 0$ for $i > m$ from m-dependence. The mean and variance of S_n are easily found to be $ES_n = n\mu$, and for $n \geq m$

$$\begin{aligned}\operatorname{var}(S_n) &= \sum_{i=1}^{n}\sum_{j=1}^{n}\operatorname{cov}(Y_i, Y_j)\\ &= n\sigma_{00} + 2(n-1)\sigma_{01} + 2(n-2)\sigma_{02} + \cdots + 2(n-m)\sigma_{0m}.\end{aligned} \tag{1}$$

We have $\operatorname{var}(S_n)/n \to \sigma^2$, where

$$\sigma^2 = \sigma_{00} + 2\sigma_{01} + 2\sigma_{02} + \cdots + 2\sigma_{0m}. \tag{2}$$

For large n, the distribution of S_n/n is approximately normal with mean μ and variance σ^2/n, as in the following theorem. For an extension to a special stationary sequence without the assumption of m-dependence, see Exercise 7.

Theorem 11. *Let $Y_1, Y_2, \ldots,$ be a stationary m-dependent sequence with finite variance and let $S_n = \sum_{i=1}^{n} Y_i$. Then*

$$(S_n - ES_n)/(\operatorname{var}(S_n))^{1/2} \xrightarrow{\mathscr{L}} \mathscr{N}(0,1),$$

or, equivalently,

$$\sqrt{n}\,(S_n/n - \mu) \xrightarrow{\mathscr{L}} \mathscr{N}(0, \sigma^2),$$

where $\mu = EY_1$, and σ^2 is given by (2).

Before presenting the proof, we give a useful lemma. First note that we may assume without loss of generality that $\mu = 0$, because we can work equally well with $Y_j - \mu$. The method of proof involves splitting the sum S_n into two parts, one a sum of independent terms to which the Central Limit Theorem may be applied, and the other a hopefully negligible dependent part. Take n very large and break S_n into s pieces of length $k + m$, where $k > m$. Write $n = s(k + m) + r$, where r is the remainder, $0 \leq r < k + m$. Let $S_n = S_n' + S_n'' + R_n$, where

$$S_n' = \sum_{j=0}^{s-1} V_{kj}, \quad S_n'' = \sum_{j=0}^{s-1} W_{kj}, \quad \text{and} \quad R_n = \sum_{i=1}^{r} Y_{s(k+m)+i},$$

where

$$V_{kj} = \sum_{i=1}^{k} Y_{j(k+m)+i} \quad \text{and} \quad W_{kj} = \sum_{i=k+1}^{k+m} Y_{j(k+m)+i}.$$

Then the V_{kj}, for $j = 1, \ldots, s$, are i.i.d. random variables with distribution depending on k. For k fixed and s large, S'_n has an approximate normal distribution with mean 0 and variance $\text{var}(S'_n) = s\,\text{var}(S_k)$. The theorem would follow if the other terms are negligible and we could take the limit first as $n \to \infty$ and then $k \to \infty$. This requires that the piece involving S''_n be negligible uniformly in n as $k \to \infty$. For this purpose the following lemma is used.

Lemma. *Suppose* $T_n = Z_{nk} + X_{nk}$ *for* $n = 1, 2, \ldots$ *and* $k = 1, 2, \ldots$. *If*

(1) $X_{nk} \xrightarrow{P} 0$ uniformly in n as $k \to \infty$,
(2) $Z_{nk} \xrightarrow{\mathscr{L}} Z_k$ as $n \to \infty$, for each k, and
(3) $Z_k \xrightarrow{\mathscr{L}} Z$ as $k \to \infty$, then

$$T_n \xrightarrow{\mathscr{L}} Z \text{ as } n \to \infty.$$

Proof. Let $\varepsilon > 0$ and let $z \in C(F_Z)$, the continuity set of F_Z. Find $\delta > 0$ such that $P(|Z - z| < \delta) < \varepsilon$ and such that $z + \delta$ and $z - \delta$ are in the continuity sets $C(F_Z)$ and $C(F_{Z_k})$ for all k. From condition (1), we may find K such that $P(|X_{nk}| \geq \delta) < \varepsilon$ for all $k > K$ and all n. From condition (3), we may find $K' \geq K$ such that for $k \geq K'$, $|P(Z_k \leq z + \delta) - P(Z \leq z + \delta)| < \varepsilon$ and $|P(Z_k \leq z - \delta) - P(Z \leq z - \delta)| > \varepsilon$. Now fix $k > K'$.

$$\begin{aligned} P(T_n \leq z) &= P(Z_{nk} + X_{nk} \leq z) \\ &\leq P(Z_{nk} \leq z + \delta) + P(|X_{nk}| \geq \delta) \\ &\leq P(Z_{nk} \leq z + \delta) + \varepsilon. \end{aligned}$$

Now apply condition (2):

$$\begin{aligned} \limsup_n P(T_n \leq z) &\leq P(Z_k \leq z + \delta) + \varepsilon \\ &\leq P(Z \leq z + \delta) + 2\varepsilon \\ &\leq P(Z \leq z) + 3\varepsilon. \end{aligned}$$

Similarly,

$$\begin{aligned} P(T_n \leq z) &= P(Z_{nk} + X_{nk} \leq z) \\ &\geq P(Z_{nk} \leq z - \delta) - P(|X_{nk}| \geq \delta) \\ &\geq P(Z_{nk} \leq z - \delta) - \varepsilon, \end{aligned}$$

and

$$\liminf_n P(T_n \le z) \ge P(Z_k \le z - \delta) - \varepsilon$$
$$\ge P(Z \le z - \delta) - 2\varepsilon$$
$$\ge P(Z \le z) - 3\varepsilon.$$

Since this holds for all $\varepsilon > 0$, we must have $\lim_n P(T_n \le z) = P(Z \le z)$. ∎

Proof of Theorem 11. We let $T_n = S_n/\sqrt{n}$, $Z_{nk} = (S'_n + R_n)/\sqrt{n}$, and $X_{nk} = S''_n/\sqrt{n}$, so that

$$T_n = \frac{S_n}{\sqrt{n}} = \frac{S'_n + R_n}{\sqrt{n}} + \frac{S''_n}{\sqrt{n}} = Z_{nk} + X_{nk},$$

and we check the conditions of the lemma. First note from the Central Limit Theorem that for fixed k, $S'_n/\sqrt{s} \xrightarrow{\mathscr{L}} \mathscr{N}(0, \text{var}(S_k))$. Then, since $s/n \to k$, we have $S'_n/\sqrt{n} = (\sqrt{s}/\sqrt{n})S'_n/\sqrt{s} \xrightarrow{\mathscr{L}} \mathscr{N}(0, \text{var}(S_k)/k)$. The term $R_n/\sqrt{n}$ has mean 0 and variance $\text{var}(S_r)/n$. Now all covariances are bounded by the variance, $|\sigma_{0j}| \le \sigma_{00}$ [$\text{var}(Y_t) = \sigma_{00}$ for all t and the correlation is bounded by 1], so $\text{var}(R_n/\sqrt{n}) \le r^2\sigma_{00}/n \le (k+m)^2\sigma_{00}/n \to 0$ for fixed k. Thus $R_n/\sqrt{n} \xrightarrow{\text{qm}} 0$, and hence Z_{nk} has the same limit law as $S'_n/\sqrt{n}$, namely, $Z_{nk} \xrightarrow{\mathscr{L}} Z_k \in \mathscr{N}(0, \text{var}(S_k)/k)$. Thus condition (2) is satisfied. Moreover, since $\text{var}(S_k)/k \to \sigma^2$ as $k \to \infty$, we have $Z_k \xrightarrow{\mathscr{L}} Z \in \mathscr{N}(0, \sigma^2)$, and condition (3) is satisfied.

To check condition (1), we note that $\text{var}(X_{nk}) = s\,\text{var}(S_m)/n \le \text{var}(S_m)/k$, independent of n, and by Chebyshev's inequality, $P(|X_{nj}| > \delta) \le \text{var}(X_{nk})/\delta^2 \le \text{var}(S_m)/(k\delta^2) \to 0$ as $k \to \infty$, uniformly in n. ∎

Application to the mth product moment. As an application, let us find the asymptotic distribution of $S_n = \sum_{i=1}^n X_i X_{i+m}$, for an i.i.d. sequence $X_0, X_1, X_2, \ldots$ with mean μ and variance τ^2. Then, $Y_i = X_i X_{i+m}$ forms an m-dependent stationary sequence so that the theorem applies. The mean of the Y_i is $EX_iX_{i+m} = \mu^2$ and the covariances are

$$\sigma_{0j} = \text{cov}(X_0 X_m, X_j X_{j+m}) = EX_0 X_m X_j X_{J+m} - \mu^4,$$

$$\sigma_{00} = (\tau^2 + \mu^2)^2 - \mu^4 = \tau^4 + 2\tau^2\mu^2,$$

$$\sigma_{0m} = \mu^2(\tau^2 + \mu^2) - \mu^4 = \tau^2\mu^2,$$

$$\sigma_{0j} = 0, \qquad \text{for } j \ne 0, \quad j \ne m.$$

Hence by the theorem, $\sqrt{n}\,(S_n/n - \mu^2) \xrightarrow{\mathscr{L}} \mathscr{N}(0, \sigma^2)$, where

$$\sigma^2 = \sigma_{00} + 2\sigma_{0m} = \tau^4 + 4\tau^2\mu^2.$$

EXERCISES

1. *Success runs.* Consider a sequence of i.i.d. Bernoulli random variables $X_0, X_1, \ldots,$ with probability p of success, $P(X = 1) = 1 - P(X = 0) = p$. For $j \geq 1$, we say a run of successes begins at j if $X_j = 1$ and $X_{j-1} = 0$. Let $Y_j = (1 - X_{j-1})X_j$ denote the indicator of the event that a run starts at j. Then $S_n = Y_1 + \cdots + Y_n$ denotes the number of runs of successes in the first n trials. We are interested in the asymptotic distribution of the number of success runs, and to simplify the algebra we have omitted the run, if any, that begins at the zeroth trial, because that will not affect the asymptotic distribution. Find the mean and variance of S_n. What is its asymptotic distribution?
2. *Runs of length r.* In a sequence of i.i.d. Bernoulli trials, $X_0, X_1, X_2, \ldots$ with probability p of success, a run of length r is a string of r consecutive 1's preceded and followed by zeros. Let Z_j denote the product $Z_j = (1 - X_{j-1})X_j \cdots X_{j+r-1}(1 - X_{j+r})$. Then $S_n = Z_1 + \cdots + Z_n$ represents the number of runs of length r in the sequence $X_0, \ldots, X_{n+r}$. Note that the Z_j form an m-dependent stationary sequence (for what m?). Find the asymptotic distribution of S_n.
3. *Badminton scoring.* Let $X_0, X_1, \ldots$ be a sequence of i.i.d. Bernoulli trials with probability p of success. Your side scores a point each time you have a success that follows a success. Let $S_n = \sum_{i=1}^{n} X_{i-1}X_i$ denote the number of points your side scores by time n. Find the asymptotic distribution of S_n.
4. *Autocovariance.* Let $X_1, X_2, \ldots$ be i.i.d. random variables with mean μ and variance τ^2. (a) Find the joint asymptotic distribution of $\overline{X}_n = (1/n)\sum_{=1}^{n} X_i$ and $\overline{Z}_n = (1/n)\sum_{i=1}^{n} X_iX_{i+1}$. (Hint: Find the asymptotic distribution of $a\overline{X}_n + b\overline{Z}_n$ for all a and b, and apply Exercise 2 from Section 3.) (b) Find the asymptotic distribution of the autocovariance, $\overline{Z}_n - \overline{X}_n^2$.
5. *Runs of increasing values.* Let $X_0, X_1, X_2, \ldots$ be i.i.d. random variables from a continuous distribution, $F(x)$. Let Z_j be one if there is a relative minimum at j, ad zero otherwise; that is, $Z_j = I\{X_{j-1} > X_j < X_{j+1}\}$. Then $S_n = \sum_{j=1}^{n} Z_j$ represents the number of relative minima in the sequence $X_0, X_1, \ldots, X_{n+1}$. It is also within one of the number of runs of increasing values in $X_0, X_1, \ldots, X_{n+1}$, because, except for the possible run starting at zero, a run of increasing values begins at j if and only if $Z_j = 1$. S_n may be used as a statistic for testing the null

hypothesis of randomness of a sequence. Find the asymptotic distribution of S_n.

6. *Autocorrelation.* Let $X_1, X_2, \ldots$ be a sequence of i.i.d. random variables with finite fourth moment. Let us define the autocorrelation of lag 1 based on the first $n+1$ observations to be

$$r_n = \frac{(1/n)\sum_{i=1}^{n} X_i X_{i+1} - \overline{X}_n^2}{(1/n)\sum_{i=1}^{n} X_i^2 - \overline{X}_n^2}.$$

Assume the mean of the distribution of the X_j is zero. (The limiting distribution of r_n does not depend on this assumption.)

(a) Let $\mathbf{Z}_i = (X_i, X_i^2, X_i X_{i+1})^T$ and show $\sqrt{n}(\overline{\mathbf{Z}}_n - \boldsymbol{\mu}) \xrightarrow{\mathscr{L}} \mathscr{N}(\mathbf{0}, \boldsymbol{\Sigma})$, where

$$\boldsymbol{\mu} = \begin{pmatrix} 0 \\ \sigma^2 \\ 0 \end{pmatrix} \quad \text{and} \quad \boldsymbol{\Sigma} = \begin{pmatrix} \sigma^2 & \mu_3 & 0 \\ \mu_3 & \mu_4 - \sigma^4 & 0 \\ 0 & 0 & \sigma^4 \end{pmatrix}.$$

(b) Show $\sqrt{n}\, r_n \xrightarrow{\mathscr{L}} \mathscr{N}(0,1)$. It is interesting to compare this robustness of the autocorrelation with the drastic nonrobustness of the correlation coefficient found in Section 8.

7. Let $\ldots, X_{-1}, X_0, X_1, \ldots$ be a sequence of unobservable i.i.d. random variables with mean ξ and variance τ^2, and let $\ldots, z_{-1}, z_0, z_1, \ldots$ be a sequence of real numbers such that $\sum_{-\infty}^{+\infty}|z_j| < \infty$. The observations are $Y_t = \sum_{j=-\infty}^{+\infty} z_j X_{t-j}$ for $t = 0, 1, 2, \ldots$. Although not m-dependent for any finite m, they form a stationary sequence with mean $\mu = EY_t = \xi \sum_{j=-\infty}^{+\infty} z_j$ and covariances

$$\sigma_{0t} = \operatorname{cov}(Y_0, Y_t) = \tau^2 \sum_{j=-\infty}^{+\infty} z_j z_{t+j}.$$

Let $S_n = \sum_{t=1}^{n} Y_t$.

Show that $\sqrt{n}(S_n/n - \mu) \xrightarrow{\mathscr{L}} \mathscr{N}(0, \sigma^2)$, where

$$\sigma^2 = \sigma_{00} + 2\sum_{t=1}^{\infty} \sigma_{0t}.$$

[Hint: The truncated version of Y_t, $Y_t^{(k)} = \sum_{|j|\le k} z_j X_{t-j}$, is a $(2k)$-dependent stationary sequence to which Theorem 11 applies. Let $S_n^{(k)} = \sum_{t=1}^{n} Y_t^{(k)}$ show that $S_n - S_n^{(k)} \xrightarrow{P} 0$ uniformly in n as $k \to \infty$, and use the lemma of this section.]

12

Some Rank Statistics

Let $R_{N1}, R_{N2}, \ldots, R_{NN}$ denote a random permutation of the integers 1 through N, with each of the $N!$ permutations being equally likely. In this section, we investigate the asymptotic distributions of sums of functions of the form

$$S_N = \sum_{J=1}^{N} z_{Nj} a_N(R_{Nj}), \tag{1}$$

where $z_{N1}, \ldots, z_{NN}$ and $a_N(1), \ldots, a_N(N)$ are given sets of numbers. To simplify the notation, we will usually drop the subscript N for z, a, and R, and so write

$$S_N = \sum_{j=1}^{N} z_j a(R_j). \tag{1'}$$

For most of the discussion to follow, N is fixed and no confusion will result. When we let N tend to infinity, we will remind you that the distribution of R depends on N and that z and a may depend on N.

Note that the distribution of S_N in (1) is unchanged if we reorder all subscripts. Thus, we may assume without loss of generality that the $a(j)$ (or the z_j or both) are arranged in increasing order. Similarly, the distribution of S_N is unchanged if we interchange $a(j)$ and z_j, because we may write $S_N = \Sigma_{J=1}^{N} a(j) z_{R'_j}$, where R'_j is the inverse permutation of R_j; that is, $R_j = i$ iff $R'_i = j$. From this, we expect the conditions for asymptotic normality of S_N to be symmetric in z and a.

Example 1. *Sampling.* Suppose that a random sample of fixed size $n \geq 1$ is drawn from a population of values $\{z_1, \ldots, z_N\}$ without replacement. If S_N denotes the sum of the sampled values, then S_N may be written in the form (1), where

$$a(j) = \begin{cases} 1, & \text{for} \quad 1 \leq j \leq n, \\ 0, & \text{for} \quad n+1 \leq j \leq N. \end{cases} \tag{2}$$

This is equivalent to including z_j in the sample if in a random permutation, $R_1, R_2, \ldots, R_N$, of $1, \ldots, N$, we have $R_j \leq n$. We may use S_N/n to estimate the population mean, or NS_N/n to estimate the population total.

Example 2. *The Two-Sample Randomization t-Test.* In the two-sample problem of comparing treatment and control, a set of N experimental units is given and a set of size $m < N$ is chosen at random, all $\binom{N}{m}$ choices being equally likely. Members of this set of size m receive the experimental treatment and the remaining $n = N - m$ units serve as controls. Let $X_1, \ldots, X_m$ denote the outcomes of the treatment group, and let $Y_1, \ldots, Y_n$ denote the outcomes of the control group. The usual test of the hypothesis of no treatment effect is based on the statistic $\overline{X}_m - \overline{Y}_n$ divided by some estimate of its variance. The randomization test is done conditionally on the values of the observations and is based only on the randomization done by the statistician. If the values of $X_1, \ldots, X_m$, $Y_1, \ldots, Y_n$ are denoted by $z_1, \ldots, z_N$, then by virtue of the randomization, each of the subsets of size m is equally like to be $X_1, \ldots, X_m$. The statistic $\overline{X}_m - \overline{Y}_n$ may then be written in the form (1) if we define

$$a(j) = \begin{cases} 1/m, & \text{for} \quad 1 \leq j \leq m, \\ -1/n, & \text{for} \quad m+1 \leq j \leq N. \end{cases} \tag{3}$$

Example 3. *The Rank-Sum Test.* The Wilcoxon rank-sum test is similar to the randomization t test, but the actual values of the observations are replaced by their ranks in the ranking of all $N = m + n$ observations. Instead of using the difference of the mean ranks, it is customary to use the sum of the ranks of the treatment observations. The rank-sum statistic under the hypothesis of no treatment effect may be written in the form (1), where

$$z_j = j \quad \text{and} \quad a(j) = \begin{cases} 1, & \text{for} \quad 1 \leq j \leq m, \\ 0, & \text{for} \quad m+1 \leq j \leq N. \end{cases} \tag{4}$$

Example 4. *Randomization Test against Trend.* When observations $X_1, \ldots, X_N$ are taken sequentially, one is often interested in testing randomness against a tendency of the observations to increase (or decrease) in time. A simple test statistic for use in this problem is based on the product moment of the observations with time, $S_N = \Sigma_{j=1}^N jX_j$. As the null hypothesis in the randomization model, it is assumed that the observations are put in random order, all $N!$ orderings being equally likely. This leads to a statistic of the form (1), where the z_j are the values of the observations in some order, and $a(j) = j$.

Example 5. *Spearman's Rho.* Another nonparametric model for testing against trend arises if, in the randomization test against trend, the observations are replaced by their ranks. The resulting statistic is $S_N = \Sigma_{j=1}^N jR_j$, where R_j is the rank of the jth observation. This is related to Spearman's rank correlation coefficient, ρ_N, which is defined as the correlation coefficient between the time of observation and the rank. Because both have mean $(N+1)/2$ and variance $(N^2-1)/12$, the correlation coefficient may be written $\rho_N = 12[(1/N)\Sigma_{j=1}^N jR_j - ((N+1)/2)^2]/(N^2-1)$. This statistic and Kendall's τ (see Exercise 7 of Section 5) are competitors used for measuring the agreement of two rankings of N objects.

Example 6. *The Hypergeometric Distribution.* If

$$z_j = \begin{cases} 1, & \text{for} \quad 1 \le j \le m, \\ 0, & \text{for} \quad m+1 \le j \le N, \end{cases} \tag{5}$$

and

$$a(j) = \begin{cases} 1, & \text{for} \quad 1 \le j \le n, \\ 0, & \text{for} \quad n+1 \le j \le N, \end{cases}$$

then the statistic (1) has a hypergeometric distribution, $\mathscr{H}(n, m, N)$.

Asymptotic Normality. The remarkably simple theorem, presented below, giving conditions under which the statistic (1) is asymptotically normal, stems from the work of Wald and Wolfowitz (1944), Noether (1949) and Hoeffding (1952). Our treatment follows the method of Hájek (1961), which gives the result as an application of the Lindenberg–Feller Theorem. See the book of Hájek and Sidák (1967) for a fuller account and for generalizations.

First we compute the mean and variance of the statistic S_n given in (1). Note that the means and variances of the $a(R_j)$ are

$$Ea(R_j) = (1/N)\sum_{i=1}^{N} a(i) = \bar{a}_N$$

and

$$\operatorname{var}\big(a(R_j)\big) = (1/N)\sum_{i=1}^{N} \big(a(i) - \bar{a}_N\big)^2 = \sigma_a^2,$$

independent of j. We use $\bar{z}_N = (1/N)\sum_{j=1}^{N} z_j$ to denote the mean of the z_j, and $\sigma_2^2 = (1/N)\sum_{j=1}^{N}(z_j - \bar{z}_N)^2$ to denote the variance.

LEMMA 1. *$ES_N = N\bar{z}_N\bar{a}_N$, and*

$$\operatorname{var} S_N = \frac{N^2}{N-1}\sigma_z^2\sigma_a^2. \tag{6}$$

Proof.

$$ES_N = \sum_{j=1}^{N} z_j Ea(R_j) = \sum_{j=1}^{N} z_j \bar{a}_N = N\bar{z}_N\bar{a}_N.$$

Note that $\operatorname{cov}(a(R_j), a(R_k))$ for $j \neq k$ is independent of j and k. Since $P(R_1 = i, R_2 = j) = 1/(N(N-1))$ for all $i \neq j$, we have

$$\begin{aligned}
\operatorname{cov}\big(a(R_1), a(R_2)\big) &= \frac{1}{N(N-1)}\sum\sum_{i\neq j}\big(a(i) - \bar{a}_N\big)\big(a(j) - \bar{a}_N\big) \\
&= -\frac{1}{N(N-1)}\sum_{i=1}^{N}\big(a(i) - \bar{a}_N\big)^2 \\
&= -\frac{1}{N-1}\sigma_a^2.
\end{aligned}$$

From this, the variance of S_N is

$$\begin{aligned}\operatorname{var} S_N &= \sum_{j=1}^{N} z_j^2 \operatorname{var} a(R_j) + \sum_{j \neq k}\sum z_j z_k \operatorname{cov}\big(a(R_j), a(R_k)\big)\\ &= \sigma_a^2\left[\sum_{j=1}^{N} z_j^2 - \frac{1}{N-1}\sum_{j \neq k}\sum z_j z_k\right]\\ &= \sigma_a^2\left[\sum z_j^2 - \frac{1}{N-1}\left(\sum z_j\right)^2 + \frac{1}{N-1}\sum z_j^2\right]\\ &= \frac{N^2}{N-1}\sigma_z^2\sigma_a^2. \quad \blacksquare\end{aligned}$$

To prove the asymptotic normality of S_N, we find a related sum S'_N of independent random variables to which the Central Limit Theorem applies and show that the normalized versions of the sums S_N and S'_N are asymptotically equivalent.

For this purpose, Let $U_1, U_2, \ldots, U_N$ be i.i.d. $\mathscr{U}(0,1)$ random variables, and let R_j denote the rank of U_j in the ordering of $U_1, \ldots, U_N$ from smallest to largest. Then $(R_1, \ldots, R_N)$ is a random permutation of the integers 1 through N and may be used in (1). Moreover, R_j/N should be fairly close to U_j. [One can show corr$(U_j, R_j/N) \to 1$ as $n \to \infty$.] Thus we may hope that in replacing the R_j in the sum (1) by $[NU_j]$ to obtain a sum of independent identically distributed terms, we have not changed the value of the sum much. We note

$$S_N - ES_N = \sum_{j=1}^{N} (z_j - \bar{z}_N)\big(a(R_j) - \bar{a}_N\big),$$

and define

$$S'_N = \sum_{j=1}^{N} (z_j - \bar{z}_N)\big(a([NU_j]) - \bar{a}_N\big).$$

Then $ES'_N = 0$, and

$$\operatorname{var}(S'_N) = \sum_{j=1}^{N} (z_j - \bar{z}_N)^2 \operatorname{var}(a(R_1)), \tag{7}$$

since the $\lceil NU_j \rceil$ are i.i.d. with the same distribution as R_1, namely, the uniform on the integers from 1 to N. The normalized versions of S_N and S'_N are asymptotically equivalent if their correlation tends to one (Exercise 4 of Section 6). We first reduce the correlation to a simpler form.

Lemma 2. $\mathrm{Corr}(S_N, S'_N) = \sqrt{N/(N-1)}\ \mathrm{corr}(a(R_1), a(\lceil NU_1 \rceil))$.

Proof.

$$\mathrm{cov}(S_N, S'_N) = \sum_{j=1}^{N} \sum_{k=1}^{N} (z_j - \bar{z}_N)(z_k - \bar{z}_N) \,\mathrm{cov}\big(a(R_j), a(\lceil NU_k \rceil)\big).$$

The value $c_1 = \mathrm{cov}(a(R_j), a(\lceil NU_j \rceil))$ is independent of j and the value $c_2 = \mathrm{cov}(a(R_j), a(\lceil NU_k \rceil))$ for $j \neq k$ is independent of j and k. We find

$$\begin{aligned}\mathrm{cov}(S_N, S'_N) &= c_1 \sum_{j=1}^{N} (z_j - \bar{z}_N)^2 + c_2 \sum_{j=1}^{N} \sum_{k=1}^{N} (z_j - \bar{z}_N)(z_k - \bar{z}_N)\\ &= (c_1 - c_2) \sum_{j=1}^{N} (z_j - \bar{z}_N)^2. \qquad (8)\end{aligned}$$

Since $\Sigma_{j=1}^{N} a(R_j)$ is a constant,

$$\begin{aligned}0 &= \mathrm{cov}\left(\sum_{j=1}^{N} a(R_j), a(\lceil NU_k \rceil) \right) = \sum_{j=1}^{N} \mathrm{cov}\big(a(R_j), a(\lceil NU_k \rceil)\big)\\ &= c_1 + (N-1)c_2.\end{aligned}$$

This shows that $c_2 = -c_1/(N-1)$. Substituting this into (8), we find

$$\mathrm{cov}(S_N, S'_N) = \frac{Nc_1}{N-1} \sum_{j=1}^{N} (z_j - \bar{z}_N)^2.$$

Using the variances found in (6) and (7), we have

$$\mathrm{corr}(S_N, S'_N) = \sqrt{N/(N-1)}\ \mathrm{corr}\big(a(R_1), a(\lceil NU_1 \rceil)\big). \quad \blacksquare$$

We wish to show that $\mathrm{corr}(S_N, S'_N)$ tends to 1, and since

$$E\big(a(R_1) - a(\lceil NU_1 \rceil)\big)^2 / \mathrm{var}(a(R_1)) = 2\big(1 - \mathrm{corr}\big(a(R_1), a(\lceil NU_1 \rceil)\big)\big),$$

it is sufficient to show $E(a(R_1) - a(\lceil NU_1 \rceil))^2/\mathrm{var}(a(R_1)) \to 0$. The following lemma of Hájek (1961, Lemma 2.1) gives a bound for this quantity. Although this result is valid in general, we give the proof only for the important special case of $a(j)$ given by (2). This allows treatment of

Examples 1, 2, 3, and 6 above. The other important special case, $a(j) = j$ found in Examples 4 and 5, is treated in Exercise 3.

Lemma 3 (Hájek). *Assume that $a(j)$ is monotone. Then*

$$E(a(R_1) - a(\lceil NU_1 \rceil))^2 \le \frac{2\sqrt{2}}{N} \max_j |a(j) - \bar{a}_N| \sqrt{\sum_{i=1}^{N} (a(i) - \bar{a}_N)^2}\,.$$

Proof. For the $a(j)$ of (2), we have $\max_j |a(j) - \bar{a}_N| = \max\{n/N, (n - N)/N\}$, and $\sum_{i=1}^{N}(a(i) - \bar{a}_N)^2 = n((n - N)/N)$, so we are to show

$$E(a(R_1) - a(\lceil NU_1 \rceil))^2 \le \frac{2\sqrt{2}}{N} \max\left\{\frac{n}{N}, 1 - \frac{n}{N}\right\}\left[n\left(1 - \frac{n}{N}\right)\right]^{1/2}.$$

We show the slightly stronger

$$E(a(R_1) - a(\lceil NU_1 \rceil))^2 \le \frac{1}{N}\left[n\left(1 - \frac{n}{N}\right)\right]^{1/2}.$$

We compute this expectation conditionally given the order statistics, $U_{(1)} < U_{(2)} < \cdots < U_{(N)}$. The key property is that the ranks $(R_1, \ldots, R_N)$ are independent of the order statistics $U_{(\cdot)} = (U_{(1)}, \ldots, U_{(N)})$. (Given the order statistics, the actual ranking of the U_j is equally likely to be any of the $N!$ rankings.) Note that if R_1 is the rank of U_1, then $U_1 = U_{(R_1)}$. Thus,

$$\begin{aligned} E(a(R_1) - a(\lceil NU_1 \rceil))^2 &= E\left[E\left\{(a(R_1) - a(\lceil NU_{(R_1)} \rceil))^2 | U_{(\cdot)}\right\}\right] \\ &= E\left[(1/N) \sum_{j=1}^{N} (a(j) - a(\lceil NU_{(j)} \rceil))^2\right]. \end{aligned}$$

Each of the terms of the sum $S = \sum_{j=1}^{N}(a(j) - a(\lceil NU_{(j)} \rceil))^2$ is 1 or 0, and S represents the number of discrepancies. If there are exactly n U_j's less than n/N, then S is zero; but as this number increases or decreases by 1, S increases by 1. Thus, $S = |K - n|$, where K is the number of $U_j \le n/N$. K has a binomial distribution with sample size N and success probability n/N. Hence,

$$\begin{aligned} E(a(R_1) - a(\lceil NU_1 \rceil))^2 &= (1/N)E[|K - n|] \\ &\le (1/N)(E(K - n)^2)^{1/2} \\ &= (1/N)(n(N - n)/N)^{1/2}. \quad \blacksquare \end{aligned}$$

We are now in a position to let N tend to infinity, so we return the subscript N to the notation.

Theorem 12. *If*

$$\delta_N = N \frac{\max_j (z_{Nj} - \bar{z}_N)^2}{\sum_{j=1}^N (z_{Nj} - \bar{z}_N)^2} \frac{\max_j (a_N(j) - \bar{a}_N)^2}{\sum_{j=1}^N (a_N(j) - \bar{a}_N)^2} \to 0, \tag{9}$$

then

$$(S_N - ES_N)/(\operatorname{var}(S_N))^{1/2} \xrightarrow{\mathscr{L}} \mathscr{N}(0,1).$$

Proof. First we note that (9) implies that

$$\frac{\max_j (a_N(j) - \bar{a}_N)^2}{\sum_{j=1}^N (a_N(j) - \bar{a}_N)^2} \to 0,$$

since

$$N \frac{\max_i (z_{Ni} - \bar{z}_N)^2}{\sum_{j=1}^N (z_{Nj} - \bar{z}_N)^2}$$

is bounded. Assuming without loss of generality that $a(j)$ is nondecreasing, this together with Lemma 3 implies that

$$E(a(R_1) - a(\lceil NU_1 \rceil))^2 / \operatorname{var}(a(R_1)) \to 0, \tag{10}$$

which from Lemma 2 and Exercise 4 of Section 6 implies that $S'_N/(\operatorname{var}(S'_N))^{1/2}$ and $(S_N - ES_N)/(\operatorname{var}(S_N))^{1/2}$ have the same asymptotic distribution. We complete the proof using the Lindeberg–Feller Theorem to show that condition (9) implies $S'_N/(\mathrm{var}(S'_N))^{1/2} \xrightarrow{\mathscr{L}} \mathscr{N}(0,1)$. We let $B_N^2 = \mathrm{var}(S'_N)$, and note that the variables $X_{Nj} = (z_{Nj} - \bar{z}_N)(a_N(\lceil NU_j \rceil) - \bar{a}_N)$ have mean 0. We check the Lindeberg condition. Let $\varepsilon > 0$.

$$\frac{1}{B_N^2} \sum_{j=1}^{N} E\left\{X_{Nj}^2 I\left(|X_{Nj}| \geq \varepsilon B_N\right)\right\}$$

$$= \frac{1}{B_N^2} \sum_{j=1}^{N} E\left\{\left(z_{Nj} - \bar{z}_N\right)^2 \left(a_N(\lceil NU \rceil) - \bar{a}_N\right)^2 \right.$$

$$\left. \times I\left(\left(z_{Nj} - \bar{z}_N\right)^2 \left(a_N(\lceil NU \rceil) - \bar{a}_N\right)^2 \geq \varepsilon^2 B_N^2\right)\right\}$$

$$\leq \frac{1}{B_N^2} \sum_{j=1}^{N} \left(z_{Nj} - \bar{z}_N\right)^2 E\left\{\left(a_N(\lceil NU \rceil) - \bar{a}_N\right)^2 I\left(\delta_N \geq \varepsilon^2\right)\right\}$$

$$= I\left(\delta_N \geq \varepsilon^2\right).$$

From (9), this is zero for N sufficiently large, completing the proof. ■

Application to Sampling. We illustrate the use of this Theorem on Example 1. The $a_N(j)$ are given by (2), where n may depend on N. So $\bar{a}_N = n/N$, and

$$(1/N) \sum_{j=1}^{N} \left(a_N(j) - \bar{a}_N\right)^2 = \mathrm{var}\left(a_N(R_1)\right)$$

$$= \mathrm{var}\left(a_N(\lceil NU_1 \rceil)\right) = (n/N)(1 - (n/N)).$$

Since $\frac{1}{4} \leq \max_j (a_N(j) - \bar{a}_N)^2 \leq 1$, condition (9) is equivalent to

$$N \frac{\max_j \left(z_{Nj} - \bar{z}_N\right)^2}{\sum_{j=1}^{N} \left(z_{Nj} - \bar{z}_N\right)^2} \frac{N}{n(N-n)} \to 0. \tag{11}$$

In particular, (9) will be satisfied if either $\min(n, N-n) \to \infty$ and

$$N \frac{\max_i \left(z_{Nj} - \bar{z}_N\right)^2}{\sum_{J=1}^{N} \left(z_{Nj} - \bar{z}_N\right)^2} \text{ is bounded,}$$

or $\min(n, N-n)/N$ is bounded away from 0 and

$$\frac{\max_j \left(z_{Nj} - \bar{z}_N\right)^2}{\sum_{j=1}^{N} \left(z_{Nj} - \bar{z}_N\right)^2} \to 0.$$

The conclusion drawn from this is that

$$\frac{S_N - ES_N}{\sqrt{\operatorname{var}(S_N)}} = \frac{(S_N/N) - \bar{z}_N}{\sqrt{s_z^2 (N-n)/(N-1)}} \xrightarrow{\mathscr{L}} \mathscr{N}(0,1).$$

This leads to the standard procedure used in sampling theory to get a confidence interval for the population mean. However, one must use some estimate of the population variance such as the sample variance. The conditions needed for approximate normality are that n and $N-n$ be large and $(N/(n(N-n)))\max_j (z_j - \bar{z}_N)^2/s_z^2$ be small. Since the latter condition involves the unobserved z's, this requires a certain amount of faith.

In the application of Theorem 12 to the two-sample randomization test of Example 2, this leap of faith is not required because we can see all the observations. The asymptotic theory for the two-sample permutation test follows directly from the above application to sampling. Namely, $(S_N - ES_N)/\sqrt{\operatorname{var}(S_N)} \xrightarrow{\mathscr{L}} \mathscr{N}(0,1)$ under the same condition (11). In addition, s_z^2 is calculable and does not need to be estimated.

EXERCISES

1. (a) For the rank-sum test statistic, S_N, of Example 3, find ES_N and $\operatorname{var}(S_N)$, and show that $(S_N - ES_N)/(\operatorname{var}(S_N))^{1/2} \xrightarrow{\mathscr{L}} \mathscr{N}(0,1)$ provided $\min(m, N-m) \to \infty$.
   (b) Suppose $m/N \to r$ as $N \to \infty$, where $0 < r < 1$. Is it true that

$$\sqrt{N}\left((S_N/N^2) - (r/2)\right) \xrightarrow{\mathscr{L}} \mathscr{N}(0, r(1-r)/12)?$$

2. Consider the hypergeometric random variable, S_N, of Example 6.
   (a) Show that $(S_N - ES_N)/(\operatorname{var}(S_N))^{1/2} \xrightarrow{\mathscr{L}} \mathscr{N}(0,1)$ provided $(n(N-n)m(N-m))/N^3 \to \infty$, in particular provided $\min(n, N-n) \to \infty$ and $\min(m, N-m)/N$ is bounded away from 0.
   (b) In the borderline case $n \to \infty$, $m \to \infty$, and $nm/N \to \lambda$, $0 < \lambda < \infty$, show that $S_N \xrightarrow{\mathscr{L}} \mathscr{P}(\lambda)$.

3. Consider Example 4 in which $a(j) = j$.
   (a) Show $E(R_1 - NU_1)^2/\text{var}(R_1) \to 0$.
   (b) Show $E(\lceil NU_1 \rceil - NU_1)^2/\text{var}(R_1) \to 0$.
   (c) Show $(x + y)^2 \leq 2x^2 + 2y^2$ for all x and y, and conclude that

$$E(R_1 - \lceil NU_1 \rceil)^2/\text{var}(R_1) \to 0,$$

   so condition (10) is satisfied.
   (d) Show for the randomization test against trend, $(S_N - ES_N)/(\text{var}(S_N))^{1/2} \xrightarrow{\mathscr{L}} \mathscr{N}(0, 1)$ provided

$$\frac{\max_j (z_{Nj} - \bar{z}_N)^2}{\sum_{J=1}^{N} (z_{Nj} - \bar{z}_N)^2} \to 0.$$

4. For the statistic $S_N = \Sigma j R_j$ of Example 5, related to Spearman's ρ, find ES_N and $\text{var}(S_N)$ and show that $(S_N - ES_N)/(\text{var}(S_N))^{1/2} \xrightarrow{\mathscr{L}} \mathscr{N}(0, 1)$.
5. What conditions on the z_j are needed to satisfy condition (9) if
   (a) $a(j) = \log(j)$.
   (b) $a(j) = 1/\sqrt{j}$.
   (c) $a(j) = 1/j$.
6. Prove the following theorem of Hájek. Let $\varphi(u)$ be a nondecreasing function defined on (0, 1) such that $0 < \sigma^2 = \int_0^1 (\varphi(u) - \bar{\varphi})^2\, du < \infty$, where $\bar{\varphi} = \int_0^1 \varphi(u)\, du$. Define $a_N(j) = \varphi(j/(N+1))$. Then, for S_N given by (1), $(S_N - ES_N)/\sqrt{\text{var}(S_N)} \xrightarrow{\mathscr{L}} \mathscr{N}(0, 1)$ provided

$$\frac{\max_j (z_{Nj} - \bar{z}_N)^2}{\sum_{j=1}^{N} (z_{Nj} - \bar{z}_N)^2} \to 0.$$

   [Hint: (a) Let $U_1, \ldots, U_N$ be i.i.d. $\mathscr{U}(0, 1)$ random variables, and let $S'_N = \Sigma_{j=1}^N (z_{Nj} - \bar{z}_N)(\varphi(U_j) - \bar{\varphi})$. Show

$$S'_N/\sqrt{\text{var}(S'_N)} \xrightarrow{\mathscr{L}} \mathscr{N}(0, 1)$$

   (Exercise 6 of Section 5).
   (b) Let R_{Nj} denote the rank of U_j in $U_1, \ldots, U_N$. Show that

$$\text{corr}(S_N, S'_N) = \sqrt{N/(N-1)}\ \text{corr}(a(R_{N1}), \varphi(U_1))$$

   (Lemma 2).
   (c) Show $R_{N1}/N \xrightarrow{\text{a.s.}} U_1$, and $a(R_{N1}) \xrightarrow{\text{a.s.}} \varphi(U_1)$ (Glivenko–Cantelli).

(d) Show $Ea(R_{N1})^2 \to E\varphi(U_1)^2$ (Riemann approximation to an integral).

(e) Show $E(a(R_{N1}) - \varphi(U_1))^2 \to 0$ (Exercise 7 of Section 2).

(f) Show the normalized versions of S_N and S'_N are asymptotically equivalent (Exercise 5 of Section 6).

7. *A k-Sample Problem.* A sample of size n_i is taken from population i for $i = 1, \ldots, k$, for a total sample size of $N = \sum_{i=1}^k n_i$. All N observations are ranked and each observation is replaced by its rank. Let S_i denote the sum of the ranks of the observations in population i. Suppose for all i that $n_i/N \to p_i$ as $n \to \infty$ for some numbers $p_i > 0$. Note that $\sum_{i=1}^k p_i = 1$. Let $\mathbf{S} = (S_1, \ldots, S_k)$, $\mathbf{p} = (p_1, \ldots, p_k)$ and $\mathbf{p}^* = (n_1, \ldots, n_k)/N$. Let $\mathbf{P}$ and $\mathbf{P}^*$ denote the matrices

$$\mathbf{P} = \begin{bmatrix} p_1 & 0 & \cdots & 0 \\ 0 & p_2 & \cdots & 0 \\ \vdots & \vdots & \ddots & \vdots \\ 0 & 0 & \cdots & p_k \end{bmatrix}$$

and

$$\mathbf{P}^* = \frac{1}{N}\begin{bmatrix} n_1 & 0 & \cdots & 0 \\ 0 & n_2 & \cdots & 0 \\ \vdots & \vdots & \ddots & \vdots \\ 0 & 0 & \cdots & n_k \end{bmatrix}$$

(a) Show

$$\sqrt{3N}\left(\frac{2}{N(N+1)}\mathbf{S} - \mathbf{p}^*\right) \xrightarrow{\mathscr{L}} \mathscr{N}(\mathbf{0}, \mathbf{P} - \mathbf{p}\mathbf{p}^T).$$

(b) Deduce

$$3(N+1)\left(\frac{2}{N(N+1)}\mathbf{S} - \mathbf{p}^*\right)^T \mathbf{P}^{*-1}\left(\frac{2}{N(N+1)}\mathbf{S} - \mathbf{p}^*\right) \xrightarrow{\mathscr{L}} \chi^2_{k-1}.$$

This is the Kruskal–Wallis statistic that generalizes the rank-sum statistic to problems of comparing more than two populations.

13

Asymptotic Distribution of Sample Quantiles

Let $X_1, \ldots, X_n$ be a sample from a distribution F on the real line and assume that F is continuous so that all observations are distinct with probability 1. We may then arrange the observations in increasing order without ties, $X_{(n:1)} < X_{(n:2)} < \cdots < X_{(n:n)}$. These variables are called the order statistics. For clarity, we will usually drop the dependence on n in the notation and write simply $X_{(k)} = X_{(n:k)}$ as the kth order statistic and let $X_{(1)} < \cdots < X_{(n)}$ denote the order statistics. For $0 < p < 1$, *the* pth *quantile* of F is defined as $x_p = F^{-1}(p)$, and *the* pth *sample quantile* is defined as $X_{(k)}$ where $k = \lceil np \rceil =$ the ceiling of np (the smallest integer greater than or equal to np). If the density $f(x)$ exists and is continuous and positive in a neighborhood of some quantiles, then the joint distribution of the corresponding sample quantiles is asymptotically normal. We give the proof for two quantiles; the extension to many quantiles is easy.

The transformation $U_{(j)} = F(X_{(j)})$ for $j = 1, \ldots, n$ gives $U_{(1)}, \ldots, U_{(n)}$ as the order statistics of a sample from a uniform distribution, $\mathscr{U}(0,1)$. We first prove the theorem for a uniform distribution and then derive the general result using the inverse transformation $g(u) = F^{-1}(u)$ in Cramér's Theorem.

The joint distribution of the order statistics $U_{(1)} \leq \cdots \leq U(n)$ from $\mathscr{U}(0,1)$ has the following well-known representation as the distribution of ratios of waiting times. The proof is left as an exercise.

Lemma 1. *Let $Y_1, Y_2, \ldots, Y_{n+1}$ be* i.i.d. *exponential random variables with mean* 1, $(\mathscr{G}(1,1))$, *and let* $S_j = \Sigma_{i=1}^{j} Y_i$ *for* $j = 1, \ldots, n+1$. *Then the conditional distribution of*

$$\left[\frac{S_1}{S_{n+1}}, \ldots, \frac{S_n}{S_{n+1}}\right]$$

given S_{n+1} *is the same as the order statistics of a sample of size n from* $\mathscr{U}(0,1)$.

This lemma implies that the joint distribution of $(U_{(k_1)}, U_{(k_2)})$ is the same as that of

$$\left[\frac{S_{k_1}}{S_{n+1}}, \frac{S_{k_2}}{S_{n+1}}\right].$$

Since the latter is a function of sums of i.i.d. random variables, it will have an asymptotic normal distribution that can be computed by the methods of Section 7.

To see this note that the Central Limit Theorem implies $\sqrt{k}((1/k)S_k - 1) \xrightarrow{\mathscr{L}} \mathscr{N}(0,1)$ as $k \to \infty$ because $\mathscr{G}(1,1)$ has mean 1 and variance 1. Hence, if $n \to \infty$ and $k_1/n \to p_1$, then

$$\sqrt{n+1}\left[\frac{1}{n+1}S_{k_1} - \frac{k_1}{n+1}\right] = \sqrt{\frac{k_1}{n+1}}\sqrt{k_1}\left[\frac{1}{k_1}S_{k_1} - 1\right]$$

$$\xrightarrow{\mathscr{L}} \sqrt{p_1}\mathscr{N}(0,1) = \mathscr{N}(0, p_1).$$

Similarly, if $n \to \infty$, $k_1/n \to p_1$, and $k_2/n \to p_2$, then

$$\sqrt{n+1}\left[\frac{1}{n+1}(S_{k_2} - S_{k_1}) - \frac{k_2 - k_1}{n+1}\right]$$

$$= \sqrt{\frac{k_2 - k_1}{n+1}}\sqrt{k_2 - k_1}\left[\frac{1}{k_2 - k_1}\sum_{k_1+1}^{k_2} Y_j - 1\right]$$

$$\xrightarrow{\mathscr{L}} \mathscr{N}(0, p_2 - p_1),$$

and

$$\sqrt{n+1}\left[\frac{1}{n+1}(S_{n+1} - S_{k_2}) - \frac{n+1-k_2}{n+1}\right] \xrightarrow{\mathscr{L}} \mathscr{N}(0, 1 - p_2).$$

Lemma 2. *If $Y_1, Y_2, \ldots$ are i.i.d. $\mathscr{G}(1,1)$, and $\sqrt{n}(k_1/n - p_1) \to 0$ and $\sqrt{n}(k_2/n - p_2) \to 0$ as $n \to \infty$, then*

$$\sqrt{n+1}\begin{bmatrix} \dfrac{1}{n+1}S_{k_1} - p_1 \\ \dfrac{1}{n+1}(S_{k_2} - S_{k_1}) - (p_2 - p_1) \\ \dfrac{1}{n+1}(S_{n+1} - S_{k_2}) - (1 - p_2) \end{bmatrix}$$

$$\xrightarrow{\mathscr{L}} \mathscr{N}\left(\mathbf{0}, \begin{bmatrix} p_1 & 0 & 0 \\ 0 & p_2 - p_1 & 0 \\ 0 & 0 & 1 - p_2 \end{bmatrix}\right).$$

Proof. Since the difference between

$$\sqrt{n+1}\left[\frac{1}{n+1}S_{k_1} - p_1\right]$$

and

$$\sqrt{n+1}\left[\frac{1}{n+1}S_{k_1} - \frac{k_1}{n+1}\right]$$

is

$$\sqrt{n+1}\left[\frac{k_1}{n+1} - p_1\right],$$

which $\to 0$, they are asymptotically equivalent. So,

$$\sqrt{n+1}\left[\frac{1}{n+1}S_{k_1} - p_1\right] \xrightarrow{\mathscr{L}} \mathscr{N}(0, p_1).$$

The situation is similar for the other two terms. Since S_{k_1}, $S_{k_2} - S_{k_1}$, and $S_{n+1} - S_{k_2}$ are independent, and each is asymptotically normal, they are jointly asymptotically independent normal. ■

Theorem 13. *If $U_{(1)} < \cdots < U_{(n)}$ are the order statistics of a sample of size n from $\mathscr{U}(0,1)$, and if $n \to \infty$, $k_1 \to \infty$, and $k_2 \to \infty$ in such a way that*

$$\sqrt{n}\left(\frac{k_1}{n} - p_1\right) \to 0$$

and

$$\sqrt{n}\left(\frac{k_2}{n} - p_2\right) \to 0,$$

where $0 < p_1 < p_2 < 1$, *then*

$$\sqrt{n}\begin{bmatrix} U_{(k_1)} - p_1 \\ U_{(k_2)} - p_2 \end{bmatrix} \xrightarrow{\mathscr{L}} \mathscr{N}\left(\mathbf{0}, \begin{bmatrix} p_1(1-p_1) & p_1(1-p_2) \\ p_1(1-p_2) & p_2(1-p_2) \end{bmatrix}\right).$$

Proof. Let

$$\mathbf{g}(x_1, x_2, x_3) = \frac{1}{x_1 + x_2 + x_3}\begin{bmatrix} x_1 \\ x_1 + x_2 \end{bmatrix}.$$

Then

$$\mathbf{g}\left(\frac{S_{k_1}}{n+1}, \frac{S_{k_2} - S_{k_1}}{n+1}, \frac{S_{n+1} - S_{k_2}}{n+1}\right) = \frac{1}{S_{n+1}}\begin{bmatrix} S_{k_1} \\ S_{k_2} \end{bmatrix},$$

which by Lemma 1 has the same distribution as $\begin{bmatrix} U_{(k_1)} \\ U_{(k_2)} \end{bmatrix}$. Then, with Theorem 7 applied to Lemma 2,

$$\sqrt{n}\begin{bmatrix} U_{(k_1)} - p_1 \\ U_{(k_2)} - p_2 \end{bmatrix} \xrightarrow{\mathscr{L}} \mathscr{N}(0, \dot{\mathbf{g}}(\boldsymbol{\mu})\boldsymbol{\Sigma}\dot{\mathbf{g}}(\boldsymbol{\mu})^T).$$

Here,

$$\dot{\mathbf{g}}(x_1, x_2, x_3) = \frac{1}{(x_1 + x_2 + x_3)^2}\begin{bmatrix} x_2 + x_3 & -x_1 & -x_1 \\ x_3 & x_3 & -(x_1 + x_2) \end{bmatrix}$$

so that

$$\dot{\mathbf{g}}(\boldsymbol{\mu}) = \dot{\mathbf{g}}(p_1, p_2 - p_1, 1 - p_2) = \begin{bmatrix} 1 - p_1 & -p_1 & -p_1 \\ 1 - p_2 & 1 - p_2 & -p_2 \end{bmatrix}.$$

Then it is merely a matter of checking that

$$\dot{\mathbf{g}}(\boldsymbol{\mu})\begin{bmatrix} p_1 & 0 & 0 \\ 0 & p_2 - p_1 & 0 \\ 0 & 0 & 1 - p_2 \end{bmatrix}\dot{\mathbf{g}}(\boldsymbol{\mu})^T = \begin{bmatrix} p_1(1-p_1) & p_1(1-p_2) \\ p_1(1-p_2) & p_2(1-p_2) \end{bmatrix}. \qquad \blacksquare$$

COROLLARY. *If $X_{(1)} < \cdots < X_{(n)}$ are order statistics of a sample of size n from a distribution F having a density $f(x)$ continuous and positive in a neighborhood of the quantiles x_{p_1} and x_{p_2} with $p_1 < p_2$, then*

$$\sqrt{n}\begin{bmatrix} X_{(\lceil np_1 \rceil)} - x_{p_1} \\ X_{(\lceil np_2 \rceil)} - x_{p_2} \end{bmatrix} \xrightarrow{\mathscr{L}} \mathscr{N}\left(\mathbf{0}, \begin{bmatrix} \dfrac{p_1(1-p_1)}{f(x_{p_1})^2} & \dfrac{p_1(1-p_2)}{f(x_{p_1})f(x_{p_2})} \\ \dfrac{p_1(1-p_2)}{f(x_{p_1})f(x_{p_2})} & \dfrac{p_2(1-p_2)}{f(x_{p_2})^2} \end{bmatrix}\right)$$

Proof. Applying the transformation $\mathbf{g}(y_1, y_2) = (F^{-1}(y_1), F^{-1}(y_2))^T$ to the variables $(U_{(\lceil np_1 \rceil)} - p_1, U_{(\lceil np_2 \rceil)} - p_2))$ of Theorem 13, and noting

$$\dot{\mathbf{g}}(y_1, y_2) = \begin{bmatrix} \dfrac{1}{f(F^{-1}(y_1))} & 0 \\ 0 & \dfrac{1}{f(F^{-1}(y_2))} \end{bmatrix}$$

the Corollary follows immediately from Theorem 7. ■

Note: For one quantile, this theorem says that

$$\sqrt{n}\,(X_{(\lceil np \rceil)} - x_p) \xrightarrow{\mathscr{L}} \mathscr{N}\left(0, \frac{p(1-p)}{f(x_p)^2}\right).$$

For a given small number, Δx, $f(x_p)\,\Delta x$ represents the approximate proportion of observations that fall within an interval of length Δx centered at x_p. These are the observations that for large n will determine the accuracy of the estimate of the pth quantile. As n increases, the number of relevant observations goes up at a rate proportional to $f(x_p)$, so the standard deviation of the estimate of x_p will be proportional to $1/f(x_p)$.

EXAMPLE 1. Let m_n represent the median of a sample of size n from a normal distribution $\mathscr{N}(\mu, \sigma^2)$. Then because $f(\mu) = 1/(\sqrt{2\pi}\,\sigma)$, $\sqrt{n}\,(m_n - \mu) \xrightarrow{\mathscr{L}} \mathscr{N}(0, (\frac{1}{4})/f(\mu)^2) = \mathscr{N}(0, \pi\sigma^2/2)$. This may be compared with $\overline{X}_n$ as an estimate of μ, $\sqrt{n}\,(\overline{X}_n - \mu) \xrightarrow{\mathscr{L}} \mathscr{N}(0, \sigma^2)$.

Asymptotic Relative Efficiency. If $\hat{\theta}_1$ and $\hat{\theta}_2$ are two estimates of a parameter θ, and if $\sqrt{n}\,(\hat{\theta}_1 - \theta) \xrightarrow{\mathscr{L}} \mathscr{N}(0, \sigma_1^2)$ and $\sqrt{n}\,(\hat{\theta}_2 - \theta) \xrightarrow{\mathscr{L}} \mathscr{N}(0, \sigma_2^2)$, then the *asymptotic efficiency of* $\hat{\theta}_1$ *relative to* $\hat{\theta}_2$ is defined to be the ratio, σ_2^2/σ_1^2. Thus, in Example 1, the asymptotic efficiency of the median, m_n, relative to the mean $\overline{X}_n$, as an estimate of the mean, μ, is $\sigma^2/(\pi\sigma^2/2) = 2/\pi = 0.6366\ldots$. This means that if you are using m_n to estimate the mean of a normal population, you may use $\overline{X}_n$ instead and get the same accuracy based on only 64% of the observations. In other words, for large samples, if you are using m_n instead of $\overline{X}_n$ to estimate μ, you are throwing away about 36% of the observations. The asymptotic relative efficiency is defined as the ratio of the variances, rather than as the ratio of standard deviations, so that it has this immediate interpretation in terms of sample size.

Example 2. The Cauchy distribution $\mathscr{C}(\mu, \sigma)$ has density

$$f(x) = \frac{1}{\pi\sigma}\frac{1}{1 + [(x-\mu)/\sigma]^2}.$$

It has median μ, first quartile $x_{1/4} = \mu - \sigma$, and third quartile $x_{3/4} = \mu + \sigma$. Thus, σ is the semi-interquartile range, $\sigma = (x_{3/4} - x_{1/4})/2$. For the sample median,

$$\sqrt{n}\,(m_n - \mu) \xrightarrow{\mathscr{L}} \mathscr{N}\left(0, \frac{\pi^2\sigma^2}{4}\right).$$

To find the asymptotic distribution of the sample semi-interquartile range, first find the asymptotic joint distribution of $X_{(n/4)}$ and $X_{(3n/4)}$. (We use the notation $X_{(t)}$ for $0 < t < n$ to represent the order statistic $X_{(\lceil t \rceil)}$). From the corollary,

$$\sqrt{n}\begin{bmatrix} X_{(n/4)} - (\mu - \sigma) \\ X_{(3n/4)} - (\mu + \sigma) \end{bmatrix} \xrightarrow{\mathscr{L}} \mathscr{N}\left(0, \pi^2\sigma^2\begin{bmatrix} \frac{3}{4} & \frac{1}{4} \\ \frac{1}{4} & \frac{3}{4} \end{bmatrix}\right).$$

Hence,

$$\sqrt{n}\left[\frac{X_{(3n/4)} - X_{(n/4)}}{2} - \sigma\right] \xrightarrow{\mathscr{L}} \mathscr{N}(0, \pi^2\sigma^2/4).$$

EXERCISES

1. Prove Lemma 1.
2. The maximum likelihood estimate of the mean of the double exponential distribution with density $f(x) = \frac{1}{2}\exp\{-|x-\mu|\}$ is the sample median. Find its asymptotic distribution.

3. Find the asymptotic distribution of the *midquartile range*, $(X_{(3n/4)} + X_{(n/4)})/2$, when sampling from the Cauchy distribution, $\mathscr{C}(\mu, \sigma)$. What is its asymptotic efficiency relative to the median?
4. Let $X_1, X_2, \ldots$ be a sample from $\mathscr{U}(0, 2\mu)$.
   (a) Find the asymptotic distribution of the median.
   (b) Find the asymptotic distribution of the midquartile range.
   (c) Find the asymptotic distribution of $\frac{2}{3}X_{(3n/4)}$.
   (d) Compare these three estimates of the mean.
5. Let $X_1, X_2, \ldots$ be a sample from the exponential distribution, $\mathscr{G}(1, \theta)$, with density $f(x) = (1/\theta)\exp\{-x/\theta\}I(x > 0)$.
   (a) For some constant c, $\sqrt{n}(cm_n - \theta) \xrightarrow{\mathscr{L}} \mathscr{N}(0, \sigma^2)$. Find c and the asymptotic variance, σ^2.
   (b) Do the same for $X_{(np)}$ in place of the median. For what value of p is the asymptotic variance a minimum? (Answer, 0.797 . . .).
6. Let $X_1, \ldots, X_n$ be a sample from the beta distribution with density, $f(x|\theta) = \theta x^{\theta-1}I(0 < x < 1)$, where $\theta > 0$.
   (a) Let M_n denote the sample median, and $m(\theta)$ denote the population median as a function of θ. What is the asymptotic distribution of $\sqrt{n}(M_n - m(\theta))$?
   (b) Let $\hat{\theta}_n = \log\frac{1}{2}/\log(M_n)$. Show $\hat{\theta}_n \xrightarrow{P} \theta$.
   (c) What is the asymptotic distribution of $\sqrt{n}(\hat{\theta}_n - \theta)$?

14

Asymptotic Theory of Extreme Order Statistics*

Let $X_1, X_2, \ldots$ be i.i.d. with *continuous* distribution function $F(x)$ and let M_n denote the maximum of the first n observations, $M_n = \max_{j \le n} X_j$. Then the distribution function of M_n is $P(M_n \le x) = F(x)^n$.

The problem is to determine if there exists an asymptotic distribution of the maximum in the sense that there are sequences a_n and $b_n > 0$ such that $(M_n - a_n)/b_n$ has some limiting distribution or, equivalently, such that

$$P\left(\frac{M_n - a_n}{b_n} \le x\right) = P(M_n \le a_n + b_n x) = F(a_n + b_n x)^n \xrightarrow{\mathscr{L}} G(x)$$

for some distribution function G. The problem for min can be treated by looking at max for $-X_j$.

It turns out that there are three different classes of limiting G's.

Definition. A function c: $[0, \infty) \to \mathbb{R}$ is *slowly varying* if for every $x > 0$,

$$\frac{c(tx)}{c(t)} \to 1, \qquad \text{as } t \to \infty.$$

Any function $c(x)$ converging to a positive finite constant as $x \to \infty$ is slowly varying. But so also are some functions that tend to 0 or ∞ as $x \to \infty$, such as $c(x) = \log x$ or even $c(x) = (\log x)^\gamma$. Not slowly varying is $c(x) = x^\gamma$ for any $\gamma \ne 0$, since $(tx)^\gamma / t^\gamma \to x^\gamma$.

*(Ref: Book of that title by J. Galambos (1978) John Wiley & Sons).

THEOREM 14. *Let $F(x)$ denote the distribution function of a random variable X, and let x_0 denote the upper boundary, possibly $+\infty$, of the distribution of X: $x_0 = \sup\{x\colon F(x) < 1\}$.*

(a) *If $x_0 = \infty$, and $1 - F(x) = x^{-\gamma}c(x)$ for some $\gamma > 0$ and some slowly varying $c(x)$, then*

$$F(b_n x)^n \to G_{1,\gamma}(x) = \begin{cases} \exp\{-x^{-\gamma}\}, & \text{for } x > 0, \\ 0, & \text{for } x \le 0, \end{cases}$$

where b_n is such that $1 - F(b_n) = 1/n$.

(b) *If $x_0 < \infty$, and $1 - F(x) = (x_0 - x)^\gamma c(1/(x_0 - x))$ for some $\gamma > 0$ and some slowly varying $c(x)$, then*

$$F(x_0 + b_n x)^n \to G_{2,\gamma}(x) = \begin{cases} \exp\{-(-x)^\gamma\}, & \text{for } x < 0, \\ 1, & \text{for } x \ge 0, \end{cases}$$

where b_n is such that $1 - F(x_0 - b_n) = 1/n$.

(c) *If there exists a function $R(t)$ such that for all x,*

$$\frac{1 - F(t + xR(t))}{1 - F(t)} \to e^{-x}$$

as $t \to x_0$ (finite or $+\infty$), then

$$F(a_n + b_n x)^n \to G_3(x) = \exp\{-e^{-x}\},$$

where $1 - F(a_n) = 1/n$ and $b_n = R(a_n)$.

Note: Part (c) is considered the general case, and G_3 the extremal distribution. Moreover, $EX^+ < \infty$ in this case and $R(t)$ can be taken to be $R(t) = E(X - t|X > t)$. The three families of distributions may be related to the exponential distribution as follows. If $Y \in \mathscr{G}(1,1)$, then $G_{1,\gamma}$ is the distribution function of $Y^{-1/\gamma}$, $G_{2,\gamma}$ is the distribution function of $-Y^{1/\gamma}$, and G_3 is the distribution function of $-\log(Y)$.

EXAMPLE 1. The t_ν distributions have density

$$f(x) = \frac{c}{(\nu + x^2)^{(\nu+1)/2}} \sim cx^{-(\nu+1)}.$$

The symbol $\sim$ stands for asymptotically equivalent and means that the ratio of the two expressions tends to 1 (here, as $x \to \infty$). Thus, $1 - F(x) = x^{-\nu}c(x)$ for some function $c(x) \to c/\nu$. Hence, case (a) holds with

$\gamma = \nu$, and

$$1 - F(b_n) \sim \frac{c}{\nu b_n^{\nu}} = \frac{1}{n} \Rightarrow b_n = \left(\frac{cn}{\nu}\right)^{1/\nu}.$$

For the Cauchy distribution, $\nu = 1$ and $c = 1/\pi$ so that

$$\frac{\pi}{n} M_n \xrightarrow{\mathscr{L}} G_{1,1}.$$

Example 2. The $\mathscr{B}e(\alpha, \beta)$ distributions have density

$$f(x) = cx^{\alpha-1}(1-x)^{\beta-1} I(0 < x < 1),$$

where $c = \Gamma(\alpha+\beta)/(\Gamma(\alpha)\Gamma(\beta))$. So $x_0 = 1$, and as $x \nearrow 1$, $f(x) \sim c(1-x)^{\beta-1}$, and

$$1 - F(x) \sim c\int_x^1 (1-u)^{\beta-1}\, du = c(1-x)^{\beta}/\beta.$$

Hence, case (b) holds with $\gamma = \beta$ and $x_0 = 1$. The equation

$$1 - F(1 - b_n) = 1/n \text{ yields } b_n^{\beta} \sim \beta/(nc),$$

so we may take

$$b_n = \left(\frac{\Gamma(\alpha)\Gamma(\beta+1)}{n\Gamma(\alpha+\beta)}\right)^{1/\beta}.$$

For the $\mathscr{U}(0,1)$ distribution, $n(M_n - 1) \xrightarrow{\mathscr{L}} G_{2,1} = -\mathscr{G}(1,1)$.

Example 3. *The Exponential Distribution.* In case (c), note that

$$\frac{1 - F(t + xR(t))}{1 - F(t)} = P(X > t + xR(t) | X > t),$$

so that the condition that this converge to e^{-x} means that there is a change of scale, $R(t)$, so that this conditional distribution is approximately exponential with parameter 1. If $F(x)$ is this exponential distribution, then $P(X > t + x | X > t) = \exp\{-x\}$ exactly, so we have $R(t) = 1$ for all t and hence $b_n = 1$ for all n. Since $1 - F(x) = \exp\{-x\}$, we may solve for a_n:

$$\exp\{-a_n\} = 1/n \Rightarrow a_n = \log n; \text{ that is, } M_n - \log n \xrightarrow{\mathscr{L}} G_3.$$

Example 4. In case (c), x_0 can also be finite. For example, let $F(t) = 1 - \exp\{1/t\}$ for $t < 0$ (so $x_0 = 0$). Then

$$\frac{1 - F(t + xR(t))}{1 - F(t)} = \exp\left\{\frac{1}{t + xR(t)} - \frac{1}{t}\right\} = \exp\left\{-\frac{xR(t)}{(t + xR(t))t}\right\}.$$

We want to choose $R(t)$ so that $R(t)/((t + xR(t))t) \to 1$ as $t \nearrow 0$. Clearly $R(t) = t^2$ works. $1/n = 1 - F(a_n) = \exp\{1/a_n\} \Rightarrow a_n = -1/\log n$ and $b_n = (1/\log n)^2$. Hence, $(\log n)^2(M_n + 1/\log n) \xrightarrow{\mathcal{L}} G_3$.

***Proof of Theorem* 14**

(a) Note that $b_n \to \infty$, so that

$$\begin{aligned}
F(b_n x)^n &= \left(1 - (b_n x)^{-\gamma} c(b_n x)\right)^n \\
&\to \exp\left\{-\lim_{n\to\infty} n(b_n x)^{-\gamma} c(b_n x)\right\} \\
&= \exp\left\{-x^{-\gamma} \lim_{n\to\infty} n b_n^{-\gamma} c(b_n x)\right\} \\
&= \exp\left\{-x^{-\gamma} \lim_{n\to\infty} n b_n^{-\gamma} c(b_n)\right\}, \text{ because } c \text{ is slowly varying} \\
&= \exp\{-x^{-\gamma}\} \text{ from the definition of } b_n.
\end{aligned}$$

(b) For $x < 0$,

$$\begin{aligned}
F(x_0 + b_n x)^n &= \left(1 - (-b_n x)^{\gamma} c(1/(-b_n x))\right)^n \\
&\to \exp\left\{-\lim_{n\to\infty} n(-b_n x)^{\gamma} c(1/(-b_n x))\right\} \\
&= \exp\left\{-(-x)^{\gamma} \lim_{n\to\infty} n b_n^{\gamma} c(1/b_n)\right\} = \exp\{-(-x)^{\gamma}\}
\end{aligned}$$

(c)

$$\begin{aligned}
F(a_n + b_n x)^n &= (1 - (1 - F(a_n + b_n x)))^n \\
&\to \exp\left\{-\lim_{n\to\infty} n(1 - F(a_n + b_n x))\right\} \\
&= \exp\left\{-\lim_{n\to\infty} n(1 - F(a_n + R(a_n)x))\right\} \\
&= \exp\left\{-\lim_{n\to\infty} n \exp\{-x\}(1 - F(a_n))\right\} \\
&= \exp\{-\exp\{-x\}\}. \quad \blacksquare
\end{aligned}$$

Note: It is a remarkable fact that the converse to Theorem 14 is true: If for some normalizing sequences a_n and b_n, $(M_n - a_n)/b_n \xrightarrow{\mathscr{L}} G$ nondegenerate, then G, up to change of location and scale, is one of the types $G_{1,\gamma}$ for some $\gamma > 0$, $G_{2,\gamma}$ for some $\gamma > 0$, or G_3. Furthermore,

(a) G is of type $G_{1,\gamma} \Leftrightarrow x_0 = \infty$ and $F(x) = 1 - x^{-\gamma}c(x)$ for some slowly varying $c(x)$;

(b) G is of type $G_{2,\gamma} \Leftrightarrow x_0 < \infty$ and $F(x) = 1 - (x_0 - x)^\gamma c(1/(x_0 - x))$ for some slowly varying $c(x)$; and

(c) G is of type $G_3 \Leftrightarrow$ for all x,

$$\frac{1 - F(t + xR(t))}{1 - F(t)} \to \exp\{-x\}$$

as $t \to x_0$, for some function, $R(t)$.

This result goes back to Fisher. See the book of Galambos for details.

Example 5. $F(x) = 1 - 1/\log x$ for $x > e$. If there exists a limit, it cannot be of type $G_{2,\gamma}$, since $x_0 = \infty$. It cannot be of type G_3, since $EX^+ = EX = \infty$, and it cannot be of type $G_{1,\gamma}$, since $1 - F(x) = 1/\log x$ is slowly varying and we must have $1 - F(x) = x^\gamma c(x)$ with γ positive. Therefore, no normalization $(M_n - a_n)/b_n$ converges in law to a nondegenerate limit.

However, we can still say something about the asymptotic distribution of M_n. Let $Y = \log X$. Then $F_Y(y) = P(\log X \le y) = P(X \le e^y) = 1 - 1/y$, for $y > 1$. This is case (a) with $\gamma = 1$ and $b_n = n$. So $(1/n)\log M_n \xrightarrow{\mathscr{L}} G_{1,1}$.

Example 6. *The Normal Distribution.* We show that the standard normal distribution falls in case (c). Let

$$F(x) = \Phi(x) = \frac{1}{\sqrt{2\pi}} \int_{-\infty}^{x} \exp\left\{-\frac{u^2}{2}\right\} du,$$

denote the distribution function of $\mathscr{N}(0,1)$.

Lemma

$$\sqrt{2\pi}(1 - \Phi(x)) = \int_x^\infty \exp\{-u^2/2\}\, du \sim \frac{1}{x}\exp\{-x^2/2\} \text{ as } x \to \infty.$$

Proof. By L'Hospital's rule, $\int_x^\infty \exp\{-u^2/2\}\, du / x^{-1}\exp\{-x^2/2\}$ has the same limit as

$$\frac{-\exp\{-x^2/2\}}{-x^{-2}\exp\{-x^2/2\} - \exp\{-x^2/2\}} = \frac{x^2}{1 + x^2} \to 1. \quad \blacksquare$$

The lemma implies that

$$\frac{1-\Phi(t+xR(t))}{1-\Phi(t)} \sim \frac{\exp\{-(t+xR(t))^2/2\}}{t+xR(t)} \cdot \frac{t}{\exp\{-t^2/2\}}$$

$$= \frac{t}{(t+xR(t))}\exp\{-txR(t) - x^2R(t)^2/2\}.$$

This converges to e^{-x} if we let $R(t) = 1/t$. Thus we have case (c) with $b_n = 1/a_n$ and $1 - \Phi(a_n) = 1/n$, and conclude that $a_n(M_n - a_n) \xrightarrow{\mathscr{L}} G_3$.

Remark. To find an asymptotic expression for a_n in this example, write $1 - \Phi(a_n) = 1/n$, using the lemma, as

$$\frac{n}{\sqrt{2\pi}\,a_n}\exp\{-a_n^2/2\} \to 1.$$

To solve this asymptotically for a_n, we first approximate by solving $\exp\{-a_n^2/2\} = 1/n$ to get $a_n = \sqrt{2\log n}$. Then we replace a_n by $\sqrt{2\log n} - a'_n$, and solve for a'_n

$$\frac{n}{\sqrt{2\pi}\,a_n}\exp\{-a_n^2/2\} = \frac{n}{\sqrt{2\pi}}\frac{\exp\{-(\log n - a'_n\sqrt{2\log n} + a_n'^2/2)\}}{\sqrt{2\log n} - a'_n}$$

$$= \frac{1}{\sqrt{2\pi}}\frac{\exp\{a'_n\sqrt{2\log n} - a_n'^2/2\}}{\sqrt{2\log n} - a'_n}.$$

If this converges to 1, then $a'_n \to 0$ in which case we may ignore the a'_n in the denominator and the $a_n'^2/2$ in the exponent. Solving

$$\exp\{a'_n\sqrt{2\log n}\} = \sqrt{2\pi 2\log n}$$

gives

$$a'_n = \left(1/\sqrt{2\log n}\right)\log\sqrt{4\pi\log n},$$

so

$$a_n = \sqrt{2\log n} - (\log\log n + \log 4\pi)/2\sqrt{2\log n}.$$

Since $b_n = 1/a_n \sim 1/\sqrt{2\log n}$, we can replace b_n (but not a_n) by this simpler form, and reduce $(M_n - a_n)/b_n$ to

$$\sqrt{2\log n}\,M_n - 2\log n + (1/2)\log\log n + 1/2\log 4\pi \xrightarrow{\mathscr{L}} G_3.$$

EXERCISES

1. For the following distributions, find the normalization such that $(M_n - a_n)/b_n$ has a nondegenerate limit if any exists.
   (a) $f(x) = e^x I\ (x < 0)$.
   (b) $f(x) = (2/x^3) I\ (x > 1)$.
   (c) $F(x) = 1 - \exp\{-x/(1-x)\}$, for $0 < x < 1$.
   (d) $f(x) = (1/\Gamma(\alpha))e^{-x}x^{\alpha-1}I(x > 0)$, the $\mathscr{G}(\alpha, 1)$ distribution. [First prove $1 - F(x) \sim (1/\Gamma(\alpha))e^{-x}x^{\alpha-1}$.]
2. Let $X_1, \ldots, X_n$ be i.i.d. with a geometric distribution with probability $\frac{1}{2}$, $P(X = j) = 1/2^{j+1}$ for $j = 0, 1, 2, \ldots$. Show that the distribution of M_n converges to a discretized version of the general case, G_3, in the following sense. Let $m(n) = \lfloor \log_2(n) \rfloor$ (the floor of $\log_2(n)$) and suppose that $n \to \infty$ along a subsequence, $n(m)$ for $m = 1, 2, \ldots,$ such that $n(m)/2^m \to \theta$ as $m \to \infty$, with $1 \leq \theta < 2$; then,
$$P(M_{n(m)} - m < j) \to \exp\{-\theta 2^{-j}\}, \qquad \text{for } j = 0, \pm 1, \pm 2, \ldots.$$
3. Let M_n denote the maximum of a sample of size n from the distribution G_3. Does there exist a normalization, $(M_n - a_n)/b_n$, with a nondegenerate limit? If so, find it.

15

Asymptotic Joint Distributions of Extrema

The following theorem is useful for finding the asymptotic distribution of the range of a sample or of the gap between the largest and next largest value of a sample.

Theorem 15. *Let $U_{(n:1)}, \ldots, U_{(n:n)}$ be order statistics of a sample of size n from $\mathscr{U}(0,1)$. Then for fixed k,*

(a)
$$n\big(U_{(n:1)}, \ldots, U_{(n:k)}\big) \xrightarrow{\mathscr{L}} (S_1, \ldots, S_k)$$

where $S_j = \Sigma_{i=1}^{j} Y_i$ and the Y_i are i.i.d. exponential, $\mathscr{G}(1,1)$.

(b) *For fixed values of $0 < p_1 < \cdots < p_n < 1$, the three vectors*

$$n\big(U_{(n:1)}, \ldots, U_{(n:k)}\big),$$

$$\sqrt{n}\,\big(U_{(n:np_1)} - p_1, \ldots, U_{(n:np_k)} - p_k\big),$$

and

$$n\big(1 - U_{(n:n)}, \ldots, 1 - U_{(n:n-k+1)}\big)$$

are asymptotically independent, with distributions of the first and third vectors as in (a), *and of the second as in Theorem* 13.

Proof. (a) Let $\mathbf{U}_{n,k} = (U_{(n:1)}, \ldots, U_{(n:k)})^T$. We show the densities of $\mathbf{U}_{n,k}$ converge and conclude the result by Scheffé's Theorem:

$$f_{\mathbf{u}_{n,k}}(\mathbf{u}) = n(n-1)\cdots(n-k+1)(1-u_k)^{n-k} \times I(0 < u_1 < \cdots < u_k < 1).$$

Let $\mathbf{S} = n\mathbf{U}_{n,k}$. Then

$$f_{\mathbf{S}}(\mathbf{s}) = \frac{n(n-1)\cdots(n-k+1)}{n^k} \times \left(1 - \frac{s_k}{n}\right)^{n-k} I(0 < s_1 < \cdots < s_k < n)$$
$$\to \exp\{-s_k\} I(0 < s_1 < \cdots < s_k < \infty),$$

which is the density of the distribution described in the theorem.

(b) Omitted.

Note: The limiting distribution of $nU_{(n:k)}$, being the sum of k independent $\mathscr{G}(1,1)$, is $\mathscr{G}(k,1)$.

Note: Part (b) of Theorem 15 holds in general (for distributions other than uniform); the lower extreme order statistics, the upper extreme order statistics, and the quantiles are asymptotically independent.

EXAMPLE 1. *The Range.* Let $R_n = U_{(n:n)} - U_{(n:1)}$ denote the range of a sample of size n from a uniform distribution, $\mathscr{U}(0,1)$. Then $n(1 - R_n) = n(1 - U_{(n:n)}) + nU_{(n:1)} \xrightarrow{\mathscr{L}} Y_1 + Y_2$, where Y_1 and Y_2 are independent $\mathscr{G}(1,1)$. Thus, $n(1 - R_n) \xrightarrow{\mathscr{L}} \mathscr{G}(2,1)$.

EXAMPLE 2. *The Midrange.* Let $M_n = \frac{1}{2}(U_{(n:1)} + U_{(n:n)})$ denote the midrange. Then

$$n\left(M_n - \tfrac{1}{2}\right) = \tfrac{1}{2}\left(nU_{(n:1)} - n(1 - U_{(n:n)})\right) \xrightarrow{\mathscr{L}} \tfrac{1}{2}(Y_1 - Y_2),$$

where Y_1 and Y_2 are as in Example 1. This has the Laplace (double exponential) distribution with density $f(z) = e^{-2|z|}$.

REMARK. If $X_{(n:1)}, \ldots, X_{(n:n)}$ are the order statistics of a sample of size n from an arbitrary continuous distribution $F(x)$, then $n(F(X_{(n:1)}), \ldots, F(X_{(n:k)})) \xrightarrow{\mathscr{L}} (S_1, \ldots, S_k)$ of part (a). Sometimes, the method of transformation of Slutsky's Theorem applied to some form of the inverse function $F^{-1}(s)$ will work to give the asymptotic distribution of $(X_{(n:1)}, \ldots, X_{(n:k)})$, as in the Example 3, below. Such considerations lead to a generalization of Theorem 14. The limiting distribution of $(X_{(n:1)}, \ldots, X_{(n:k)})$ properly normalized is as $(-S_1^{-1/\gamma}, \ldots, -S_k^{-1/\gamma})$ for case (a), as $(S_1^{1/\gamma}, \ldots, S_k^{1/\gamma})$ for case (b), and as $(\log S_1, \ldots, \log S_k)$ for case (c).

Example 3. Let $Z_{1,n}$ be the largest, and $Z_{2,n}$ the second largest, of a sample of size n from a Cauchy distribution, $\mathscr{C}(0,1)$. To find the large sample joint distribution of $Z_{1,N}$ and $Z_{2,n}$, we first note that $n((1 - F(Z_{1,n})), (1 - F(Z_{2,n}))) \xrightarrow{\mathscr{L}} (S_1, S_2)$, where S_1 and S_2 are as described in Theorem 15, and F is the distribution function of $\mathscr{C}(0,1)$. Then, since

$$1 - F(x) = \frac{1}{\pi}\int_x^\infty \frac{1}{1+t^2}\,dt \sim \frac{1}{\pi x}, \qquad \text{as } x \to \infty,$$

we conclude that $n((1 - F(Z_{1,n})), (1 - F(Z_{2,n})))$, and

$$\frac{n}{\pi}\left(\frac{1}{Z_{1,n}}, \frac{1}{Z_{2,n}}\right)$$

are asymptotically equivalent, and so have the same limiting distribution, namely, that of (S_1, S_2). Finally, an application of Slutsky's Theorem using the reciprocal transformation shows that

$$\frac{\pi}{n}(Z_{1,n}, Z_{2,n}) \xrightarrow{\mathscr{L}} \left(\frac{1}{S_1}, \frac{1}{S_2}\right).$$

From this, we may deduce an interesting property for the top two record values of a sample from a Cauchy distribution, namely, that the ratio $R_n = Z_{2,n}/Z_{1,n}$, of the second largest to the largest observation converges in law to S_1/S_2, which has a uniform distribution, $\mathscr{U}(0,1)$. Moreover, R_n and $Z_{2,n}/n$ are asymptotically independent (since S_1/S_2 and S_2 are independent).

EXERCISES

1. Let $X_{(n:1)}, \ldots, X_{(n:n)}$ be order statistics of a sample of size n from $\mathscr{N}(\mu, 1)$. Find the proper location and scale normalization (using Example 6 of Section 13) of the midrange such that the limit distribution exists, and find the limit (logistic). What is its asymptotic efficiency relative to $\overline{X}_n$?

2. Let $Z_{1,n}$ and $Z_{2,n}$ be the largest and second-largest record values (order statistics), respectively, of a sample of size n from the exponential distribution, $\mathscr{G}(1,1)$. (a) Find the density of the limiting joint distribution of $Z_{1,n}$ and $Z_{2,n}$, properly normalized, as $n \to \infty$. (b) Note that (asymptotically) $Z_{1,n} - Z_{2,n}$ and $Z_{2,n}$ are independent, and that $Z_{1,n} - Z_{2,n}$ has an exponential distribution.
3. Let $X_1, \ldots, X_n$ be a sample from a uniform distribution on the interval $(\theta - 0.5, \theta + 0.5)$. Among the various estimates of θ, one may use the median, $\hat{\theta}_1 = X_{([n/2])}$, and one may use the midrange, $\hat{\theta}_2 = (\max(X_i) + \min(X_i))/2$. Compare the 95% confidence intervals for θ obtained from these two estimates, when $n = 100$.
4. Let $Z_{1,n}$ and $Z_{2,n}$ be the largest and second-largest order statistics from a sample of size n from the normal distribution, $\mathscr{N}(0,1)$, and let a_n be defined by $1 - \Phi(a_n) = 1/n$. Show that

$$a_n(Z_{1n} - a_n, Z_{2n} - a_n) \xrightarrow{\mathscr{L}} (-\log S_1, -\log S_2),$$

where S_1 and S_2 are defined as in Theorem 15. Conclude that $U_n = \exp\{a_n(Z_{2n} - Z_{1n})\}$ has asymptotically a $\mathscr{U}(0,1)$ distribution, and that U_n and $a_n(Z_{2n} - a_n)$ are asymptotically independent.

4

Efficient Estimation and Testing

16

A Uniform Strong Law of Large Numbers

Certain important statistical problems have the following form. Let $X_1, X_2, \ldots$ be a sequence of i.i.d. random variables with common distribution function $F(x)$, and let $U(x, \theta)$ be a measurable function of x for all θ in some parameter space Θ. The statistic of interest for purposes of estimation or testing hypotheses is $(1/n)\sum_{i=1}^{n} U(X_i, \theta)$. If it is assumed that

$$\mu(\theta) = EU(X, \theta) = \int U(x, \theta)\, dF(x) \tag{1}$$

exists and is finite for all $\theta \in \Theta$, then by the Strong Law of Large Numbers

$$\frac{1}{n}\sum_{1}^{n} U(X_j, \theta) \xrightarrow{\text{a.s.}} \mu(\theta), \qquad \text{as } n \to \infty \tag{2}$$

for each $\theta \in \Theta$. It is important to strengthen this conclusion so that the convergence is uniform in θ in the sense that

$$\sup_{\theta \in \Theta} \left| \frac{1}{n}\sum_{1}^{n} U(X_j, \theta) - \mu(\theta) \right| \xrightarrow{\text{a.s.}} 0, \qquad \text{as } n \to \infty. \tag{3}$$

As an example of the use of (3), suppose we have a sequence $\hat{\theta}_n$ of estimates of θ (possibly dependent on $X_1, \ldots, X_n$) such that $\hat{\theta}_n \xrightarrow{\text{a.s.}} \theta_0$ as

$n \to \infty$, where θ_0 can be considered the true value. Suppose also that $\mu(\theta)$ is continuous in θ. We would like to conclude that

$$\frac{1}{n}\sum_1^n U(X_j, \hat{\theta}_n) \xrightarrow{\text{a.s.}} \mu(\theta_0), \qquad \text{as } n \to \infty. \tag{4}$$

By itself, (2) is not strong enough to give this result. However, (4) follows easily from (3):

$$\begin{aligned}
&\left|\frac{1}{n}\sum_1^n U(X_j, \hat{\theta}_n) - \mu(\theta_0)\right| \\
&\quad \le \left|\frac{1}{n}\sum_1^n U(X_j, \hat{\theta}_n) - \mu(\hat{\theta}_n)\right| + \left|\mu(\hat{\theta}_n) - \mu(\theta_0)\right| \\
&\quad \le \sup_{\theta\in\Theta}\left|\frac{1}{n}\sum_1^n U(X_j, \theta) - \mu(\theta)\right| + \left|\mu(\hat{\theta}_n) - \mu(\theta_0)\right| \\
&\quad \xrightarrow{\text{a.s.}} 0, \qquad \text{as } n \to \infty,
\end{aligned} \tag{5}$$

using $\hat{\theta}_n \xrightarrow{\text{a.s.}} \theta_0$, continuity of $\mu(\theta)$ and Slutsky's Theorem.

The theorems below, due to Le Cam, give conditions on U and the distribution F under which (3) holds. If Θ were finite, then (3) follows directly from (2), because the intersection of a finite number of sets of probability 1 has probability 1. So one expects (3) to hold also if Θ is compact and $U(x, \theta)$ is continuous in θ for all x. Under a uniform boundedness condition, this is so.

Theorem 16(a). *If*

(1) Θ *is compact,*
(2) $U(x, \theta)$ *is continuous in* θ *for all* x,
(3) *There exists a function* $K(x)$ *such that* $EK(X) < \infty$ *and* $|U(x, \theta)| \le K(x)$, *for all* x *and* θ.

Then

$$P\left\{\lim_{n\to\infty}\sup_{\theta\in\Theta}\left|\frac{1}{n}\sum_1^n U(X_j, \theta) - \mu(\theta)\right| = 0\right\} = 1.$$

We also prove a one-sided version of this theorem for use in the next section. A real-valued function, $f(\theta)$, defined on Θ is said to be *upper semicontinuous* (u.s.c.) on Θ, if for all θ in Θ and for any sequence θ_n in Θ such that $\theta_n \to \theta$, we have $\limsup_{n\to\infty} f(\theta_n) \le f(\theta)$ or, equivalently, if for all θ in Θ, $\sup_{|\theta'-\theta|<\rho} f(\theta') \to f(\theta)$ as $\rho \to 0$.

Theorem 16(b). *If*

(1) Θ *is compact,*
(2) $U(x, \theta)$ *is upper semicontinuous in* θ *for all* x,
(3) *there exists a function* $K(x)$ *such that* $EK(X) < \infty$ *and* $U(x, \theta) \le K(x)$ *for all* x *and* θ,
(4) *for all* θ *and for all sufficiently small* $\rho > 0$, $\sup_{|\theta' - \theta| < \rho} U(x, \theta')$ *is measurable in* x,

Then

$$P\left\{ \limsup_{n \to \infty} \sup_{\theta \in \Theta} \frac{1}{n} \sum_1^n U(X_j, \theta) \le \sup_{\theta \in \Theta} \mu(\theta) \right\} = 1.$$

Proof of part (b). Let

$$\varphi(x, \theta, \rho) = \sup_{|\theta' - \theta| < \rho} U(x, \theta').$$

Then φ is measurable in x for all sufficiently small $\rho > 0$ by (4), φ is bounded above by an integrable function by (3), and $\varphi(x, \theta, \rho) \searrow U(x, \theta)$ as $\rho \searrow 0$ by (2).

Therefore, by the Monotone Convergence Theorem, as $\rho \searrow 0$.

$$\int \varphi(x, \theta, \rho)\, dF(x) \searrow \int U(x, \theta)\, dF(x) = \mu(\theta)$$

Let $\varepsilon > 0$. For each θ, find ρ_θ so that $\int \varphi(x, \theta, \rho_\theta)\, dF(x) < \mu(\theta) + \varepsilon$. The spheres $S(\theta, \rho_\theta) = \{\theta' \colon |\theta - \theta'| < \rho_\theta\}$ cover Θ so by (1) there exists a finite subcover, say, $\Theta \subset \bigcup_1^m S(\theta_j, \rho_{\theta_j})$. For each $\theta \in \Theta$ there exists an index j such that $\theta \in S(\theta_j, \rho_{\theta_j})$. From the definition of φ, $U(x, \theta) \le \varphi(x, \theta_j, \rho_{\theta_j})$ for all x. Hence,

$$\frac{1}{n} \sum_1^n U(X_j, \theta) \le \frac{1}{n} \sum_1^n \varphi(X_j, \theta_j, \rho_{\theta_j}),$$

so that

$$\sup_{\theta \in \Theta} \frac{1}{n} \sum_1^n U(X_j, \theta) \le \sup_{1 \le j \le m} \frac{1}{n} \sum_1^n \varphi(X_j, \theta_j, \rho_{\theta_j}).$$

Now apply the strong law of large numbers to $(1/n)\Sigma_1^n \varphi(X_j, \theta_j, \rho_{\theta_j})$:

$$P\left\{\lim_{n\to\infty} \frac{1}{n}\sum_1^n \varphi(X_j, \theta_j, \rho_{\theta_j}) \le \mu(\theta_j) + \varepsilon, \text{ for } j = 1, 2, \ldots, m\right\} = 1,$$

$$P\left\{\limsup_{n\to\infty} \sup_{1\le j\le m} \frac{1}{n}\sum_1^n \varphi(X_j, \theta_j, \rho_{\theta_j}) \le \sup_{1\le j\le m} \mu(\theta_j) + \varepsilon\right\} = 1,$$

$$P\left\{\limsup_{n\to\infty} \sup_{\theta\in\Theta} \frac{1}{n}\sum_1^n U(X_j, \theta) \le \sup_{\theta\in\Theta} \mu(\theta) + \varepsilon\right\} = 1.$$

Because it is true for all $\varepsilon > 0$, it is true for $\varepsilon = 0$. ■

Proof of (a). First note that, $U(x, \theta)$ being continuous in θ, condition (4) of part (b) is automatically satisfied because

$$\sup_{|\theta'-\theta|<\rho} U(x, \theta') = \sup_{\theta'\in D} U(x, \theta')$$

for any denumerable set D, dense in $\{\theta': |\theta' - \theta| < \rho\}$.

Next note that $\mu(\theta)$ is continuous:

$$\lim_{\theta'\to\theta} \mu(\theta') = \lim_{\theta'\to\theta} \int U(x, \theta')\, dF(x) = \int U(x, \theta)\, dF(x) = \mu(\theta)$$

by the Lebesgue Dominated Convergence Theorem, since U is bounded by K, an integrable function. Therefore, if Theorem 16(a) were true for $\mu(\theta) = 0$, it would follow for arbitrary $\mu(\theta)$ by considering $U(x, \theta) - \mu(\theta)$, continuous in θ and bounded by $K(x) + EK(X)$. Thus, we assume $\mu(\theta) = 0$. From the one-sided theorem applied to $U(x, \theta)$ and $-U(x, \theta)$,

$$P\left\{\limsup_{n\to\infty} \sup_{\theta\in\Theta} \frac{1}{n}\sum_1^n U(X_j, \theta) \le 0\right\} = 1$$

and

$$P\left\{\limsup_{n\to\infty} \sup_{\theta\in\Theta} -\frac{1}{n}\sum_1^n U(X_j, \theta) \le 0\right\} = 1.$$

The conclusion follows from this because for an arbitrary function g,

$$0 \le \sup_\theta |g(\theta)| = \max\left\{\sup_\theta g(\theta), \sup_\theta -g(\theta)\right\}. \quad ■$$

Remark. We note for use in the next section that under the conditions of Theorem 16(b) the function $\mu(\theta)$ is upper semicontinuous (i.e., for every $\theta \in \Theta$, $\limsup_{\theta' \to \theta} \mu(\theta') \le \mu(\theta)$). The proof is analogous to the proof of continuity of $\mu(\theta)$ for Theorem 16(a), namely,

$$\begin{aligned}\limsup_{\theta' \to \theta} \mu(\theta') &= \limsup_{\theta' \to \theta} EU(X, \theta') \\ &\le E \limsup_{\theta' \to \theta} U(X, \theta') \le EU(X, \theta) = \mu(\theta)\end{aligned}$$

using the Fatou–Lebesgue Theorem (the one-sided dominated convergence theorem) since $U(x, \theta)$ is bounded above by an integrable function, $K(x)$.

17

Strong Consistency of Maximum-Likelihood Estimates

A sequence of estimates $\{\tilde{\theta}_n\}$ of a parameter $\theta \in \Theta$ is said to be *weakly consistent* (resp. *strongly consistent*) *for* $\theta \in \Theta$ if for every $\theta \in \Theta$, $\tilde{\theta}_n \xrightarrow{\text{P}} \theta$ (resp. $\tilde{\theta}_n \xrightarrow{\text{a.s.}} \theta$) when θ is the true value of the parameter. In this section, we show that under fairly general conditions, the maximum-likelihood estimates are strongly consistent as the sample size tends to infinity.

Let $X_1, \ldots, X_n$ be i.i.d. with density $f(x|\theta)$ with respect to some σ-finite measure ν (usually Lebesgue measure or counting measure), where $\theta \in \Theta$.

The likelihood function is defined as

$$L_n(\theta) = \mathbf{L}_n(\theta|x_1, \ldots, x_n) = \prod_1^n f(x_j|\theta)$$

when the observed values of $X_1, \ldots, X_n$ are $x_1, \ldots, x_n$. The *log likelihood function* is denoted by $l_n(\theta) = \log L_n(\theta)$.

A *maximum-likelihood estimate* (MLE) of θ is any function, $\hat{\theta}_n = \hat{\theta}_n(x_1, \ldots, x_n)$, such that $L_n(\hat{\theta}_n) = \sup_{\theta \in \Theta} L_n(\theta)$ or, equivalently, $l_n(\hat{\theta}_n) = \sup_{\theta \in \Theta} l_n(\theta)$. A MLE may not exist. When it does, it may not be measurable and it may be consistent. It certainly exists if Θ is compact and $f(x|\theta)$ is upper semicontinuous in θ for all x, since then $L_n(\theta)$ is upper semicontinuous on a compact set, and an upper semicontinuous function on a compact set achieves its maximum.

The proof of consistency of the MLE is based on the following lemma. Let $f_0(x)$ and $f_1(x)$ be densities with respect to a σ-finite measure ν. The

Kullback–Leibler information number is defined as

$$K(f_0, f_1) = E_0 \log \frac{f_0(X)}{f_1(X)} = \int \log \frac{f_0(x)}{f_1(x)} f_0(x)\, d\nu(x).$$

In this expression, $\log(f_0(x)/f_1(x))$ is defined as $+\infty$ if $f_1(x) = 0$ and $f_0(x) > 0$, so the expectation could be $+\infty$. Although $\log(f_0(x)/f_1(x))$ is defined as $-\infty$ when $f_1(x) > 0$ and $f_0(x) = 0$, the integrand, $\log(f_0(x)/f_1(x)) f_0(x)$, is defined as zero in this case. $K(f_0, f_1)$ is a measure of the ability of the likelihood ratio to distinguish between f_0 and f_1 when f_0 is true.

Lemma (Shannon–Kolmogorov Information Inequality). *Let $f_0(x)$ and $f_1(x)$ be densities with respect to ν. Then*

$$K(f_0, f_1) = E_0 \log \frac{f_0(X)}{f_1(X)} = \int \log \frac{f_0(x)}{f_1(x)} f_0(x)\, d\nu(x) \geq 0,$$

with equality if and only if $f_1(x) = f_0(x)$ (a.e. $d\nu$).

Proof. Since $\log x$ is strictly convex, Jensen's inequality implies

$$-K(f_0, f_1) = E_0 \log \frac{f_1(X)}{f_0(X)} \leq \log E_0 \frac{f_1(X)}{f_0(X)},$$

with equality if and only if $f_1(X)/f_0(X)$ is a constant with probability 1 when X has density f_0. But

$$E_0 \frac{f_1(X)}{f_0(X)} = \int \frac{f_1(x)}{f_0(x)} f_0(x)\, d\nu(x) = \int_{S_0} f_1(x)\, d\nu(x) \leq 1,$$

where $S_0 = \{x\colon f_0(x) > 0\}$, with equality if and only if S_0 has probability 1 under $f_1(x)$. The combination of these two inequalities gives the result. ∎

This lemma is used in the proof of consistency of the MLE as follows. Let θ_0 denote the true value of θ. The MLE is the value of θ that maximizes

$$l_n(\theta) - l_n(\theta_0) = \log L_n(\theta) - \log L_n(\theta_0)$$
$$= \sum_1^n \bigl(\log f(X_j|\theta) - \log f(X_j|\theta_0)\bigr).$$

From the Strong Law of Large Numbers and the lemma,

$$\frac{1}{n}\log\frac{L_n(\theta)}{L_n(\theta_0)} = \frac{1}{n}\sum_1^n \log\frac{f(X_j|\theta)}{f(X_j|\theta_0)} \xrightarrow{\text{a.s.}} E_{\theta_0}\log\frac{f(X|\theta)}{f(X|\theta_0)} = -K(\theta_0,\theta) < 0,$$

unless $f(x|\theta) = f(x|\theta_0)$. So eventually the likelihood function will be larger at θ_0 than at any specific value θ provided different θ correspond to different distributions (the condition of identifiability). This gives a meaning to the numerical value of the Kullback–Leibler information number. When θ_0 is the true value, the likelihood ratio, $L_n(\theta)/L_n(\theta_0)$, converges to zero exponentially fast, at rate $\exp\{-nK(\theta_0,\theta)\}$.

This already implies that if Θ is finite the MLE is strongly consistent. In the following theorem, this observation is extended to compact Θ when $f(x|\theta)$ is upper semicontinuous in θ.

Theorem 17. *Let $X_1, X_2, \ldots$ be i.i.d. with density $f(x|\theta)$, $\theta \in \Theta$, and let θ_0 denote the true value of θ. If*

(1) *Θ is compact,*
(2) *$f(x|\theta)$ is upper semicontinuous in θ for all x,*
(3) *there exists a function $K(x)$ such that $E_{\theta_0}|K(X)| < \infty$ and*

$$U(x,\theta) = \log f(x|\theta) - \log f(x|\theta_0) \le K(x), \qquad \text{for all } x \text{ and } \theta,$$

(4) *for all $\theta \in \Theta$ and sufficiently small $\rho > 0$, $\sup_{|\theta'-\theta|<\rho} f(x|\theta')$ is measurable in x,*
(5) *(identifiability) $f(x|\theta) = f(x|\theta_0)$ (a.e. $d\nu$) $\Rightarrow \theta = \theta_0$,*

then, for any sequence of maximum-likelihood estimates $\hat{\theta}_n$ of θ,

$$\hat{\theta}_n \xrightarrow{\text{a.s.}} \theta_0.$$

Proof. The conditions of Theorem 16(b) are satisfied for the function $U(x,\theta)$. Let $\rho > 0$ and $S = \{\theta\colon |\theta - \theta_0| \ge \rho\}$. Then S is compact and from Theorem 16(b),

$$P_{\theta_0}\left\{\limsup_{n\to\infty}\sup_{\theta\in S}\frac{1}{n}\sum_1^n U(X_j,\theta) \le \sup_{\theta\in S}\mu(\theta)\right\} = 1,$$

where $\mu(\theta) = -K(\theta_0, \theta) = \int U(x, \theta) f(x|\theta_0))\, d\nu(x) < 0$ for $\theta \in S$ from the lemma. Furthermore, $\mu(\theta)$ is upper semicontinuous (Section 16) and hence achieves it is maximum value on S. Let $\delta = \sup_{\theta \in S} \mu(\theta)$; then $\delta < 0$, and

$$P_{\theta_0}\left\{ \limsup_{n \to \infty} \sup_{\theta \in S} \frac{1}{n} \sum_1^n U(X_j, \theta) \leq \delta \right\} = 1.$$

Thus, with probability 1, there exists an N such that for all $n > N$,

$$\sup_{\theta \in S} \frac{1}{n} \sum_1^n U(X_j, \theta) \leq \delta/2 < 0,$$

say. But

$$\frac{1}{n} \sum_1^n U\left(X_j, \hat{\theta}_n\right) = \sup_{\theta \in \Theta} \frac{1}{n} \sum_1^n U(X_j, \theta) \geq 0,$$

since the sum is equal to 0 for $\theta = \theta_0$. This implies that $\hat{\theta}_n \notin S$ for $n > N$; that is, $|\hat{\theta}_n - \theta| < \rho$. Since ρ is arbitrary, the theorem follows. This proof is due to Wald (1948). ■

Note: Allowing $f(x|\theta)$ to be upper semicontinuous in θ (rather than requiring continuity) covers cases like the uniform, $U(\theta, \theta + 1)$. In such a case, the density is chosen to be the upper semicontinuous version, $f(x|\theta) = I(\theta \leq x \leq \theta + 1)$. We note that if $f(x|\theta)$ is continuous in θ, then condition (4) is automatically satisfied.

Note: Nothing in the theorem requires $\hat{\theta}_n$ to be measurable. In this theorem, MLEs are strongly consistent even if they are not random variables! (Here, convergence almost surely does not imply convergence in probability.) In general, $\hat{\theta}_n$ can be chosen to be measurable according to the following result which follows from a selection theorem of von Neumann (1949). (See for example Parathasarathy (1972), Section 8.) *If $\mathscr{X}$ is a Borel subset of a Euclidean space, and if Θ is a compact subset of a Euclidean space, and if $\varphi(x, \theta)$ is jointly measurable in (x, θ) and upper semicontinuous in θ for each $x \in \mathscr{X}$, then there exists a Lebesgue measurable selection $\hat{\theta}(x)$ such that*

$$\varphi\left(x, \hat{\theta}\ (x)\right) = \sup_{\theta \in \Theta} \varphi(x, \theta), \qquad \text{for all } x.$$

Counterexample to the removal of condition (3). Consider the following densities on $[-1, 1]$ with parameter space $\Theta = [0, 1]$,

$$f(x|\theta) = (1-\theta)\frac{1}{\delta(\theta)}\left(1 - \frac{|x-\theta|}{\delta(\theta)}\right)I(|x-\theta| \le \delta(\theta)) + \theta\frac{1}{2}I(|x| \le 1),$$

where $\delta(\theta)$ is continuous decreasing with $\delta(0) = 1$ and $0 < \delta(\theta) < 1 - \theta$. This provides a continuous parametrization between the triangular distribution when $\theta = 0$, and the uniform distribution, when $\theta = 1$.

Clearly, conditions (1), (2), (4), and (5) of Theorem 17 are satisfied. We show that if $\delta(\theta) \to 0$ sufficiently fast as $\theta \to 1$, then $\hat{\theta}_n \xrightarrow{\text{a.s.}} 1$ whatever be the true value of $\theta \in \Theta$.

Given a sample $X_1, \ldots, X_n$ from f, $\hat{\theta}_n$ is that value of θ that maximizes

$$\begin{aligned} l_n(\theta) &= \sum_1^n \log f(x_j|\theta) \\ &= n_\theta \log\frac{\theta}{2} + \sum_{|x_i-\theta|<\delta(\theta)} \log\left[\frac{1-\theta}{\delta(\theta)}\left(1 - \frac{|x_i-\theta|}{\delta(\theta)}\right) + \frac{\theta}{2}\right], \end{aligned}$$

where n_θ is the number of X_i not in $\{x\colon |x-\theta| < \delta(\theta)\}$. For every fixed number $\alpha < 1$,

$$\max_{0\le\theta\le\alpha} \frac{1}{n} l_n(\theta) \le \max_{0\le\theta\le\alpha} \log\left[\frac{1-\theta}{\delta(\theta)} + \frac{\theta}{2}\right] \le \log\left[\frac{1}{\delta(\alpha)} + \frac{1}{2}\right].$$

We will show that $\hat{\theta}_n \xrightarrow{\text{a.s.}} 1$ whatever be the true value of θ if $\delta(\theta) \to 0$ sufficiently fast as $\theta \to 1$ by showing

$$\max_{0\le\theta\le 1} \frac{1}{n} l_n(\theta) \xrightarrow{\text{a.s.}} \infty.$$

Let $M_n = \max\{X_1, \ldots, X_n\}$. Then $M_n \xrightarrow{\text{a.s.}} 1$ whatever be the true value of θ, and

$$\max_{0\le\theta\le 1} \frac{1}{n} l_n(\theta) \ge \frac{1}{n} l_n(M_n) \ge \frac{n-1}{n} \log\frac{M_n}{2} + \frac{1}{n}\log\left[\frac{1-M_n}{\delta(M_n)} + \frac{M_n}{2}\right].$$

Therefore,

$$\liminf_{n\to\infty} \max_{0\le\theta\le 1} \frac{1}{n} l_n(\theta) \ge \liminf_{n\to\infty} \frac{1}{n} \log \frac{1-M_n}{\delta(M_n)} - \log 2.$$

Whatever be the value of θ, M_n converges a.s. to 1 at a certain rate the slowest rate being for the triangular distribution ($\theta = 0$). Thus we can choose $\delta(\theta) \to 0$ sufficiently fast as $\theta \to 1$, so that $(1/n)\log((1 - M_n)/\delta(M_n)) \xrightarrow[S]{\text{a.s.}} \infty$. ■

How fast? First note that $(n)^{1/4}(1 - M_n) \xrightarrow{\text{a.s.}} 0$, because for $\theta = 0$,

$$\begin{aligned}
&\sum P_0\left(n^{1/4}(1 - M_n) > \varepsilon\right) \\
&\quad = \sum P_0\left(M_n < 1 - \varepsilon/n^{1/4}\right) = \sum \left(1 - \varepsilon^2/(2\sqrt{n}\,)\right)^n \\
&\quad \le \sum \left(\exp\{-\varepsilon^2/(2\sqrt{n}\,)\}\right)^n = \sum \exp\{\varepsilon^2\sqrt{n}\,/2\} < \infty,
\end{aligned}$$

and the Borel–Cantelli Lemma implies $P_0\{n^{1/4}(1 - M_n) > \varepsilon \text{ i.o.}\} = 0$. Then, for

$$\delta(\theta) = (1-\theta)\exp\left\{-(1-\theta)^{-4}\right\},$$

we find

$$\frac{1}{n}\log\frac{1-M_n}{\delta(M_n)} = \frac{1}{n}\log\exp\left\{(1-M_n)^{-4}\right\} = \frac{1}{n(1-M_n)^4} \xrightarrow{\text{a.s.}} \infty.$$

EXERCISES

1. Check the conditions of Theorem 17 for the $\mathscr{U}(0, \theta)$ distribution, $f(x|\theta) = (1/\theta)I_{[0,\theta]}(x)$, when $\Theta = [1, 2]$.
2. [Oliver, (1972)] Let $X_1, \ldots, X_n$ be a sample from the triangular distribution on [0, 1] with mode θ,

$$f(x|\theta) = 2\left(\frac{x}{\theta}I_{[0,\theta]}(x) + \frac{1-x}{1-\theta}I_{[\theta,1]}(x)\right),$$

   and let $X_{(0)} = 0, X_{(1)}, \ldots, X_{(n)}, X_{(n+1)} = 1$ denote the order statistics.
   (a) Show that for $X_{(k)} \le \theta \le X_{(k+1)}$ the likelihood function is decreasing if $\theta < k/n$ and increasing if $\theta > k/n$.
   (b) Conclude that the maximum likelihood estimate is equal to one of the $X(k)$ for which $(k-1)/n \le X_{(k)} \le k/n$. In fact, the likelihood function has a local maximum at each such $X_{(k)}$.

3. [Neyman and Scott (1948)] Suppose we have a sample of size d from each of n normal populations with common unknown variance but possibly different unknown means

$$X_{ij} \in \mathcal{N}(\mu_i, \sigma^2), \qquad I = 1, \ldots, n, \quad j = 1, \ldots, d,$$

where all the X_{ij} are independent.
(a) Find the maximum-likelihood estimate of σ^2.
(b) Show that for d fixed, the MLE of σ^2 is not consistent as $n \to \infty$. Why doesn't Theorem 17 apply?
(c) Find a consistent estimate of σ^2.

18

Asymptotic Normality of the Maximum-Likelihood Estimate

To obtain asymptotic normality of the MLE, more restrictive conditions on $f(x|\boldsymbol{\theta})$ are needed. In particular, it will be assumed that $(\partial^2/\partial\theta^2)f(x|\boldsymbol{\theta})$ exists and is continuous. This will rule out cases like the uniform distribution on the interval $(0, \theta)$, $\theta > 0$, where the maximum-likelihood estimate is the maximum of the sample, converges to the true value at the much faster rate of $1/n$, and is not asymptotically normal. (See Example 2 of Section 14.)

When $(\partial/\partial\boldsymbol{\theta})f(x|\boldsymbol{\theta})$ exists, one can seek the MLE, $\hat{\boldsymbol{\theta}}_n$, as a solution of the *likelihood equation*,

$$\dot{l}_n(\boldsymbol{\theta}) = \frac{\partial}{\partial\boldsymbol{\theta}} \log L_n(\boldsymbol{\theta}) = \sum_1^n \frac{\partial}{\partial\boldsymbol{\theta}} \log f(x_j|\boldsymbol{\theta}) = \mathbf{0}.$$

There may be many solutions to $\dot{l}_n(\boldsymbol{\theta}) = \mathbf{0}$ even if the MLE is unique, however, there generally exist solutions of this equation that are strongly consistent even if the MLE is not consistent! The reason for this is as follows. If the true value $\boldsymbol{\theta}_0$ lies in the interior of $\Theta \subset \mathbb{R}^k$, if $(\partial/\partial\boldsymbol{\theta})\log f(x|\boldsymbol{\theta})$ exists and is continuous in $\boldsymbol{\theta}$ for all x, and if the conditions of Theorem 17 are satisfied for some compact neighborhood Θ' of $\boldsymbol{\theta}_0$, $\Theta' \subset \Theta$, then the MLE within Θ', call it $\hat{\boldsymbol{\theta}}_n$, converges a.s. to $\boldsymbol{\theta}_0$, and once $\hat{\boldsymbol{\theta}}_n$ is in the interior of Θ', it will satisfy $\dot{l}(\hat{\boldsymbol{\theta}}_n) = \mathbf{0}$.

Let

$$\boldsymbol{\Psi}(x,\boldsymbol{\theta}) = \left(\frac{\partial}{\partial\boldsymbol{\theta}} \log f(x|\boldsymbol{\theta})\right)^T, \qquad \text{a } k \text{ vector,}$$

and

$$\dot{\mathbf{\Psi}}(x,\boldsymbol{\theta}) = \frac{\partial^2}{\partial\boldsymbol{\theta}^2} \log f(x|\boldsymbol{\theta}), \qquad \text{a } k \text{ by } k \text{ matrix.}$$

Then, *Fisher Information* is defined as

$$\mathscr{I}(\boldsymbol{\theta}) = E_{\boldsymbol{\theta}}\mathbf{\Psi}(X,\boldsymbol{\theta})\mathbf{\Psi}(X,\boldsymbol{\theta})^T, \qquad \text{a } k \text{ by } k \text{ matrix.}$$

Assuming that the partial derivative with respect to $\boldsymbol{\theta}$ can be passed under the integral sign in $\int f(x|\boldsymbol{\theta})\, d\nu(x) = 1$, we find

$$E_{\boldsymbol{\theta}}\mathbf{\Psi}(X,\boldsymbol{\theta}) = \int\left[\frac{(\partial/\partial\boldsymbol{\theta})f(x|\boldsymbol{\theta})}{f(x|\boldsymbol{\theta})}\right]f(x\boldsymbol{\theta})\, d\nu(x) = \int\frac{\partial}{\partial\boldsymbol{\theta}}f(x|\boldsymbol{\theta})\, d\nu(x) = \mathbf{0},$$

so that $\mathscr{I}(\boldsymbol{\theta})$ is in fact the covariance matrix of $\mathbf{\Psi}$,

$$\mathscr{I}(\boldsymbol{\theta}) = \operatorname{var}_{\boldsymbol{\theta}}(\mathbf{\Psi}(X,\boldsymbol{\theta})).$$

If the second partial derivatives with respect to $\boldsymbol{\theta}$ can be passed under the integral sign, then $\int(\partial^2/\partial\boldsymbol{\theta}^2)f(x|\boldsymbol{\theta})\, d\nu(x) = \mathbf{0}$, and

$$\begin{aligned} E_{\boldsymbol{\theta}}\dot{\mathbf{\Psi}}(X,\boldsymbol{\theta}) &= \int\left[\frac{\partial}{\partial\boldsymbol{\theta}}\frac{(\partial/\partial\boldsymbol{\theta})f(x|\boldsymbol{\theta})}{f(x|\boldsymbol{\theta})}\right]f(x|\boldsymbol{\theta})\, d\nu(x) \\ &= \int\frac{f(x|\boldsymbol{\theta})(\partial^2/\partial\boldsymbol{\theta}^2)f(x|\boldsymbol{\theta}) - ((\partial/\partial\boldsymbol{\theta})f(x|\boldsymbol{\theta}))^T((\partial/\partial\boldsymbol{\theta})f(x|\boldsymbol{\theta}))}{f(x|\boldsymbol{\theta})^2} \\ &\qquad \times f(x|\boldsymbol{\theta})\, d\nu(x) \\ &= \mathbf{0} - \int\mathbf{\Psi}(x,\boldsymbol{\theta})\mathbf{\Psi}(x,\boldsymbol{\theta})^T f(x|\boldsymbol{\theta})\, d\nu(x). \end{aligned}$$

Thus,

$$\mathscr{I}(\boldsymbol{\theta}) = -E_{\boldsymbol{\theta}}\dot{\mathbf{\Psi}}(X,\boldsymbol{\theta}).$$

Example 1. *The Poisson distributions,* $\mathscr{P}(\theta)$. $f(x|\theta) = e^{-\theta}\theta^x/x!$ $x = 0, 1, 2, \ldots$, $\log f(x|\theta) = c - \theta + x\log\theta$, and $\psi(x,\theta) = -1 + x/\theta$. Therefore, $\mathscr{I}(\theta) = \operatorname{var}_\theta(-1 + X/\theta) = \theta/\theta^2 = 1/\theta$. We may also compute $\mathscr{I}(\theta)$ using $\dot\psi(x|\theta) = -x/\theta^2$, so $\mathscr{I}(\theta) = E_\theta X/\theta^2 = \theta/\theta^2 = 1/\theta$. Derivatives may be passed under the integral sign since the Poisson distributions form an exponential family.

Example 2. *The normal distributions, $\mathcal{N}(\mu, \sigma^2)$.*

$$\log f(x|\mu, \sigma) = -\log\sqrt{2\pi}\,\sigma - (1/2\sigma^2)(x-\mu)^2.$$

$$\boldsymbol{\Psi}(x, (\mu, \sigma)) = \begin{bmatrix} (x-\mu)/\sigma^2 \\ -1/\sigma + (x-\mu)^2/\sigma^3 \end{bmatrix}$$

$$\dot{\boldsymbol{\Psi}}(x, (\mu, \sigma)) = \begin{bmatrix} -1/\sigma^2 & -2(x-\mu)/\sigma^3 \\ -2(x-\mu)/\sigma^3 & 1/\sigma^2 - 3(x-\mu)^2/\sigma^4 \end{bmatrix}.$$

Hence,

$$\mathcal{I}(\mu, \sigma) = \begin{bmatrix} 1/\sigma^2 & 0 \\ 0 & 2/\sigma^2 \end{bmatrix}.$$

Theorem 18 (Cramér). *Let $X_1, X_2, \ldots$ be i.i.d. with density $f(x|\boldsymbol{\theta})$ (with respect to $d\nu$), and let $\boldsymbol{\theta}_0$ denote the true value of the parameter. If*

(1) *Θ is an open subset of $\mathbb{R}^k$,*
(2) *second partial derivatives of $f(x|\boldsymbol{\theta})$ with respect to $\boldsymbol{\theta}$ exist and are continuous for all x, and may be passed under the integral sign in $\int f(x|\boldsymbol{\theta})\, d\nu(x)$,*
(3) *there exists a function $K(x)$ such that $E_{\boldsymbol{\theta}_0} K(X) < \infty$ and each component of $\dot{\boldsymbol{\Psi}}(x, \boldsymbol{\theta})$ is bounded in absolute value by $K(x)$ uniformly in some neighborhood of $\boldsymbol{\theta}_0$,*
(4) *$\mathcal{I}(\boldsymbol{\theta}_0) = -E_{\boldsymbol{\theta}_0} \dot{\boldsymbol{\Psi}}(X, \boldsymbol{\theta}_0)$ is positive definite,*
(5) *$f(x|\boldsymbol{\theta}) = f(x|\boldsymbol{\theta}_0)$ a.e. $d\nu \Rightarrow \boldsymbol{\theta} = \boldsymbol{\theta}_0$,*

Then there exists a strongly consistent sequence $\hat{\boldsymbol{\theta}}_n$ of roots of the likelihood equation such that

$$\sqrt{n}\left(\hat{\boldsymbol{\theta}}_n - \boldsymbol{\theta}_0\right) \xrightarrow{\mathcal{L}} \mathcal{N}\left(\mathbf{0}, \mathcal{I}(\boldsymbol{\theta}_0)^{-1}\right).$$

Proof.

1. *Existence of consistent roots.* Let $S_\rho = \{\boldsymbol{\theta}: |\boldsymbol{\theta} - \boldsymbol{\theta}_0| \le \rho\}$ for some $\rho > 0$ be a compact neighborhood of $\boldsymbol{\theta}_0$ on which components of $\dot{\boldsymbol{\Psi}}(x, \boldsymbol{\theta})$ are uniformly bounded by $K(x)$ as in (3). The existence of a strongly consistent sequence $\hat{\boldsymbol{\theta}}_n$ of roots of $\dot{l}_n(\boldsymbol{\theta}) = \mathbf{0}$ follows from Theorem 17 with $\Theta = S_\rho$. Conditions (1), (2), and (5) of that theorem are automatic;

condition (4) follows from continuity of $f(x|\boldsymbol{\theta})$ in $\boldsymbol{\theta}$. To check condition (3) expand $U(x,\boldsymbol{\theta})$ as

$$U(x,\boldsymbol{\theta}) = U(x,\boldsymbol{\theta}_0) + \boldsymbol{\Psi}(x,\boldsymbol{\theta}_0)^T(\boldsymbol{\theta}-\boldsymbol{\theta}_0)$$
$$+(\boldsymbol{\theta}-\boldsymbol{\theta}_0)^T\int_0^1\int_0^1 \lambda\dot{\boldsymbol{\Psi}}(x,\boldsymbol{\theta}_0+\lambda\mu(\boldsymbol{\theta}-\boldsymbol{\theta}_0))\,d\lambda\,d\mu(\boldsymbol{\theta}-\boldsymbol{\theta}_0).$$

That $U(x,\boldsymbol{\theta})$ is bounded, uniformly on S_ρ, by an integrable function follows, because $U(x,\boldsymbol{\theta}_0)=0$, $\boldsymbol{\Psi}(x,\boldsymbol{\theta}_0)$ is integrable, and the components of $\dot{\boldsymbol{\Psi}}$ are bounded by $K(x)$ uniformly on S_ρ.

2. *Asymptotic normality*. Note $\dot{l}_n(\boldsymbol{\theta}) = \sum_1^n \boldsymbol{\Psi}(X_i,\boldsymbol{\theta})$. Expand $\dot{l}_n$ as

$$\dot{l}_n(\boldsymbol{\theta}) = \dot{l}_n(\boldsymbol{\theta}_0) + \int_0^1 \sum_1^n \dot{\boldsymbol{\Psi}}(X_i,\boldsymbol{\theta}_0+\lambda(\boldsymbol{\theta}-\boldsymbol{\theta}_0))\,d\lambda(\boldsymbol{\theta}-\boldsymbol{\theta}_0).$$

Now let $\boldsymbol{\theta}=\hat{\boldsymbol{\theta}}_n$ where $\hat{\boldsymbol{\theta}}_n$ is any strongly consistent sequence satisfying $\dot{l}_n(\hat{\boldsymbol{\theta}}_n)=\mathbf{0}$, and divide by $\sqrt{n}$:

$$\frac{1}{\sqrt{n}}\dot{l}_n(\boldsymbol{\theta}_0) = \mathbf{B}_n\sqrt{n}\left(\hat{\boldsymbol{\theta}}_n-\boldsymbol{\theta}_0\right),$$

where

$$\mathbf{B}_n = -\int_0^1 \frac{1}{n}\sum_1^n \dot{\boldsymbol{\Psi}}\left(X_i,\boldsymbol{\theta}_0+\lambda\left(\hat{\boldsymbol{\theta}}_n-\boldsymbol{\theta}_0\right)\right)d\lambda.$$

From the Central Limit Theorem, because $E_{\boldsymbol{\theta}_0}\boldsymbol{\Psi}(X,\boldsymbol{\theta}_0)=\mathbf{0}$ and $\mathrm{var}_{\boldsymbol{\theta}_0}\,\boldsymbol{\Psi}(X,\boldsymbol{\theta}_0)=\mathscr{I}(\boldsymbol{\theta}_0)$, we find that

$$\frac{1}{\sqrt{n}}\dot{l}_n(\boldsymbol{\theta}_0) = \sqrt{n}\left(\frac{1}{n}\sum_1^n \boldsymbol{\Psi}(X_i,\boldsymbol{\theta}_0)\right) \xrightarrow{\mathscr{L}} \mathbf{Z}\in\mathscr{N}(\mathbf{0},\mathscr{I}(\boldsymbol{\theta}_0)).$$

If we show $\mathbf{B}_n \xrightarrow{\text{a.s.}} \mathscr{I}(\boldsymbol{\theta}_0)$, then eventually $\mathbf{B}_n^{-1}$ will exist and by Slutsky's Theorem.

$$\sqrt{n}\left(\hat{\boldsymbol{\theta}}_n-\boldsymbol{\theta}_0\right) = \mathbf{B}_n^{-1}\frac{1}{\sqrt{n}}\dot{l}_n(\boldsymbol{\theta}_0) \xrightarrow{\mathscr{L}} \mathscr{I}(\boldsymbol{\theta}_0)^{-1}\mathbf{Z}\in\mathscr{N}\left(0,\mathscr{I}(\boldsymbol{\theta}_0)^{-1}\right).$$

Let $\varepsilon>0$. To show $\mathbf{B}_n \xrightarrow{\text{a.s.}} \mathscr{I}(\boldsymbol{\theta}_0)$, first note that $E_{\boldsymbol{\theta}_0}\dot{\boldsymbol{\Psi}}(X,\boldsymbol{\theta})$ is continuous in $\boldsymbol{\theta}$ from condition (3), so there is a $\rho>0$ such that $|\boldsymbol{\theta}-\boldsymbol{\theta}_0|<\rho$ implies

$$\left|E_{\boldsymbol{\theta}_0}\dot{\boldsymbol{\Psi}}(X,\boldsymbol{\theta})+\mathscr{I}(\boldsymbol{\theta}_0)\right|<\varepsilon.$$

Next note from the Uniform Strong Law of Large Numbers, Theorem 16(a), that with probability 1 there is an integer N such that

$$n > N \text{ implies } \sup_{\boldsymbol{\theta} \in S_\rho} \left| \frac{1}{n} \sum_1^n \dot{\boldsymbol{\Psi}}(X_j, \boldsymbol{\theta}) - E_{\boldsymbol{\theta}_0} \dot{\boldsymbol{\Psi}}(X, \boldsymbol{\theta}) \right| < \varepsilon.$$

Then, assuming N is so large that $n > N \Rightarrow |\hat{\boldsymbol{\theta}}_n - \boldsymbol{\theta}_0| < \rho$,

$$n > N \Rightarrow |\mathbf{B}_n - \mathscr{I}(\boldsymbol{\theta}_0)| \le \int_0^1 \left| \frac{1}{n} \sum_1^n \dot{\boldsymbol{\Psi}}\left(X_i, \boldsymbol{\theta}_0 + \lambda(\hat{\boldsymbol{\theta}}_n - \boldsymbol{\theta}_0)\right) + \mathscr{I}(\boldsymbol{\theta}_0) \right| d\lambda$$

$$\le \int_0^1 \sup_{\boldsymbol{\theta} \in S_\rho} \left[\left| \frac{1}{n} \sum_1^n \dot{\boldsymbol{\Psi}}(X_j, \boldsymbol{\theta}) - E_{\boldsymbol{\theta}_0} \dot{\boldsymbol{\Psi}}(X, \boldsymbol{\theta}) \right| + \left| E_{\boldsymbol{\theta}_0} \dot{\boldsymbol{\Psi}}(X, \boldsymbol{\theta}) + \mathscr{I}(\boldsymbol{\theta}_0) \right| \right] d\lambda$$

$$\le 2\varepsilon. \quad \blacksquare$$

Remarks. One often says that this theorem states that the maximum likelihood estimate is asymptotically normal. However, that is a rather loose interpretation. All it really claims is that, under the conditions stated, there is a consistent sequence of roots of the likelihood equation that is asymptotically normal with Fisher information as its variance. Under these same conditions, the MLE may not be one of these roots; even if it is, it may not be consistent. An example similar to that found at the end of the previous section may be constructed that satisfies the conditions of Theorem 18, so that the MLE will be inconsistent even though it is one of the roots of the likelihood equation. Even so, in such an example, there will exist a consistent sequence of roots. This theorem gives no hint as to which root one should use as the estimate. Exercise 5 gives a simple example in which there may exist many roots of the likelihood equation, and many maxima of the likelihood.

However, under the conditions of Theorem 18, if there is a unique root of the likelihood equation for every n, as in many applications, this sequence of roots will be consistent and asymptotically normal.

Passing the derivative under the integral sign.

Lemma. *If* $(\partial/\partial\theta)\, g(x,\theta)$ *exists and is continuous in* θ *for all* x *and all* θ *in an open interval* S, *and if* $|(\partial/\partial\theta)\, g(x,\theta)| \le K(x)$ *on* S *where* $\int K(x)\, d\nu(x) < \infty$, *and if* $\int g(x,\theta)\, d\nu(x)$ *exists on* S, *then*

$$\frac{d}{d\theta}\int g(x,\theta)\, d\nu(x) = \int \frac{\partial}{\partial\theta} g(x,\theta)\, d\nu(x).$$

Proof. From the Mean-Value Theorem,

$$\left|\frac{g(x,\theta+\delta) - g(x,\theta)}{\delta}\right| \le \int_0^1 \left|\frac{\partial}{\partial\theta} g(x,\theta+\lambda\delta)\right| d\lambda \le K(x),$$

so that the result follows from the Lebesgue Dominated Convergence Theorem by taking the limit as $\delta \to 0$ on both sides of

$$\frac{\int g(x,\theta+\delta)\, d\nu(x) - \int g(x,\theta)\, d\nu(x)}{\delta} = \int \frac{g(x,\theta+\delta) - g(x,\theta)}{\delta}\, d\nu(x). \qquad \blacksquare$$

EXERCISES

1. Find the MLE and its asymptotic distribution for
   (a) $f(x|\theta) = \theta x^{\theta-1} I(0 < x < 1)$, $\Theta = (0, \infty)$.
   (b) $f(x|\theta) = (1-\theta)\theta^x$, $x = 0, 1, 2, \ldots$, $\Theta = (0, 1)$.
2. Find the likelihood equations and the asymptotic distribution of the MLE for the parameters of the gamma distribution, $\mathscr{G}(\alpha, \beta)$,
   $$f(x|\alpha,\beta) = \frac{1}{\Gamma(\alpha)\beta^\alpha} x^{\alpha-1} \exp\{-x/\beta\} I(x > 0),$$
   $$\Theta = \{(\alpha,\beta)\colon \alpha > 0,\ \beta > 0\}.$$
   [Note: In the solution, you should encounter the digamma function, $\digamma(\alpha) = d/d\alpha \log \Gamma(\alpha)$, and the trigamma function, $\digamma'(\alpha) = (d/d\alpha)\digamma(\alpha)$.]
3. Find the likelihood equations and the asymptotic distribution of the MLE for the parameters of $f(x|\theta_1,\theta_2) = \exp\{-\theta_2 \cosh(x-\theta_1) - \zeta(\theta_2)\}$ where the parameter space is $\Theta = \{(\theta_1,\theta_2)\colon \theta_2 > 0\}$, and where ζ is the normalizing constant, $\zeta(\theta_2) = \log \int_{-\infty}^{\infty} \exp\{-\theta_2 \cosh(x)\}\, dx$.
4. *Additivity of Information for Independent Random Variables.* Let X and Y be independent random variables with densities depending on θ and

assume that Fisher information, $\mathcal{I}_X(\theta)$ and $\mathcal{I}_Y(\theta)$, exists for both X and Y. Show that Fisher information for the pair, (X,Y), is given by $\mathcal{I}_{X,Y}(\theta) = \mathcal{I}_X(\theta) + \mathcal{I}_Y(\theta)$.

5. Let $X_1, \ldots, X_n$ be a sample from the Cauchy distribution, $\mathscr{C}(\theta, 1)$, and let $X_{(1)}, \ldots, X_{(n)}$ denote the corresponding order statistics.
   (a) Show that if $X_{(n)} > X_{(n-1)} + 2n$, then $\dot{l}_n(\theta)$ has a root in the interval $(X_{(n)} - 1, X_{(n)})$.
   (b) Show that $P(X_{(n)} > X_{(n-1)} + 2n)$ converges to a positive limit as n tends to infinity. (See Example 3 of Section 15.)
6. What was thought to be a certain species of moth is attracted to a capture tank at rate λ per day. One the first day, the number X of moths caught was recorded. It is assumed that X has a Poisson distribution with mean λ. Later, it was pointed out that this species is, in fact, two different similar species, so a second day of capture was undertaken. This time, the numbers Y_1 and Y_2 of moths caught of these species separately were noted. It is assumed that these are Poisson random variables with means λ_1 and λ_2, where $\lambda_1 + \lambda_2 = \lambda$, and it is assumed that X, Y_1, and Y_2 are independent.
   (a) Using X, Y_1, and Y_2, find the maximum likelihood estimate of λ_1 and λ_2.
   (b) Assuming λ_1 and λ_2 large, what is the approximate variance of your estimate of λ_1, as a function of λ_1 and λ_2?
7. Let $X_1, \ldots, X_n$ be a sample from the distribution with density

$$f(x|\theta_1, \theta_2) = \frac{1}{\theta_1 + \theta_2} \begin{cases} \exp\{-x/\theta_1\}, & \text{if } x > 0, \\ \exp\{+x/\theta_2\}, & \text{if } x < 0, \end{cases}$$

   where $\theta_j > 0$ and $\theta_2 > 0$ are unknown parameters.
   (a) Find the likelihood function in terms of the sufficient statistics, $S_1 = \Sigma X_j I(X_j > 0)$ and $S_2 = -\Sigma X_j I(X_j < 0)$. Note $S_1 \geq 0$ and $S_2 \geq 0$ but $S_1 = 0$ or $S_2 = 0$ with positive probability.
   (b) Find the maximum likelihood estimates $\hat{\theta}_1$ and $\hat{\theta}_2$ as solutions of the likelihood equations.
   (c) Find the Fisher information matrix.
   (d) What is the joint asymptotic distribution of $\hat{\theta}_1$ and $\hat{\theta}_2$?

19

The Cramér–Rao Lower Bound

In this section, we prove the information inequality. This inequality relates the variance of an arbitrary statistic to Fisher Information. When applied to an estimate of a parameter based on a sample from a distribution, this inequality is known as the Cramér–Rao lower bound. If an unbiased estimate attains the Cramér–Rao bound, it is automatically a best unbiased estimate. We will see that the bound for unbiased estimates may not be achievable, and even if it is achieved, the achieving estimate may not be admissible. In the investigation of the inequality for a vector parameter, we note the effect of not knowing the values of nuisance parameters.

We start with the simplest case, that of a one-dimensional parameter space, Θ. Let X (possibly a vector of observations) have density $f(x|\theta)$ with respect to $d\nu(x)$ for $\theta \in \Theta$, an open interval in $\mathbb{R}^1$. When $(\partial/\partial\theta) f(x|\theta)$ exists as a random variable, Fisher Information may be defined as

$$\mathscr{I}(\theta) = \operatorname{var}_\theta\left(\frac{\partial}{\partial\theta} \log f(X, \theta)\right). \tag{1}$$

THEOREM 19. *The Information Inequality. Let $\hat{\theta}(x)$ be an estimate of θ with finite expectation, $g(\theta) = E_\theta \hat{\theta}(X)$. Assume that $(\partial/\partial\theta) f(x|\theta)$ exists and that $\partial/\partial\theta$ can be passed under the integral sign in $\int f(x|\theta)\, d\nu(x) = 1$ and in $\int \hat{\theta}(x) f(x|\theta)\, d\nu(x) = g(\theta)$. Assume that $0 < \mathscr{I}(\theta)$, where $\mathscr{I}(\theta)$ is Fisher Information. Then for all θ,*

$$\operatorname{var}_\theta \hat{\theta}\,(X) \geq \frac{g'(\theta)^2}{\mathscr{I}(\theta)}. \tag{2}$$

Moreover, equality holds in (2) for some value θ if and only if $(\partial/\partial\theta)\log f(x|\theta)$ and $\hat{\theta}(x)$ are linearly related.

Proof. Let $\Psi(x, \theta) = (\partial/\partial\theta)\log f(x, \theta)$. Then, by the regularity conditions,

$$E_\theta \Psi(X, \theta) = \int \frac{\partial}{\partial\theta} f(x|\theta)\, d\nu(x) = 0$$

for all θ, and

$$\begin{aligned} g'(\theta) &= \int \hat{\theta}\,(x) \frac{\partial}{\partial\theta} f(x|\theta)\, d\nu(x) \\ &= E_\theta \hat{\theta}\,(X)\Psi(X, \theta) = \operatorname{cov}_\theta\big(\hat{\theta}\,(X), \Psi(X, \theta)\big). \end{aligned}$$

Now using the inequality $\operatorname{cov}(U, V)^2 \le \operatorname{var} U \cdot \operatorname{var} V$ (the correlation c-efficient is between -1 and $+1$) with equality if and only if U and V are linearly related, we find

$$g'(\theta)^2 \le \operatorname{var}_\theta \hat{\theta}\,(X) \cdot \operatorname{var}_\theta \Psi(X, \theta),$$

which completes the proof because $\mathscr{I}(\theta) = \operatorname{var}_\theta \Psi(X, \theta)$. ■

Remark 1. The moreover part of this theorem, that equality holds in (2) if and only if $(\partial/\partial\theta)\log f(x|\theta)$ and $\hat{\theta}(x)$ are linearly related, means that there is equality in (2) for some fixed θ if and only if for that θ there are constants, a' and b', depending on θ, such that $\Psi(x, \theta) = b'\hat{\theta}(x) + a'$. There is equality in (2) for all θ if ad only if $\Psi(x, \theta)$ has this form for all θ; that is (after integrating on θ), $\log f(x|\theta) = \hat{\theta}(x)b(\theta) + a(\theta) + c(x)$. In other words, $\hat{\theta}(x)$ achieves equality for all θ in the information inequality if and only if $\hat{\theta}(x)$ is a natural sufficient statistic of an exponential family

$$f(x|\theta) = \exp\{\hat{\theta}\,(x)b(\theta) + a(\theta)\}h(x) \tag{3}$$

with respect to some measure $d\nu(x)$.

As an example, the density of the beta distribution, $\mathscr{B}e(\alpha, 1)$, written in exponential form is $f(x|\alpha) = \alpha \exp\{(\alpha - 1)\log(x) + \log(\alpha)\}I\,(0 < x < 1)$ for $\alpha > 0$. Thus, $\hat{\theta}(x) = -\log(x)$ is an unbiased estimate of its expectation, $\theta(\alpha) = E_\alpha(-\log(X)) = 1/\alpha$, that achieves equality in (2) for all α. (See Exercise 1.) Moreover, $-\log(X)$ is the only function of X, up to addition and multiplication by scalars, that achieves equality in (2) for all α.

Remark 2. It is interesting to view this inequality in terms of the bias of the estimate. The bias of $\hat{\theta}(X)$ as an estimate of θ is defined as $b(\theta) = E_\theta \hat{\theta}(X) - \theta = g(\theta) - \theta$. Then, because $g'(\theta) = 1 + b'(\theta)$, we have as a lower bound on the variance of $\hat{\theta}$,

$$\operatorname{var}_\theta \hat{\theta}\ (X) \geq (1 + b'(\theta))^2 / \mathscr{I}(\theta).$$

If $\hat{\theta}(X)$ is an unbiased estimate of θ, then $b(\theta) \equiv 0$, so that

$$\operatorname{var}_\theta \hat{\theta}\ (X) \geq \mathscr{I}(\theta)^{-1}$$

provides a lower bound for the variance of an unbiased estimate of θ.

If $X_1, \ldots, X_n$ is a sample of size n from $f(x|\theta)$, then the Fisher Information computed from $\prod f(x_i|\theta)$ is n times the Fisher Information based on a sample of size 1,

$$\mathscr{I}_n(\theta) = \operatorname{var}_\theta\left(\frac{\partial}{\partial\theta} \log \prod_1^n f(X_j|\theta)\right) = \sum_1^n \operatorname{var}_\theta\left(\frac{\partial}{\partial\theta} \log f(X_j|\theta)\right) = n\mathscr{I}_1(\theta).$$

Combining these observations, we obtain a lower bound for the variance of an estimate $\hat{\theta}(X_1, \ldots, X_n)$ of θ based on a sample size n from $f(x|\theta)$,

$$\operatorname{var}_\theta \hat{\theta}\ (X_1, \ldots, X_n) \geq \frac{(1 + b'(\theta))^2}{n\mathscr{I}(\theta)},$$

where $b(\theta)$ is the bias of $\hat{\theta}$, and $\mathscr{I}(\theta)$ is Fisher information in a sample of size 1. This inequality is known as *the Cramér–Rao lower bound.*

Example 1. Given a sample $X_1, \ldots, X_n$ from the gamma distribution, $\mathscr{G}(\alpha, \beta)$, with α known, we obtain as a lower bound for the variance of an unbiased estimate $\hat{\beta}$ of β,

$$\operatorname{var}_\beta \hat{\beta}\ (X_1, \ldots, X_n) \geq \frac{1}{n(\alpha/\beta^2)} = \frac{\beta^2}{n\alpha},$$

because $\mathscr{I}(\beta) = \alpha/\beta^2$ as computed in Exercise 2, Section 18. In this problem, $S_n = \sum_1^n X_i$ is a sufficient statistic for β and $S_n \in \mathscr{G}(n\alpha, \beta)$ so that $ES_n = n\alpha\beta$, and $\operatorname{var} S_n = n\alpha\beta^2$. Hence, $\hat{\beta} = S_n/n\alpha$ is an unbiased estimate of β and $\operatorname{var}_\beta \hat{\beta} = (\operatorname{var} S_n)/n^2\alpha^2 = n\alpha\beta^2/n^2\alpha^2 = \beta^2/n\alpha$. Thus, $\hat{\beta} = \overline{X}_n/\alpha$ is a best unbiased estimate of β. This result also follows from the fact that $\overline{X}_n$ is a complete sufficient statistic for β, and any function of a complete sufficient statistic is a best unbiased estimate of its expectation.

Example 2. Suppose in Example 1 we want to find a bound on the variance of an unbiased estimate of $\theta = 1/\beta$. We may use the information inequality directly with $g(\beta) = 1/\beta$ or, equivalently, we may change parameters to $\theta = 1/\beta$ and apply Cramér–Rao. The former gives $(-1/\beta^2)^2\beta^2/n\alpha = 1/n\alpha\beta^2$ as a lower bound for the variance of an unbiased estimate of $g(\beta) = 1/\beta$. Straightforward computations give $E(1/S_n) = 1/(n\alpha - 1)\beta$ and $\text{var}(1/S_n) = 1/(n\alpha - 1)^2(n\alpha - 2)\beta^2$. Since $\hat{\theta} = (n\alpha - 1)/S_n$ is an unbiased estimate of $\theta = 1/\beta$ and a function of a complete sufficient statistic, $\hat{\theta}$ is a best unbiased estimate of $\theta = 1/\beta$, yet

$$\text{var}\,\hat{\theta} = (n\alpha - 1)^2 \,\text{var}\left(\frac{1}{S_n}\right) = \frac{1}{(n\alpha - 2)\beta^2}.$$

This is strictly greater than the Cramér–Rao lower bound. This shows the Cramér–Rao bound may not be attainable.

Example 3. Let $X_1, \ldots, X_n$ be a sample from $\mathcal{N}(\mu, \sigma^2)$ with μ known. To estimate $g(\sigma) = \sigma^2$, Example 2 of Section 18 and the information inequality with $g'(\sigma) = 2\sigma$ give $(2\sigma)^2/n(2/\sigma^2) = 2\sigma^4/n$ as a lower bound for the variance of an unbiased estimate of σ^2. Since $\hat{\sigma}^2 = (1/n)\sum_1^n (X_i - \mu)^2$ is a complete sufficient statistic and an unbiased estimate of σ^2, it is a best unbiased estimate of σ^2. Moreover,

$$\text{var}\,\hat{\sigma}^2 = (1/n^2) \sum_1^n \text{var}(X_i - \mu)^2 = n \cdot 2\sigma^4/n^2 = 2\sigma^4/n,$$

so the lower bound is attained. However, there a biased estimate that is better; that is, there is an estimate with uniformly smaller mean-squared error, namely $\tilde{\sigma}^2 = (1/(n+2))\sum_1^n (X_i - \mu)^2$. Because the mean-squared error is the variance plus the square of the bias, we have

$$\text{MSE}_\sigma(\tilde{\sigma}^2) = 2n\sigma^4/(n+2)^2 + \left((n\sigma^2/(n+2) - \sigma^2\right)^2 = 2\sigma^4/(n+2).$$

This is less than $\text{MSE}_\sigma(\hat{\sigma}^2) = 2\sigma^4/n$. Just because an unbiased estimate has a variance that achieves the Cramér–Rao lower bound does not mean it is any good.

Generalization to a Vector Parameter. The generalization of the information inequality to k-dimensional Θ requires comparison of covariance matrices. Given two $k \times k$ covariance matrices $\mathbf{\Sigma}_1$ and $\mathbf{\Sigma}_2$, we say $\mathbf{\Sigma}_1 \geq \mathbf{\Sigma}_2$ if $\mathbf{\Sigma}_1 - \mathbf{\Sigma}_2$ is nonnegative definite, that is, if $\mathbf{a}'(\mathbf{\Sigma}_1 - \mathbf{\Sigma}_2)\mathbf{a} \geq 0$ for all k-vectors $\mathbf{a}$.

Theorem 19′. *Let X have density $f(x|\boldsymbol{\theta})$ with respect to $d\nu(x)$ for $\boldsymbol{\theta} \in \Theta$ an open set in $\mathbb{R}^k$, and assume that Fisher information, $\mathscr{I}(\boldsymbol{\theta})$, exists and is nonsingular for all $\boldsymbol{\theta} \in \Theta$. Let $\hat{\boldsymbol{\theta}}(x)$ be an r-dimensional vector such that $\mathbf{g}(\boldsymbol{\theta}) = E_{\boldsymbol{\theta}}\hat{\boldsymbol{\theta}}(X)$ exists on Θ. Assume that $(\partial/\partial\boldsymbol{\theta})f(x|\boldsymbol{\theta})$ exists and that $\partial/\partial\boldsymbol{\theta}$ can be passed under the integral sign in $\int f(x|\boldsymbol{\theta})\,d\nu(x)$ and $\int\hat{\boldsymbol{\theta}}(x)f(x|\boldsymbol{\theta})\,d\nu(x)$. Then,*

$$\operatorname{var}_{\boldsymbol{\theta}} \hat{\boldsymbol{\theta}}(X) \geq \dot{\mathbf{g}}(\boldsymbol{\theta})\mathscr{I}(\boldsymbol{\theta})^{-1}\dot{\mathbf{g}}(\boldsymbol{\theta})^T,$$

where $\mathscr{I}(\boldsymbol{\theta})$ is the Fisher information matrix and $\dot{\mathbf{g}}(\boldsymbol{\theta})$ is the $r \times k$ matrix of partial derivatives of $\mathbf{g}(\boldsymbol{\theta})$.

Proof. Let $\boldsymbol{\Psi}(x,\boldsymbol{\theta}) = ((\partial/\partial\boldsymbol{\theta})\log f(x|\boldsymbol{\theta}))^T$, a k vector. As before,

$$E_{\boldsymbol{\theta}}\boldsymbol{\Psi}(X,\boldsymbol{\theta}) = \mathbf{0}, \quad \text{and} \quad \dot{\mathbf{g}}(\boldsymbol{\theta}) = \operatorname{cov}_{\boldsymbol{\theta}}\big(\hat{\boldsymbol{\theta}}(X), \boldsymbol{\Psi}(X,\boldsymbol{\theta})\big).$$

Hence

$$\begin{aligned}
&\operatorname{var}_{\boldsymbol{\theta}}\big(\hat{\boldsymbol{\theta}} - \dot{\mathbf{g}}\mathscr{I}(\boldsymbol{\theta})^{-1}\boldsymbol{\Psi}\big)\\
&\quad = \operatorname{var}_{\boldsymbol{\theta}} \hat{\boldsymbol{\theta}} - 2\operatorname{cov}_{\boldsymbol{\theta}}\big(\hat{\boldsymbol{\theta}}, \dot{\mathbf{g}}\mathscr{I}(\boldsymbol{\theta})^{-1}\boldsymbol{\Psi}\big) + \operatorname{var}_{\boldsymbol{\theta}}\big(\dot{\mathbf{g}}\mathscr{I}(\boldsymbol{\theta})^{-1}\boldsymbol{\Psi}\big)\\
&\quad = \operatorname{var}_{\boldsymbol{\theta}} \hat{\boldsymbol{\theta}} - 2\operatorname{cov}_{\boldsymbol{\theta}}(\hat{\boldsymbol{\theta}}, \boldsymbol{\Psi})\mathscr{I}(\boldsymbol{\theta})^{-1}\dot{\mathbf{g}}^T + \dot{\mathbf{g}}\mathscr{I}^{-1} \operatorname{var}_{\boldsymbol{\theta}} \boldsymbol{\Psi}\mathscr{I}(\boldsymbol{\theta})^{-1}\dot{\mathbf{g}}^T\\
&\quad = \operatorname{var}_{\boldsymbol{\theta}} \hat{\boldsymbol{\theta}} - 2\dot{\mathbf{g}}\mathscr{I}(\boldsymbol{\theta})^{-1}\dot{\mathbf{g}}^T + \dot{\mathbf{g}}\mathscr{I}(\boldsymbol{\theta})^{-1}\mathscr{I}(\boldsymbol{\theta})\mathscr{I}(\theta)^{-1}\dot{\mathbf{g}}^T\\
&\quad = \operatorname{var}_{\boldsymbol{\theta}} \hat{\boldsymbol{\theta}} - \dot{\mathbf{g}}\mathscr{I}(\boldsymbol{\theta})^{-1}\dot{\mathbf{g}}^T \geq \mathbf{0}. \quad \blacksquare
\end{aligned}$$

Remark 3. The Cramér–Rao lower bound for the variance of an *unbiased* estimate of a vector $\boldsymbol{\theta}$ based on a sample of size n is, since $\dot{\mathbf{g}}(\boldsymbol{\theta}) = \mathbf{I}$,

$$\operatorname{var}_{\boldsymbol{\theta}} \hat{\boldsymbol{\theta}}(X_1,\ldots,X_n) \geq \frac{1}{n}\mathscr{I}(\boldsymbol{\theta})^{-1}.$$

Note the effect of nuisance parameters. If it is desired to estimate θ_1 and the rest of the parameters are known, the lower bound is $1/(n\mathscr{I}_{11}(\boldsymbol{\theta}))$ where $\mathscr{I}_{11}(\boldsymbol{\theta})$ is the upper left component of $\mathscr{I}(\boldsymbol{\theta})$. If the other parameters are unknown, the lower bound is $\mathscr{I}^{11}(\boldsymbol{\theta})/n$ where $\mathscr{I}^{11}(\boldsymbol{\theta})$ is the upper left component of $\mathscr{I}(\boldsymbol{\theta})^{-1}$. It may or may not happen that $\mathscr{I}^{11}(\boldsymbol{\theta}) = 1/\mathscr{I}_{11}(\boldsymbol{\theta})$.

Example 4. In the $\mathscr{N}(\mu, \sigma^2)$ Example 2 of Section 18, we found

$$\mathscr{I}(\mu, \sigma) = \begin{bmatrix} 1/\sigma^2 & 0 \\ 0 & 2/\sigma^2 \end{bmatrix}.$$

Hence,

$$\mathscr{I}(\mu, \sigma)^{-1} = \begin{bmatrix} \sigma^2 & 0 \\ 0 & \sigma^2/2 \end{bmatrix}.$$

In this case, there is an unbiased estimate of μ, namely, $\overline{X}_n$, whose variance achieves the lower bound of σ^2/n, this bound being the same whether or not σ^2 is known.

Example 5. In the $\mathscr{G}(\alpha, \beta)$ example of this section, we saw that for α known, $\hat{\beta} = \overline{X}_n/\alpha$ is a best unbiased estimate of β achieving the Cramér–Rao bound. If α is unknown we cannot use this estimate. In fact, because the inverse of Fisher information (Exercise 2 of Section 18) is

$$\mathscr{I}(\boldsymbol{\theta})^{-1} = \begin{bmatrix} Ŧ(\alpha) & 1/\beta \\ 1/\beta & \alpha/\beta^2 \end{bmatrix}^{-1} = \frac{\beta^2}{\alpha Ŧ(\alpha) - 1} \begin{bmatrix} \alpha/\beta^2 & -1/\beta \\ -1/\beta & Ŧ(\alpha) \end{bmatrix},$$

no unbiased estimate of β can have a variance smaller than $\beta^2 Ŧ(\alpha)/n(\alpha Ŧ(\alpha) - 1)$, which is greater than $\beta^2/n\alpha$, the bound when α is known, obtained by using $\overline{X}_n/\alpha$.

=

Ŧ

EXERCISES

1. Let $X_1, \ldots, X_n$ be a sample from the beta distribution, $\mathscr{B}e(\theta, 1)$, $f(x|\theta) = \theta x^{\theta-1} I(0 < x < 1)$. (a) Find the MLE of $1/\theta$. Show it is unbiased and achieves the Cramér–Rao lower bound. (b) Show $\overline{X}_n$ is an unbiased estimate of $\theta/(\theta+1)$. Compare its variance to the Cramér–Rao or information inequality bound.
2. Consider the bivariate normal with density

$$f(x, y|\boldsymbol{\theta}) = \frac{1}{2\pi\sqrt{1-\rho^2}\,\sigma_1\sigma_2} \exp\left\{ -\frac{1}{2(1-\rho^2)} \left[\left(\frac{x-\mu_1}{\sigma_1}\right)^2 - 2\rho\left(\frac{x-\mu_1}{\sigma_1}\right)\left(\frac{y-\mu_2}{\sigma_2}\right) + \left(\frac{y-\mu_2}{\sigma_2}\right)^2 \right] \right\}$$

where $\boldsymbol{\theta} = (\mu_1, \mu_2, \sigma_1, \sigma_2, \rho)$. Checking my computations:

$$\mathscr{I}(\boldsymbol{\theta}) = \frac{1}{1-\rho^2}$$

$$\times \begin{bmatrix} 1/\sigma_1^2 & -\rho/\sigma_1\sigma_2 & 0 & 0 & 0 \\ -\rho/\sigma_1\sigma_2 & 1/\sigma_2^2 & 0 & 0 & 0 \\ 0 & 0 & (2-\rho^2)/\sigma_1^2 & -\rho^2/\sigma_1\sigma_2 & -\rho/\sigma_1 \\ 0 & 0 & -\rho^2/\sigma_1\sigma_2 & (2-\rho^2)/\sigma_2^2 & -\rho/\sigma_2 \\ 0 & 0 & -\rho/\sigma_1 & -\rho/\sigma_2 & (1+\rho^2)/(1-\rho^2) \end{bmatrix},$$

$$\mathscr{I}(\boldsymbol{\theta})^{-1} = \begin{bmatrix} \sigma_1^2 & \rho\sigma_1\sigma_2 & 0 & 0 & 0 \\ \rho\sigma_1\sigma_2 & \sigma_2^2 & 0 & 0 & 0 \\ 0 & 0 & \sigma_1^2/2 & \rho^2\sigma_1\sigma_2/2 & \rho\sigma_1(1-\rho^2)/2 \\ 0 & 0 & \rho^2\sigma_1\sigma_2/2 & \sigma_2^2/2 & \rho\sigma_2(1-\rho^2)/2 \\ 0 & 0 & \rho\sigma_1(1-\rho^2)/2 & \rho\sigma_2(1-\rho^2)/2 & (1-\rho^2)^2 \end{bmatrix}.$$

3. Assuming this is correct, find a lower bound for a sample of size n, for the variance of an unbiased estimate of:
   (a) $\mu_1 - \mu_2$,
   (b) μ_1/σ_1,
   (c) $\sigma_{12} = \rho\sigma_1\sigma_2$.
4. Let $X_1, \ldots, X_n$ be independent random variables having Poisson distributions with means $\exp\{\theta z_1\}, \ldots, \exp\{\theta z_n\}$, respectively, where $z_1, \ldots, z_n$ are known real numbers. Find the Cramér–Rao lower bound for the variance of an unbiased estimate of θ based on $X_1, \ldots, X_n$.
5. Suppose that X has a uniform distribution on the interval $(0, \theta)$, where $\theta \in \Theta = (0, \infty)$.
   (a) Note that $\partial/\partial\theta$ cannot be passed under the integral sign in $\int f(x|\theta)\,d\nu(x) = 1$.
   (b) Show that $\text{var}_\theta((\partial/\partial\theta)\log f(X, \theta)) = 0$, so that the Cramér–Rao bound is infinite.
   (c) Note that $2X$ is an unbiased estimate of θ and has finite variance.

20

Asymptotic Efficiency

In this section, we define a sequence of estimates to be asymptotically efficient if the Cramér–Rao lower bound to the variance is achieved in the limit. In an aside, we note the phenomenon of superefficiency. But our main objective is to see how to improve a subefficient sequence of estimates by the method of scoring, and to show that one application of scoring is usually enough to achieve asymptotic efficiency.

Under the conditions of Theorem 18, the MLE $\hat{\boldsymbol{\theta}}_n$ was seen to be asymptotically unbiased in a reasonably strong sense, because whatever be the true value of $\boldsymbol{\theta}$, $\sqrt{n}(\hat{\boldsymbol{\theta}}_n - \boldsymbol{\theta})$ is asymptotically normal with mean zero. In addition, the asymptotic variance of the MLE is $(1/n)\mathscr{I}(\boldsymbol{\theta})^{-1}$ which is the Cramér–Rao lower bound for the variance of any unbiased estimate of $\boldsymbol{\theta}$ based on a sample of size n.

Definition. Let $X_1, X_2, \ldots$ be i.i.d. random variables with distribution depending upon a parameter $\boldsymbol{\theta} \in \Theta$. A sequence of estimates $\{\tilde{\boldsymbol{\theta}}_n\}$ of $\boldsymbol{\theta}$, with $\tilde{\boldsymbol{\theta}}_n$ a function of $X_1, \ldots, X_n$, such that $\sqrt{n}(\tilde{\boldsymbol{\theta}}_n - \boldsymbol{\theta}) \xrightarrow{\mathscr{L}} \mathscr{N}(\mathbf{0}, \boldsymbol{\Sigma}(\boldsymbol{\theta}))$ whatever be the true value of $\boldsymbol{\theta}$, is said to be *asymptotically efficient* if $\boldsymbol{\Sigma}(\boldsymbol{\theta}) = \mathscr{I}(\boldsymbol{\theta})^{-1}$ for all $\boldsymbol{\theta} \in \Theta$.

By definition, the MLE is asymptotically efficient under the conditions of Theorem 18. Certainly, no sequence of unbiased estimates can have a smaller variance asymptotically for any $\boldsymbol{\theta}$. We would like to say that no sequence of estimates satisfying the asymptotic normality condition can have a smaller variance asymptotically for any $\boldsymbol{\theta}$. That this is not quite true is seen in the following example due to J. L. Hodges. (See Le Cam (1953).)

Example 1. [J. L. Hodges] Let $\hat{\theta}_n$ be MLEs (in one dimension), such that $\sqrt{n}(\hat{\theta}_n - \theta) \xrightarrow{\mathscr{L}} \mathscr{N}(0, \mathscr{I}(\theta)^{-1})$, whatever be the true value of θ, and let θ_0 be an arbitrary value of θ. Define

$$\tilde{\theta}_n = \begin{cases} \theta_0, & \text{if } \sqrt[4]{n}\,|\hat{\theta}_n - \theta_0| \le 1, \\ \hat{\theta}_n, & \text{if } \sqrt[4]{n}\,|\hat{\theta}_n - \theta_0| > 1. \end{cases}$$

If $\theta \neq \theta_0$, then

$$\begin{aligned} P_\theta\left(\hat{\theta}_n \neq \tilde{\theta}_n\right) &\le P_\theta\left(\sqrt[4]{n}\,|\hat{\theta}_n - \theta_0| \le 1\right) \\ &\le P_\theta\left(|\theta - \theta_0| - |\hat{\theta}_n - \theta| \le 1/\sqrt[4]{n}\right) \\ &= P_\theta\left(|\hat{\theta}_n - \theta| \ge |\theta - \theta_0| - 1/\sqrt[4]{n}\right) \\ &= P_\theta\left(\sqrt{n}\,|\hat{\theta}_n - \theta| \ge \sqrt{n}\,|\theta - \theta_0| - \sqrt[4]{n}\right) \to 0. \end{aligned}$$

Hence, $\hat{\theta}_n$ and $\tilde{\theta}_n$ are asymptotically equal, and

$$\sqrt{n}\left(\tilde{\theta}_n - \theta\right) \xrightarrow{\mathscr{L}} \mathscr{N}\left(0, \mathscr{I}(\theta)^{-1}\right).$$

If $\theta = \theta_0$, then

$$\begin{aligned} P_{\theta_0}\left(\tilde{\theta}_n = \theta_0\right) &= P_{\theta_0}\left(\sqrt[4]{n}\,|\hat{\theta}_n - \theta_0| \le 1\right) \\ &= P_{\theta_0}\left(\sqrt{n}\,|\hat{\theta}_n - \theta_0| \le \sqrt[4]{n}\right) \to 1. \end{aligned}$$

Hence, when $\theta = \theta_0$, $\sqrt{n}(\tilde{\theta}_n - \theta_0) \to \mathscr{N}(0, 0)$. We find $\sqrt{n}(\tilde{\theta}_n - \theta) \xrightarrow{\mathscr{L}} \mathscr{N}(0, \sigma^2(\theta))$ where

$$\sigma^2(\theta) = \begin{cases} \mathscr{I}(\theta)^{-1}, & \theta \neq \theta_0, \\ 0, & \theta = \theta_0. \end{cases}$$

Thus, $\tilde{\theta}_n$ is a *superefficient* estimate.

Improving Subefficient Estimates. The method of moments ordinarily provides asymptotically normal estimates. Sometimes these estimates are asymptotically efficient [for example, in estimating θ in $\mathscr{P}(\theta)$ by $\overline{X}_n$, and (μ, σ^2) in $\mathscr{N}(\mu, \sigma^2)$ by $(\overline{X}_n, s_x^2)$, the method of moments and MLE coincide] but usually they are not. One would like to use MLE, but this has the disadvantage of being difficult to evaluate in general. The likelihood equations, $\dot{l}_n(\boldsymbol{\theta}) = \mathbf{0}$, are generally highly nonlinear and one must resort to numerical approximation methods to solve them. One good strategy is to use *Newton's method* with one of the simply computed estimates based on the method of moments or sample quantiles as the initial guess. This method takes the initial guess, $\hat{\boldsymbol{\theta}}^{(0)}$, and inductively generates a sequence of hopefully better and better estimates by

$$\hat{\boldsymbol{\theta}}^{(k+1)} = \hat{\boldsymbol{\theta}}^{(k)} - \ddot{l}_n(\boldsymbol{\theta}^{(k)})^{-1}\dot{l}_n(\hat{\boldsymbol{\theta}}^{(k)}), \qquad k = 0, 1, 2, \dots .$$

One simplification of this strategy can be made if the Fisher information matrix is available. Ordinarily, $(1/n)\ddot{l}_n(\hat{\boldsymbol{\theta}}^{(k)})$ will converge as $n \to \infty$ to $-\mathscr{I}(\boldsymbol{\theta})$ and so can be replaced by $-\mathscr{I}(\hat{\boldsymbol{\theta}}^{(k)})$ in the iterations.

$$\hat{\boldsymbol{\theta}}^{(k+1)} = \hat{\boldsymbol{\theta}}^{(k)} + \mathscr{I}(\hat{\boldsymbol{\theta}}^{(k)})^{-1}(1/n)\dot{l}_n(\hat{\boldsymbol{\theta}}^{(k)}), \qquad k = 0, 1, 2, \dots .$$

This is the *method of scoring*. The *scores*, $\mathscr{I}(\hat{\boldsymbol{\theta}}^{(k)})^{-1}(1/n)\dot{l}_n(\boldsymbol{\theta}^{(k)})$, are the increments added to an estimate to improve it.

Example 2. (*Logistic*) Let $X_1, X_2, \dots, X_n$ be a sample from density

$$f(x|\theta) = \frac{\exp\{-(x-\theta)\}}{(1+\exp\{-(x-\theta)\})^2}.$$

The log-likelihood function is

$$l_n(\theta) = -\sum_1^n (X_j - \theta) - 2\sum_1^n \log\big(1 + \exp\{-(X_j - \theta)\}\big),$$

and the likelihood equations are

$$\dot{l}_n(\theta) = n - 2\sum_1^n \frac{\exp\{-(X_j-\theta)\}}{1+\exp\{-(X_j-\theta)\}} = 0 \quad \text{or} \quad \frac{1}{n}\sum_1^n \frac{1}{1+\exp\{X_j-\theta\}} = \frac{1}{2}.$$

Newton's method is easy to apply here because

$$\ddot{l}_n(\theta) = -2\sum_1^n \frac{\exp\{X_j-\theta\}}{\left(\exp\{X_j-\theta\}+1\right)^2}.$$

Even easier is the method of scoring, since $\mathscr{I}(\boldsymbol{\theta}) = \frac{1}{3}$ [$\mathscr{I}(\boldsymbol{\theta})$ is a constant for location parameter families of distributions.] As an initial guess we may use the sample median, m_n, or the sample mean, $\overline{X}_n$. The asymptotic distributions are

$$\sqrt{n}\,(m_n - \theta) \xrightarrow{\mathscr{L}} \mathscr{N}\left(0, \frac{1}{4f(\theta|\theta)^2}\right) = \mathscr{N}(0,4),$$

$$\sqrt{n}\,(\overline{X}_n - \theta) \xrightarrow{\mathscr{L}} \mathscr{N}\left(0, \frac{\pi^2}{3}\right) = \mathscr{N}(0, 3.2899\ldots).$$

Since for the MLE, $\hat{\theta}_n$,

$$\sqrt{n}\,(\hat{\theta}_n - \theta) \xrightarrow{\mathscr{L}} \mathscr{N}(0, \mathscr{I}(\theta)^{-1}) = \mathscr{N}(0,3),$$

it would seem worthwhile to improve m_n or $\overline{X}_n$ by an iteration or two of

$$\hat{\theta}^{(k+1)} = \hat{\theta}^{(k)} + 3\left[1 - \frac{2}{n}\sum_1^n \frac{1}{\exp\{X_j - \hat{\theta}^{(k)}\} + 1}\right].$$

Example 3. (*Gamma*) Let $X_1, \ldots, X_n$ be a sample from density

$$f(x|\alpha, \beta) = 1/(\Gamma(\alpha)\beta^\alpha)\exp\{-x/\beta\}x^{\alpha-1}I(x > 0),$$

where $\alpha > 0$ and $\beta > 0$ are unknown. The log-likelihood function is

$$l_n(\alpha, \beta) = -n \log \Gamma(\alpha) - n\alpha \log \beta - (1/\beta)\sum_1^n X_j + (\alpha - 1)\log \prod X_j.$$

The likelihood equations are

$$-n\digamma(\alpha) - n \log \beta + \sum_1^n \log X_j = 0,$$

$$-\frac{n\alpha}{\beta} + \frac{1}{\beta^2}\sum_1^n X_j = 0,$$

where $\digamma(\alpha)$ is the digamma function. This simplifies to

$$\alpha\beta = \overline{X}_n$$

$$\digamma(\alpha) + \log \beta = \frac{1}{n}\sum_1^n \log X_j.$$

To solve these equations, we may use Newton's method with

$$\ddot{l}_n(\alpha,\beta) = -n\begin{bmatrix} \text{Ŧ}(\alpha) & \dfrac{1}{\beta} \\ \dfrac{1}{\beta} & \dfrac{2\overline{X}_n - \alpha\beta}{\beta^3} \end{bmatrix},$$

where $\text{Ŧ}(\alpha)$ is the trigamma function, or the method of scoring with

$$\mathscr{I}(\alpha,\beta) = \begin{bmatrix} \text{Ŧ}(\alpha) & \dfrac{1}{\beta} \\ \dfrac{1}{\beta} & \dfrac{\alpha}{\beta^2} \end{bmatrix}.$$

The scores are

$$\mathscr{I}(\alpha,\beta)^{-1}\frac{1}{n}\dot{l}_n(\alpha,\beta)$$

$$= \frac{1}{\alpha\text{Ŧ}(\alpha) - 1}\begin{bmatrix} \alpha & -\beta \\ -\beta & \beta^2\text{Ŧ}(\alpha) \end{bmatrix}\begin{bmatrix} \dfrac{1}{n}\sum_1^n \log X_j - \digamma(\alpha) - \log\beta \\ \dfrac{1}{\beta^2}\overline{X}_n - \dfrac{\alpha}{\beta} \end{bmatrix}$$

$$= \frac{1}{\alpha\text{Ŧ}(\alpha) - 1}\begin{bmatrix} \dfrac{\alpha}{n}\sum_1^n \log X_j - \alpha\digamma(\alpha) - \alpha\log\beta - \dfrac{1}{\beta}\left(\overline{X}_n - \alpha\beta\right) \\ -\dfrac{\beta}{n}\sum_1^n \log X_j + \beta\digamma(\alpha) + \beta\log\beta + \text{Ŧ}(\alpha)\left(\overline{X}_n - \alpha\beta\right) \end{bmatrix}.$$

As initial values, the method of moments may be used. This entails solving $\overline{X}_n = \alpha\beta$ and $s_x^2 = \alpha\beta^2$ for α and β: $\tilde{\alpha} = \overline{X}_n^2/s_x^2$ and $\tilde{\beta} = s_x^2/\overline{X}_n$.

In this example, one of the likelihood equations can be solved easily, $\alpha\beta = \overline{X}_n$, for β in terms of α say, $\beta = (1/\alpha)\overline{X}_n$, which may be substituted into the other equation. This gives one equation to be solved for α: $\Gamma\text{-}(\alpha) - \log\alpha = (1/n)\sum_1^n \log X_j - \log\overline{X}_n$. Newton's method on this equation leads to the iteration:

$$\alpha^{(k+1)} = \alpha^{(k)} + \frac{(1/n)\sum_1^n \log X_j - \log\overline{X}_n - \digamma(\alpha^{(k)}) + \log\alpha^{(k)}}{\text{Ŧ}(\alpha^{(k)}) - 1/\alpha^{(k)}}$$

Starting with $\alpha^{(0)} = \bar{X}_n^2/s_x^2$, this leads to the same sequence of estimates as above with initial values as given, since we will always have $\alpha^{(k)}\beta^{(k)} = \bar{X}_n$.

Once is Enough. In improving asymptotically normal estimates by scoring, one iteration is generally enough to achieve asymptotic efficiency!

Theorem 20. *Let $\tilde{\boldsymbol{\theta}}_n$ be a strongly consistent sequence such that $\sqrt{n}(\tilde{\boldsymbol{\theta}}_n - \boldsymbol{\theta}) \xrightarrow{\mathscr{L}} \mathscr{N}(\mathbf{0}, \boldsymbol{\Sigma}(\boldsymbol{\theta}))$ when $\boldsymbol{\theta}$ is the true value of the parameter, where $\boldsymbol{\Sigma}(\boldsymbol{\theta}) < \infty$ for all $\boldsymbol{\theta}$. Then under the assumptions of Theorem* 18, *both estimates*

$$\tilde{\boldsymbol{\theta}}_n^{(1)} = \tilde{\boldsymbol{\theta}}_n - \ddot{l}_n(\tilde{\boldsymbol{\theta}}_n)^{-1}\dot{l}_n(\tilde{\boldsymbol{\theta}}_n) \quad \text{and} \quad \boldsymbol{\theta}_n^* = \tilde{\boldsymbol{\theta}}_n + \mathscr{I}(\tilde{\boldsymbol{\theta}}_n)^{-1}(1/n)\dot{l}_n(\tilde{\boldsymbol{\theta}}_n)$$

are asymptotically equivalent to the MLE, and hence are asymptotically efficient.

Proof. Let $\hat{\boldsymbol{\theta}}_n$ be a strongly consistent sequence satisfying $\dot{l}_n(\hat{\boldsymbol{\theta}}_n) = \mathbf{0}$. Expanding $\dot{l}_n(\tilde{\boldsymbol{\theta}}_n)$ about $\hat{\boldsymbol{\theta}}_n$,

$$\dot{l}_n(\tilde{\boldsymbol{\theta}}_n) = \dot{l}_n(\hat{\boldsymbol{\theta}}_n) + \int_0^1 \ddot{l}_n\left(\hat{\boldsymbol{\theta}}_n + v(\tilde{\boldsymbol{\theta}}_n - \hat{\boldsymbol{\theta}}_n)\right) dv(\tilde{\boldsymbol{\theta}}_n - \hat{\boldsymbol{\theta}}_n),$$

and using

$$(\tilde{\boldsymbol{\theta}}_n^{(1)} - \hat{\boldsymbol{\theta}}_n) = (\tilde{\boldsymbol{\theta}}_n - \hat{\boldsymbol{\theta}}_n) - \ddot{l}_n(\tilde{\boldsymbol{\theta}}_n)^{-1}\dot{l}_n(\tilde{\boldsymbol{\theta}}_n),$$

we find

$$\sqrt{n}(\tilde{\boldsymbol{\theta}}_n^{(1)} - \hat{\boldsymbol{\theta}}_n) = \left[\mathbf{I} - \ddot{l}_n(\tilde{\boldsymbol{\theta}}_n)^{-1}\int_0^1 \ddot{l}_n\left(\hat{\boldsymbol{\theta}}_n + v(\tilde{\boldsymbol{\theta}}_n - \hat{\boldsymbol{\theta}}_n)\right) dv\right]\sqrt{n}(\tilde{\boldsymbol{\theta}}_n - \hat{\boldsymbol{\theta}}_n).$$

Because as in the proof of Theorem 18, $(1/n)\ddot{l}_n(\tilde{\boldsymbol{\theta}}_n) \xrightarrow{\text{a.s.}} -\mathscr{I}(\boldsymbol{\theta})$ and

$$\frac{1}{n}\int_0^1 \ddot{l}_n\left(\hat{\boldsymbol{\theta}}_n + v(\tilde{\boldsymbol{\theta}}_n - \hat{\boldsymbol{\theta}}_n)\right) dv \xrightarrow{\text{a.s.}} -\mathscr{I}(\boldsymbol{\theta})$$

from the Uniform Strong Law of Large Numbers, the term in square brackets converges to zero almost surely. The last term, $\sqrt{n}(\tilde{\boldsymbol{\theta}}_n - \hat{\boldsymbol{\theta}}_n) = \sqrt{n}(\tilde{\boldsymbol{\theta}}_n - \boldsymbol{\theta}) - \sqrt{n}(\hat{\boldsymbol{\theta}}_n - \boldsymbol{\theta})$, is bounded in probability because both terms are asymptotically normal. Hence, $\sqrt{n}(\tilde{\boldsymbol{\theta}}^{(1)} - \hat{\boldsymbol{\theta}}_n) \xrightarrow{\text{P}} \mathbf{0}$ as $n \to \infty$. The argument for $\boldsymbol{\theta}_n^*$ is identical. ■

EXERCISES

1. Show that Fisher Information is
   (a) $\mathscr{I}(\theta) = \frac{1}{3}$ for the logistic distribution $\mathscr{L}(\theta, 1)$.
   (b) $\mathscr{I}(\theta) = \frac{1}{2}$ for the Cauchy distribution $\mathscr{C}(\theta, 1)$.
2. Let $X_1, \ldots, X_n$ be a sample from the Cauchy distribution, $\mathscr{C}(\theta, 1)$. Find the likelihood equations. Find the scores. What is the asymptotic distribution of the median? What is the asymptotic distribution of the median improved by scoring?
3. Let $X_1, \ldots, X_n$ be a sample from a mixture of gamma distributions:
$$f(x \mid \theta) = [(1 - \theta)e^{-x} + \theta x e^{-x}]I \qquad (x > 0),$$
   where $0 < \theta < 1$. What is the estimate of θ given by the method of moments? What is its asymptotic distribution? Show how to improve this estimate by one iteration of Newton's method applied to the likelihood equation.
4. Let $X_1, \ldots, X_n$ be a sample from an exponential distribution with density $f(x \mid \theta) = \theta e^{-\theta x} I(x > 0)$, where $\theta > 0$ is an unknown parameter to be estimated.
   (a) Find the asymptotic efficiency of $\tilde{\theta}_n$, the estimate of θ given by the method of moments.
   (b) Show that, out of all distributions with mean $1/\theta$ and variance $1/\theta^2$ that satisfy the conditions of the Cramér–Rao inequality, Fisher Information is minimized by the above exponential distribution.

21

Asymptotic Normality of Posterior Distributions

Bayes estimates provide another class of asymptotically efficient estimates. We assume that $\boldsymbol{\theta}$ is chosen from Θ an open subset of $\mathbb{R}^k$ according to a prior density $g(\boldsymbol{\theta})$ with respect to Lebesgue measure, $d\boldsymbol{\theta}$, and that $g(\boldsymbol{\theta})$ is continuous and positive on Θ. The posterior density of $\boldsymbol{\theta}$, given a sample $X_1, \ldots, X_n$ from $f(x|\boldsymbol{\theta})$, is

$$g(\boldsymbol{\theta}|x_1,\ldots,x_n) = \frac{\left(\prod_1^n f(x_j|\boldsymbol{\theta})\right)g(\boldsymbol{\theta})}{\int_\Theta \left(\prod_1^n f(x_j|\boldsymbol{\theta})\right)g(\boldsymbol{\theta})\,d\boldsymbol{\theta}} = \frac{L_n(\boldsymbol{\theta})g(\boldsymbol{\theta})}{\int_\Theta L_n(\boldsymbol{\theta})g(\boldsymbol{\theta})\,d\boldsymbol{\theta}}.$$

The conclusion of the Bernstein–von Mises Theorem below is that this posterior density is close to a normal density centered at $\hat{\boldsymbol{\theta}}_n$, the MLE of Theorem 18, with variance $(1/n)\mathscr{I}(\boldsymbol{\theta}_0)^{-1}$ when $\boldsymbol{\theta}_0$ is the true value. More precisely, the conditional density of $\boldsymbol{\vartheta} = \sqrt{n}\,(\boldsymbol{\theta} - \hat{\boldsymbol{\theta}}_n)$ given the data,

$$f_n(\boldsymbol{\vartheta}|x_1,\ldots,x_n) = \frac{L_n\left((1/\sqrt{n}\,)\boldsymbol{\vartheta} + \hat{\boldsymbol{\theta}}_n\right)g\left(\frac{1}{\sqrt{n}}\boldsymbol{\vartheta} + \hat{\boldsymbol{\theta}}_n\right)}{\int L_n\left((1/\sqrt{n}\,)\boldsymbol{\vartheta} + \hat{\boldsymbol{\theta}}_n\right)g\left((1/\sqrt{n}\,)\boldsymbol{\vartheta} + \hat{\boldsymbol{\theta}}_n\right)d\boldsymbol{\vartheta}},$$

approaches the density of $\mathscr{N}(\mathbf{0}, \mathscr{I}(\boldsymbol{\theta}_0)^{-1})$ as $n \to \infty$,

$$\varphi(\boldsymbol{\vartheta}) = \frac{|\det \mathscr{I}(\boldsymbol{\theta}_0)|^{1/2}}{(2\pi)^{k/2}} \exp\left\{-\tfrac{1}{2}\boldsymbol{\vartheta}^T\mathscr{I}(\boldsymbol{\theta}_0)\boldsymbol{\vartheta}\right\}.$$

Note that this limiting posterior distribution is independent of the prior distribution, $g(\boldsymbol{\theta})$. This version of the theorem is due to Le Cam (1953).

Theorem 21 (Bernstein–von Mises). *Assume that $g(\boldsymbol{\theta})$ is continuous and that $g(\boldsymbol{\theta}) > 0$ for all $\boldsymbol{\theta} \in \Theta$. Under the assumptions of Theorem* 18,

$$\frac{L_n(\hat{\boldsymbol{\theta}}_n + \boldsymbol{\vartheta}/\sqrt{n})}{L_n(\hat{\boldsymbol{\theta}}_n)} g(\hat{\boldsymbol{\theta}}_n + \boldsymbol{\vartheta}/\sqrt{n}) \xrightarrow{\text{a.s.}} \exp\{-\tfrac{1}{2}\boldsymbol{\vartheta}^T \mathcal{I}(\boldsymbol{\theta}_0)\boldsymbol{\vartheta}\} g(\boldsymbol{\theta}_0),$$

where $\hat{\boldsymbol{\theta}}_n$ is the strongly consistent sequence of roots of the likelihood equation of Theorem 18. *If, in addition,*

$$\int \frac{L_n(\hat{\boldsymbol{\theta}}_n + \boldsymbol{\vartheta}/\sqrt{n})}{L_n(\hat{\boldsymbol{\theta}}_n)} g(\hat{\boldsymbol{\theta}}_n + \boldsymbol{\vartheta}/\sqrt{n})\, d\boldsymbol{\vartheta} \xrightarrow{\text{a.s.}} \int \exp\{-\tfrac{1}{2}\boldsymbol{\vartheta}^T \mathcal{I}(\boldsymbol{\theta}_0)\boldsymbol{\vartheta}\}\, d\boldsymbol{\vartheta}\, g(\boldsymbol{\theta}_0),$$

then

$$\int |f_n(\boldsymbol{\vartheta}|x_1, \ldots, x_n) - \varphi(\boldsymbol{\vartheta})|\, d\boldsymbol{\vartheta} \xrightarrow{\text{a.s.}} 0.$$

Proof. $L_n(\boldsymbol{\theta}) = \exp\{l_n(\boldsymbol{\theta})\}$. Expand $l_n(\boldsymbol{\theta})$ about $\hat{\boldsymbol{\theta}}_n$:

$$l_n(\boldsymbol{\theta}) = l_n(\hat{\boldsymbol{\theta}}_n) + \dot{l}_n(\boldsymbol{\theta})(\boldsymbol{\theta} - \hat{\boldsymbol{\theta}}_n) - n(\boldsymbol{\theta} - \hat{\boldsymbol{\theta}}_n)^T \mathbf{I}_n(\boldsymbol{\theta})(\boldsymbol{\theta} - \hat{\boldsymbol{\theta}}_n),$$

where

$$\mathbf{I}_n(\boldsymbol{\theta}) = -\frac{1}{n}\int_0^1\int_0^1 v\ddot{l}(\hat{\boldsymbol{\theta}}_n + uv(\boldsymbol{\theta} - \hat{\boldsymbol{\theta}}_n))\, du\, dv.$$

With probability 1, $\dot{l}_n(\hat{\boldsymbol{\theta}}_n) = \mathbf{0}$ for n sufficiently large, so

$$\frac{L_n(\boldsymbol{\theta})}{L_n(\hat{\boldsymbol{\theta}}_n)} = \exp\left\{-n(\boldsymbol{\theta} - \hat{\boldsymbol{\theta}}_n)^T \mathbf{I}_n(\boldsymbol{\theta})(\boldsymbol{\theta} - \hat{\boldsymbol{\theta}}_n)\right\}.$$

Since $(1/n)\ddot{l}_n(\boldsymbol{\theta})$ converges uniformly to $E_{\boldsymbol{\theta}_0}\dot{\boldsymbol{\psi}}(X, \boldsymbol{\theta})$ in a neighborhood of $\boldsymbol{\theta}_0$ (as in the proof of Theorem 18), and $E_{\boldsymbol{\theta}_0}\dot{\boldsymbol{\psi}}(X, \boldsymbol{\theta})$ is continuous in $\boldsymbol{\theta}$ and equal to $-\mathcal{I}(\boldsymbol{\theta}_0)$ at $\boldsymbol{\theta} = \boldsymbol{\theta}_0$,

$$I_n(\hat{\boldsymbol{\theta}}_n + \boldsymbol{\vartheta}/\sqrt{n}) = -\frac{1}{n}\int_0^1\int_0^1 v\ddot{l}(\hat{\boldsymbol{\theta}}_n + uv\boldsymbol{\vartheta}/\sqrt{n})\, du\, dv \to \tfrac{1}{2}\mathcal{I}(\boldsymbol{\theta}_0).$$

Hence,

$$\begin{aligned}
&\frac{L_n(\hat{\boldsymbol{\theta}}_n + \boldsymbol{\vartheta}/\sqrt{n})}{L_n(\hat{\boldsymbol{\theta}}_n)} g(\hat{\boldsymbol{\theta}}_n + \boldsymbol{\vartheta}/\sqrt{n}) \\
&\quad = \exp\left\{-\tfrac{1}{2}\boldsymbol{\vartheta}^T \mathbf{I}_n(\hat{\boldsymbol{\theta}}_n + \boldsymbol{\vartheta}/\sqrt{n})\boldsymbol{\vartheta}\right\} g(\hat{\boldsymbol{\theta}}_n + \boldsymbol{\vartheta}/\sqrt{n}) \\
&\quad \xrightarrow{\text{a.s.}} \exp\{-\tfrac{1}{2}\boldsymbol{\vartheta}^T \mathcal{I}(\boldsymbol{\theta}_0)\boldsymbol{\vartheta}\} g(\boldsymbol{\theta}_0).
\end{aligned}$$

The final sentence of the theorem follows directly from Scheffé's Theorem. ■

Example. Let $X_1, \dots, X_n$ be i.i.d. $\mathscr{G}(1, 1/\theta)$, $f(x|\theta) = \theta e^{-\theta x} I\ (x > 0)$ and let the prior distribution be $\mathscr{G}(1, 1)$, $g(\theta) = e^{-\theta} I\ (\theta > 0)$. The posterior distribution is

$$g(\theta | x_1, \dots, x_n) \propto \theta^n \exp\left\{ -\theta \left(\sum_1^n X_i + 1 \right) \right\} I(\theta > 0),$$

namely $\mathscr{G}(n+1, 1/(\Sigma_1^n X_i + 1))$. Because $l_n(\theta) = n \log \theta - \theta \Sigma_1^n X_i$, and $\dot{l}_n(\theta) = (n/\theta) - \Sigma_1^n X_i$, the MLE is $\hat{\theta}_n = 1/\overline{X}_n$. Fisher Information is $\mathscr{I}(\theta) = 1/\theta^2$, so the Bernstein–von Mises Theorem says that the posterior distribution of $\sqrt{n}(\theta - 1/\overline{X}_n)$ should be asymptotically $\mathscr{N}(0, \theta_0^2)$. This can be seen directly. In $\mathscr{G}(\alpha, \beta)$, β is a scale parameter, so the distribution of $(\Sigma_1^n X_i + 1)\theta$ given $X_1, \dots, X_n$ is $\mathscr{G}(n+1, 1)$, which being the sum of $n+1$ independent $\mathscr{G}(1,1)$s is asymptotically normal with mean $n+1$ and variance $n+1$, from the Central Limit Theorem. That is,

$$\frac{\left((n\overline{X}_n + 1)\theta - (n+1) \right)}{\sqrt{n+1}} \xrightarrow{\mathscr{L}} \mathscr{N}(0, 1).$$

Since $\overline{X}_n \xrightarrow{\text{a.s}} 1/\theta_0$, we may conclude almost surely,

$$\sqrt{n}\,\overline{X}_n \left(\theta - \frac{1 + 1/n}{\overline{X}_n + 1/n} \right) \xrightarrow{\mathscr{L}} \mathscr{N}(0, 1),$$

and hence

$$\sqrt{n} \left(\theta - \frac{1}{\overline{X}_n} \right) \xrightarrow{\mathscr{L}} \mathscr{N}(0, \theta_0^2).$$

The Bernstein–von Mises Theorem concludes something slightly stronger, namely, that the density of $\sqrt{n}(\theta - (1/\overline{X}_n))$ converges almost surely to the density of $\mathscr{N}(0, \theta_0^2)$.

Asymptotic Efficiency of Bayes Estimates. Suppose the loss is squared error, $L(\boldsymbol{\theta}, \mathbf{a}) = (\boldsymbol{\theta} - \mathbf{a})^T(\boldsymbol{\theta} - \mathbf{a})$, so that the Bayes estimate given a sample $X_1, \dots, X_n$ is $\tilde{\boldsymbol{\theta}}_n = E(\boldsymbol{\theta} | X_1, \dots, X_n)$. Assume we can interchange expectation and the limit in the Bernstein–von Mises Theorem; that is, assume that the conditional expectation of $\boldsymbol{\vartheta} = \sqrt{n}(\boldsymbol{\theta} - \hat{\boldsymbol{\theta}}_n)$ given $X_1, \dots, X_n$ converges almost surely to zero. Then $\sqrt{n}(\tilde{\boldsymbol{\theta}}_n - \hat{\boldsymbol{\theta}}_n) \to \mathbf{0}$ so that the Bayes estimate and the MLE are asymptotically equivalent ($\tilde{\boldsymbol{\theta}}_n$ is much closer to $\hat{\boldsymbol{\theta}}_n$ than to $\boldsymbol{\theta}_0$). Hence,

$$\sqrt{n}\left(\tilde{\boldsymbol{\theta}}_n - \boldsymbol{\theta}_0\right) \xrightarrow{\mathscr{L}} \mathscr{N}\left(\mathbf{0}, \mathscr{I}(\boldsymbol{\theta}_0)^{-1}\right);$$

that is, the Bayes estimate is asymptotically efficient.

Using this, we can give a stronger version of the asymptotic optimality of asymptotically efficient estimates. Although an asymptotically efficient sequence of estimates can be improved asymptotically at a single parameter point by the method of Hodges, and similarly for any finite set of points or even a countable set of points, such estimates cannot be improved on a set of positive measure. Suppose that $\boldsymbol{\theta}_n^*$ is a sequence of estimates such that $\sqrt{n}\,(\boldsymbol{\theta}_n^* - \boldsymbol{\theta}_0) \xrightarrow{\mathscr{L}} \mathscr{N}(\mathbf{0}, \boldsymbol{\Sigma}(\boldsymbol{\theta}_0))$ when $\boldsymbol{\theta}_0$ is the true value of $\boldsymbol{\theta}$ and that $\boldsymbol{\Sigma}(\boldsymbol{\theta}) \leq \mathscr{I}(\boldsymbol{\theta})^{-1}$ for all $\boldsymbol{\theta}$ and $\boldsymbol{\Sigma}(\boldsymbol{\theta}) < \mathscr{I}(\boldsymbol{\theta})^{-1}$ for $\boldsymbol{\theta}$ in a set of positive measure. Then again assuming interchange of expectation and limit,

$$\int E_{\boldsymbol{\theta}}(\boldsymbol{\theta}_n^* - \boldsymbol{\theta})^2 g(\boldsymbol{\theta})\, d\boldsymbol{\theta} < \int E_{\boldsymbol{\theta}}\left(\tilde{\boldsymbol{\theta}}_n - \boldsymbol{\theta}\right)^2 g(\boldsymbol{\theta})\, d\boldsymbol{\theta}$$

for n sufficiently large, contradicting the assumption that $\tilde{\boldsymbol{\theta}}_n$ is Bayes with respect to $g(\boldsymbol{\theta})\, d\boldsymbol{\theta}$. In other words, no sequence of estimates can improve asymptotically on the MLE (or any asymptotically efficient estimate) on a set of positive measure.

EXERCISES

1. Let $X_1, \ldots, X_n$ be a sample from the Poisson distribution with probability mass function, $f(x|\theta) = e^{-\theta}\theta^x/x!$ for $x = 0, 1, 2, \ldots$, where $\theta > 0$. Suppose that the prior distribution of θ is the inverse power distribution with density, $g(\theta) = 1/(\theta + 1)^2$ for $\theta > 0$. What approximately is the posterior density of θ, $g(\theta|X_1, \ldots, X_n)$, for large n? In what sense is this approximation valid?
2. (A Bernstein–von Mises type of result for a nonregular distribution.) Let $X_1, \ldots, X_n$ be a sample from the uniform distribution on the interval $(0, \theta)$, where $\theta \in \Theta = (0, \infty)$. Assume that the prior distribution of θ has a density, $g(\theta)$, that is bounded, continuous, and positive on Θ. Let θ_0 denote the true value of θ, and let $M_n = \max\{X_1, \ldots, X_n\} =$ MLE of θ. Show that the posterior density of $\vartheta = n(\theta - M_n)$ given $X_1, \ldots, X_n$ converges to the density of the exponential distribution with mean θ_0.

22

Asymptotic Distribution of the Likelihood Ratio Test Statistic

Let $X_1, \ldots, X_n$ be a sample from density $f(x|\boldsymbol{\theta})$ where $\boldsymbol{\theta} \subset \Theta \subset \mathbb{R}^k$. The likelihood ratio test provides a general method for testing H_0: $\boldsymbol{\theta} \in \Theta_0$ versus H_1: $\boldsymbol{\theta} \in \Theta - \Theta_0$ for a given subset Θ_0 of Θ. This tests rejects H_0 when the likelihood ratio test statistic,

$$\lambda_n = \frac{\sup_{\boldsymbol{\theta} \in \Theta_0} \prod_1^n f(x_j|\boldsymbol{\theta})}{\sup_{\boldsymbol{\theta} \in \Theta} \prod_1^n f(x_j|\boldsymbol{\theta})} = \frac{L_n(\boldsymbol{\theta}_n^*)}{L_n(\hat{\boldsymbol{\theta}}_n)} \tag{1}$$

is too small, where $\boldsymbol{\theta}_n^*$ is the MLE over Θ_0, and $\hat{\boldsymbol{\theta}}_n$ is the MLE over Θ. When the sample size is large, evaluation of a cutoff point can be facilitated in many important situations by the following theorem. These situations occur when Θ_0 is a $(k - r)$-dimensional subspace of Θ. Writing the components of the vector $\boldsymbol{\theta} \in \mathbb{R}^k$ as $\boldsymbol{\theta}^T = (\theta^1, \theta^2, \ldots, \theta^k)$, we assume the null hypothesis is of the form

$$H_0: \qquad \theta^1 = \theta^2 = \cdots = \theta^r = 0 \tag{2}$$

where $1 \le r \le k$. More general situations, in which H_0 is of the form H_0: $g_1(\boldsymbol{\theta}) = \cdots = g_r(\boldsymbol{\theta}) = 0$ for some smooth real-valued functions $g_1, \ldots, g_r$, can be put into this form by a reparametrization. The integer r represents the number of restrictions under the null hypothesis.

Theorem 22 [Wilks (1938)]. *Suppose the assumptions of Theorem* 18 *are satisfied and that* H_0: $\theta^1 = \theta^2 = \cdots = \theta^r = 0$ *where* $1 \le r \le k$. *Suppose that the true value* $\boldsymbol{\theta}_0$ *satisfies* H_0. *Then*

$$-2\log\lambda_n \xrightarrow{\mathscr{L}} \chi_r^2. \tag{3}$$

Proof. $-2\log\lambda_n = 2[l_n(\hat{\boldsymbol{\theta}}_n) - l_n(\boldsymbol{\theta}_n^*)]$ where $\hat{\boldsymbol{\theta}}_n$ = MLE over Θ, and $\boldsymbol{\theta}_n^*$ = MLE over Θ_0. Expand $l_n(\boldsymbol{\theta}_n^*)$ about $\hat{\boldsymbol{\theta}}_n$:

$$l_n(\boldsymbol{\theta}_n^*) = l_n(\hat{\boldsymbol{\theta}}_n) + \dot{l}_n(\hat{\boldsymbol{\theta}}_n)(\boldsymbol{\theta}_n^* - \hat{\boldsymbol{\theta}}_n) - n(\boldsymbol{\theta}_n^* - \hat{\boldsymbol{\theta}}_n)^T \mathbf{I}_n(\boldsymbol{\theta}_n^*)(\boldsymbol{\theta}_n^* - \hat{\boldsymbol{\theta}}_n),$$

where

$$\mathbf{I}_n(\boldsymbol{\theta}_n^*) = -\frac{1}{n}\int_0^1\int_0^1 v\ddot{l}_n\big(\hat{\boldsymbol{\theta}}_n + uv(\boldsymbol{\theta}_n^* - \hat{\boldsymbol{\theta}}_n)\big)\,du\,dv \xrightarrow{\text{a.s.}} \frac{1}{2}\mathscr{I}(\boldsymbol{\theta}_0),$$

as in the proof of Theorem 18. For sufficiently large n, $\dot{l}_n(\hat{\boldsymbol{\theta}}_n) = \mathbf{0}$, so

$$\begin{aligned} -2\log\lambda_n &= 2n(\boldsymbol{\theta}_n^* - \hat{\boldsymbol{\theta}}_n)^T \mathbf{I}_n(\boldsymbol{\theta}_n^*)(\boldsymbol{\theta}_n^* - \hat{\boldsymbol{\theta}}_n) \\ &\sim n(\boldsymbol{\theta}_n^* - \hat{\boldsymbol{\theta}}_n)^T \mathscr{I}(\boldsymbol{\theta}_0)(\boldsymbol{\theta}_n^* - \hat{\boldsymbol{\theta}}_n). \end{aligned} \tag{4}$$

If H_0 were simple, say H_0: $\boldsymbol{\theta} = \boldsymbol{\theta}_0$, then $\boldsymbol{\theta}_n^* = \boldsymbol{\theta}_0$ and we would be finished, because we know $\sqrt{n}(\hat{\boldsymbol{\theta}}_n - \boldsymbol{\theta}_0) \xrightarrow{\mathscr{L}} \mathscr{N}(\mathbf{0}, \mathscr{I}(\boldsymbol{\theta}_0)^{-1})$. To find the asymptotic distribution of $\sqrt{n}(\boldsymbol{\theta}_n^* - \hat{\boldsymbol{\theta}}_n)$ in general, expand $\dot{l}_n(\boldsymbol{\theta}_n^*)$ about $\hat{\boldsymbol{\theta}}_n$:

$$\begin{aligned} \frac{1}{\sqrt{n}}\dot{l}_n(\boldsymbol{\theta}_n^*) &= \frac{1}{\sqrt{n}}\dot{l}_n(\hat{\boldsymbol{\theta}}_n) + \frac{1}{n}\int_0^1 \ddot{l}_n\big(\hat{\boldsymbol{\theta}}_n + v(\boldsymbol{\theta}_n^* - \hat{\boldsymbol{\theta}}_n)\big)\,dv\sqrt{n}\,(\boldsymbol{\theta}_n^* - \hat{\boldsymbol{\theta}}_n) \\ &\sim -\mathscr{I}(\theta_0)\sqrt{n}\,(\boldsymbol{\theta}_n^* - \hat{\boldsymbol{\theta}}_n) \end{aligned}$$

Thus

$$\sqrt{n}\,(\boldsymbol{\theta}_n^* - \hat{\boldsymbol{\theta}}_n) \sim -\mathscr{I}(\theta_0)^{-1}\frac{1}{\sqrt{n}}\dot{l}_n(\boldsymbol{\theta}_n^*) \tag{5}$$

and

$$-2\log\lambda_n \sim \frac{1}{\sqrt{n}}\dot{l}_n(\boldsymbol{\theta}_n^*)^T \mathscr{I}(\theta_0)^{-1}\frac{1}{\sqrt{n}}\dot{l}_n(\boldsymbol{\theta}_n^*). \tag{6}$$

To find the asymptotic distribution of $\dot{l}_n(\boldsymbol{\theta}_n^*)$, expand about $\boldsymbol{\theta}_0$:

$$\frac{1}{\sqrt{n}}\dot{l}_n(\boldsymbol{\theta}_n^*) = \frac{1}{\sqrt{n}}\dot{l}_n(\boldsymbol{\theta}_0) + \frac{1}{n}\int_0^1 \ddot{l}_n(\boldsymbol{\theta}_0 + v(\boldsymbol{\theta}_n^* - \boldsymbol{\theta}_0))\, dv \sqrt{n}\,(\boldsymbol{\theta}_n^* - \boldsymbol{\theta}_0). \tag{7}$$

Partition $\mathscr{I}(\boldsymbol{\theta}_0)$ into four matrices,

$$\mathscr{I}(\boldsymbol{\theta}_0) = \begin{bmatrix} \underset{\mathbf{G}_1}{r \times r} & \underset{\mathbf{G}_2}{r \times (k-r)} \\ \underset{\mathbf{G}_2^T}{(k-r) \times r} & \underset{\mathbf{G}_3}{(k-r) \times (k-r)} \end{bmatrix},$$

and let

$$\mathbf{H} = \begin{bmatrix} \mathbf{0} & \mathbf{0} \\ \mathbf{0} & \mathbf{G}_3^{-1} \end{bmatrix}.$$

Note that the last $k - r$ components of $\dot{l}_n(\boldsymbol{\theta}_n^*)$ are zero, so that $\mathbf{H}\dot{l}_n(\boldsymbol{\theta}_n^*) = \mathbf{0}$ and

$$\mathbf{H}\frac{1}{\sqrt{n}}\dot{l}_n(\boldsymbol{\theta}_0) \sim \mathbf{H}\mathscr{I}(\theta_0)\sqrt{n}\,(\boldsymbol{\theta}_n^* - \boldsymbol{\theta}_0) = \sqrt{n}\,(\boldsymbol{\theta}_n^* - \boldsymbol{\theta}_0)$$

since the first r components of $\boldsymbol{\theta}_n^*$ and $\boldsymbol{\theta}_0$ are zero. Substituting into Eq. (7), we find

$$\frac{1}{\sqrt{n}}\dot{l}_n(\boldsymbol{\theta}_n^*) \sim [\mathbf{I} - \mathscr{I}(\boldsymbol{\theta}_0)\mathbf{H}]\frac{1}{\sqrt{n}}\dot{l}_n(\boldsymbol{\theta}_0).$$

From the Central Limit Theorem,

$$\frac{1}{\sqrt{n}}\dot{l}_n(\boldsymbol{\theta}_0) = \sqrt{n}\left(\frac{1}{n}\dot{l}_n(\boldsymbol{\theta}_0)\right) \xrightarrow{\mathscr{L}} \mathscr{N}(\mathbf{0}, \mathscr{I}(\boldsymbol{\theta}_0)).$$

Hence,

$$\frac{1}{\sqrt{n}}\dot{l}_n(\boldsymbol{\theta}_n^*) \xrightarrow{\mathscr{L}} [\mathbf{I} - \mathscr{I}(\boldsymbol{\theta}_0)\mathbf{H}]\mathbf{Y}, \qquad \text{where } \mathbf{Y} \in \mathscr{N}(\mathbf{0}, \mathscr{I}(\boldsymbol{\theta}_0)),$$

so that from Eq. (6),

$$-2\log\lambda_n \xrightarrow{\mathscr{L}} \mathbf{Y}^T[\mathbf{I}-\mathscr{I}(\boldsymbol{\theta}_0)\mathbf{H}]^T\mathscr{I}(\boldsymbol{\theta}_0)^{-1}[\mathbf{I}-\mathscr{I}(\boldsymbol{\theta}_0)\mathbf{H}]\mathbf{Y}$$

$$= \mathbf{Y}^T\left[\mathscr{I}(\boldsymbol{\theta}_0)^{-1}-\mathbf{H}\right]\mathbf{Y} \qquad [\text{because } \mathbf{H}\mathscr{I}(\boldsymbol{\theta}_0)\mathbf{H}=\mathbf{H}]$$

$$= \mathbf{Z}^T\mathscr{I}(\boldsymbol{\theta}_0)^{1/2}\left[\mathscr{I}(\boldsymbol{\theta}_0)^{-1}-\mathbf{H}\right]\mathscr{I}(\boldsymbol{\theta}_0)^{1/2}\mathbf{Z},$$

where $\mathbf{Z}=\mathscr{I}(\boldsymbol{\theta}_0)^{-1/2}\mathbf{Y}\in\mathscr{N}(\mathbf{0},\mathbf{I})$). It is easily checked that the matrix $\mathbf{P}=\mathscr{I}(\boldsymbol{\theta}_0)^{1/2}[\mathscr{I}(\boldsymbol{\theta}_0)^{-1}-\mathbf{H}[\mathscr{I}(\boldsymbol{\theta}_0)^{1/2}$ is a projection and that $\text{rank}(\mathbf{P})=\text{trace}(\mathbf{P})=\text{trace}(\mathscr{I}(\boldsymbol{\theta}_0)[\mathscr{I}(\boldsymbol{\theta}_0)^{-1}-\mathbf{H}])=\text{trace}(\mathbf{I}-\mathscr{I}(\boldsymbol{\theta}_0)\mathbf{H})=r$. Therefore $-2\log\lambda_n\xrightarrow{\mathscr{L}}\mathbf{Z}^T\mathbf{P}\mathbf{Z}\in\chi_r^2$, as was to be shown. ■

Note: The maximum-likelihood estimates that appear in the definition of λ_n may be replaced by any of the efficient estimates, such as those of Sections 18 and 19, without disturbing the asymptotic distribution of $-2\log\lambda_n$.

Example 1. Let $X_1,\ldots,X_n$ be a sample from $\mathscr{N}(\mu,\sigma^2)$. Find the likelihood ratio test of the hypothesis H_0: $\mu=0$, $\sigma=1$. Here $r=2$ and

$$L_n(\mu,\sigma)=\left[\frac{1}{\sqrt{2\pi}\,\sigma}\right]^n\exp\left\{-\frac{1}{2\sigma^2}\sum_1^n(X_j-\mu)^2\right\},$$

so that

$$\lambda_n=\frac{L_n(0,1)}{L_n(\overline{X},s)}=\frac{\exp\left\{-\frac{1}{2}\sum_1^n X_j^2\right\}}{s^{-n}\exp\{-n/2\}},$$

since the maximum-likelihood estimates of (μ,σ) under Θ are $\hat{\mu}=\overline{X}$, and $\hat{\sigma}^2=s^2=(1/n)\Sigma_1^n(X_i-\overline{X})^2$. Hence,

$$-2\log\lambda_n=-n\log s^2+\sum_1^n X_j^2-n\xrightarrow{\mathscr{L}}\chi_2^2$$

when H_0 is true. At the 5% level, we reject H_0 if

$$-2\log\lambda_n>\chi^2_{2;\,0.05}=2\log 20=5.99\ldots.$$

Example 2. Let $X_1, \ldots, X_c$ have a multinomial distribution based on n trials, each resulting in one of c outcomes (cells) with respective probabilities $p_1, \ldots, p_c$, where $p_i > 0$ for all i, and $\sum_1^c p_i = 1$. Thus,

$$L_n(p_1, \ldots, p_c) = \binom{n}{x_1 \ldots x_c} \prod_1^c p_j^{x_j}$$

provided X_i are integers ≥ 0, and $\sum_1^c X_i = n$. Consider testing the hypothesis H_0: $p_1 = \cdots = p_c = 1/c$. Even though it appears that there are c restrictions, we have $r = c - 1$ because of the original constraint $\sum_1^c p_i = 1$. The maximum-likelihood estimates of the p_i under Θ are $\hat{p}_i = X_i/n$ for $i = 1, \ldots, c$. Hence,

$$\lambda_n = \frac{\binom{n}{x_1 \cdots x_c} \prod_1^c (1/c)^{x_j}}{\binom{n}{x_1 \cdots x_c} \prod_1^c (x_j/n)^{x_j}} = \prod_1^c \left(\frac{n}{cx_j}\right)^{x_j}$$

and

$$-2 \log \lambda_n = 2 \sum_1^c x_j \log\left(\frac{cx_j}{n}\right) \xrightarrow{\mathscr{L}} \chi^2_{c-1}$$

under H_0. The usual test of H_0 in this situation is of course Pearson's χ^2.

Power. We may also find an approximation to the power of the likelihood ratio test at an alternative close to the null hypothesis. Suppose that $\boldsymbol{\theta}$ is the true value and that $\boldsymbol{\theta}_0$ is the parameter point in H_0 that is closest to $\boldsymbol{\theta}$. Define $\boldsymbol{\delta} = \sqrt{n}(\boldsymbol{\theta} - \boldsymbol{\theta}_0)$. As in the discussion of the power of Pearson's χ^2 test, we take $\boldsymbol{\theta}$ to be converging to $\boldsymbol{\theta}_0$ in such a way that $\boldsymbol{\delta}$ is fixed. In the proof of Theorem 22, this changes the limiting distribution of $(1/\sqrt{n})\dot{l}_n(\boldsymbol{\theta}_0)$. It may be found by the expansion,

$$\frac{1}{\sqrt{n}}\dot{l}_n(\boldsymbol{\theta}_0) = \frac{1}{\sqrt{n}}\dot{l}_n(\boldsymbol{\theta}) + \frac{1}{n}\ddot{l}_n(\boldsymbol{\theta})\sqrt{n}(\boldsymbol{\theta}_0 - \boldsymbol{\theta})$$

$$\xrightarrow{\mathscr{L}} \mathbf{Y} = \mathscr{N}(\mathbf{0}, \mathscr{I}(\boldsymbol{\theta}_0)) + \mathscr{I}(\boldsymbol{\theta}_0)\boldsymbol{\delta} = \mathscr{N}(\mathscr{I}(\boldsymbol{\theta}_0)\boldsymbol{\delta}, \mathscr{I}(\boldsymbol{\theta}_0)).$$

As before, if we let $\mathbf{Z} = \mathscr{I}(\boldsymbol{\theta}_0)^{-1/2}\mathbf{Y}$, then $-2\log\lambda_n \xrightarrow{\mathscr{L}} \mathbf{Z}^T\mathbf{P}\mathbf{Z}$, where $\mathbf{P} = \mathscr{I}(\boldsymbol{\theta}_0)^{1/2}[\mathscr{I}(\boldsymbol{\theta}_0)^{-1} - \mathbf{H}[\mathscr{I}(\boldsymbol{\theta}_0)^{1/2}$ is a projection of rank r, but this time $\mathbf{Z} \in \mathscr{N}(\mathscr{I}(\boldsymbol{\theta}_0)^{1/2}\boldsymbol{\delta}, \mathbf{I}))$ so that (see Exercise 4),

$$-2\log\lambda_n \xrightarrow{\mathscr{L}} \mathbf{Z}^T\mathbf{P}\mathbf{Z} \in \chi_r^2(\varphi),$$

where the noncentrality parameter φ is

$$\varphi = \boldsymbol{\delta}^T \mathscr{I}(\boldsymbol{\theta}_0)^{1/2} \mathbf{P} \mathscr{I}(\boldsymbol{\theta}_0)^{1/2} \boldsymbol{\delta} = \boldsymbol{\delta}^T \mathscr{I}(\boldsymbol{\theta}_0) \left[\mathscr{I}(\boldsymbol{\theta}_0)^{-1} - \mathbf{H} \right] \mathscr{I}(\boldsymbol{\theta}_0) \boldsymbol{\delta}.$$

If we use the form of $\mathscr{I}(\boldsymbol{\theta})$ in terms of the matrices $\mathbf{G}_1$, $\mathbf{G}_2$, and $\mathbf{G}_3$, the noncentrality parameter φ reduces to the simpler form,

$$\varphi = \boldsymbol{\delta}_r^T (\mathbf{G}_1 - \mathbf{G}_2 \mathbf{G}_3^{-1} \mathbf{G}_2^T) \boldsymbol{\delta}_r,$$

where $\boldsymbol{\delta}_r$ is the vector of the first r components of $\boldsymbol{\delta}$. Note the effect of nuisance parameters. If $\theta_{r+1}, \ldots, \theta_k$ were known, the noncentrality parameter would be $\boldsymbol{\delta}_r^T \mathbf{G}_1 \boldsymbol{\delta}_r$.

Example 1 (continued). Let us find the approximate power at the alternative $\mu = 0.2$, $\sigma = 1.2$, when $n = 50$ and the test is conducted at the 5% level. First we compute $\boldsymbol{\delta}^T = \sqrt{n}\,(0.2, 0.2)$. To compute φ, recall that Fisher Information for the normal distribution is

$$\mathscr{I}(\mu, \sigma) = \begin{bmatrix} 1/\sigma^2 & 0 \\ 0 & 2/\sigma^2 \end{bmatrix}.$$

In this problem the matrix $\mathbf{H}$ is empty, so that $\varphi = \boldsymbol{\delta}^T \mathscr{I}(0, 1) \boldsymbol{\delta} = 6$. From the Fix Tables (Table 3) of the power of χ_2^2, we find a power of approximately $\beta = 0.58$. To get a power of 0.9 at this alternative, we need φ to be about 12.655, so we must increase n to about 106.

Note that in the calculation of the information matrix in φ we used the null hypothesis value, $\sigma = 1$, but from the point of view of the asymptotic theory, the true value, $\sigma = 1.2$, should serve as well. However, this would give a smaller value of φ, $\varphi = 4.167$, and a power of about $\beta = 0.43$. The sample size is not yet large enough to smooth out this difference. Perhaps a better approximation to the power would be given using the compromise value, $\sigma = 1.1$ ($\beta = 0.50$).

EXERCISES

1. Let $X_1, \ldots, X_n$ be a sample from $\mathscr{N}(\mu_x, \sigma_x^2)$ and $Y_1, \ldots, Y_n$ be an independent sample from $\mathscr{N}(\mu_y, \sigma_y^2)$. Find the likelihood ratio test for testing H_0: $\mu_x = \mu_y$ and $\sigma_x^2 = \sigma_y^2$ and state its asymptotic distribution.
2. Let $X_1, \ldots, X_n$ be a sample from the exponential distribution with density $f(x|\theta) = \theta \exp\{-\theta x\} I\ (x > 0)$ and $Y_1, \ldots, Y_n$ be an independent sample from $f(y|\mu) = \mu \exp\{-\mu y\} I\ (y > 0)$. Find the likelihood ratio test and its asymptotic distribution for testing H_0: $\mu = 2\theta$.

3. For $i = 1, \ldots, k$, let $X_{i1}, X_{i2}, \ldots, X_{in}$ be independent samples from Poisson distributions, $\mathscr{P}(\theta_i)$, respectively. Find the likelihood ratio test and its asymptotic distribution, for testing H_0: $\theta_1 = \theta_2 = \cdots = \theta_k$.
4. Show that if $\mathbf{Z} \in \mathscr{N}(\boldsymbol{\delta}, \mathbf{I}))$ and if $\mathbf{P}$ is a symmetric projection of rank r, then $\mathbf{Z}^T\mathbf{P}\mathbf{Z} \in \chi_r^2(\boldsymbol{\delta}^T\mathbf{P}\boldsymbol{\delta})$.
5. (a) Consider the likelihood ratio test of H_0: $\mu = 0$ against all alternatives based on a sample of size $n = 1000$ from a normal distribution with mean μ and unknown standard deviation σ. What is the approximate distribution of $-2\log\lambda_n$ if the true values of the parameters are $\mu = 0.1$ and $\sigma = \sigma_0$ for some fixed σ_0?
   (b) Suppose instead the distribution is $\mathscr{G}(\alpha, \beta)$ and H_0: $\alpha = 1$ with β unknown. What is the approximate distribution of $-2\log\lambda_n$ if the true values of the parameters are $\alpha = 1.1$ and $\beta = \beta_0$? (Note that this distribution is independent of β_0.)
6. *One-Sided Likelihood Ratio Tests.* The likelihood ratio test against one-sided alternatives is more complex and is no longer asymptotically distribution-free under the null hypothesis. This may be illustrated in testing H_0: $\boldsymbol{\theta} = \boldsymbol{\theta}_0$ when $\boldsymbol{\theta}$ is two-dimensional. Make the same assumptions as in Theorem 22, with $k = r = 2$ and take $\boldsymbol{\theta}_0 = \mathbf{0}$.
   (a) Let λ_n denote the likelihood ratio test statistic for testing H_0: $\boldsymbol{\theta} = \mathbf{0}$ against H_1: $\theta_1 > 0$, θ_2 unrestricted. Show that under the null hypothesis, $-2\log\lambda_n \xrightarrow{\mathscr{L}} 0.5\chi_1^2 + 0.5\chi_2^2$ (the mixture of a χ_1^2 and a χ_2^2 with probability 0.5 each).
   (b) In testing H_0: $\boldsymbol{\theta} = \mathbf{0}$ against H_1: $\theta_1 \geq 0$, $\theta_2 \geq 0$, $\boldsymbol{\theta} \neq \mathbf{0}$, show that $-2\log\lambda_n \xrightarrow{\mathscr{L}} p\delta_0 + 0.5\chi_1^2 + (0.5 - p)\chi_2^2$ under H_0, where δ_0 is the distribution degenerate at 0, and $p = \arccos(\rho)/2\pi$, where ρ is the correlation coefficient of the variables whose covariance matrix is $\mathscr{I}(\boldsymbol{\theta}_0)$. Thus the limiting distribution of $-2\log\lambda_n$ depends on the correlation of the underlying distribution.

23

Minimum Chi-Square Estimates

In this section we treat estimation problems by minimum distance methods, using a general theory of quadratic forms in asymptotically normal variables. This theory contains minimum χ^2 methods as a particular case.

We observe a sequence of d-dimensional random vectors $\mathbf{Z}_n$ whose distribution depends upon a k-dimensional parameter $\boldsymbol{\theta}$ lying in a parameter space Θ assumed to be a nonempty open subset of $\mathbb{R}^k$ where $k \le d$. It is given that the $\mathbf{Z}_n$ are asymptotically normal;

$$\sqrt{n}\,(\mathbf{Z}_n - \mathbf{A}(\boldsymbol{\theta})) \xrightarrow{\mathscr{L}} \mathscr{N}(\mathbf{0}, \mathbf{C}(\boldsymbol{\theta})), \tag{1}$$

where $\mathbf{A}(\boldsymbol{\theta})$ is a d vector and $\mathbf{C}(\boldsymbol{\theta})$ is a $d \times d$ covariance matrix for all $\boldsymbol{\theta} \in \Theta$. We make two assumptions on $\mathbf{A}(\boldsymbol{\theta})$:

$$\mathbf{A}(\boldsymbol{\theta}) \text{ is } \textit{bicontinuous} \text{ (that is, } \boldsymbol{\theta}_n \to \boldsymbol{\theta} \Leftrightarrow \mathbf{A}(\boldsymbol{\theta}_n) \to \mathbf{A}(\boldsymbol{\theta})), \tag{2}$$

$$\mathbf{A}(\boldsymbol{\theta}) \textit{ has a continuous first partial derivative, } \mathbf{A}(\boldsymbol{\theta}), \textit{ of full rank } k. \tag{3}$$

We measure the distance of $\mathbf{Z}_n$ to $\mathbf{A}(\boldsymbol{\theta})$ through a quadratic form of the type

$$Q_n(\boldsymbol{\theta}) = n(\mathbf{Z}_n - \mathbf{A}(\boldsymbol{\theta}))^T \mathbf{M}(\boldsymbol{\theta})(\mathbf{Z}_n - \mathbf{A}(\boldsymbol{\theta})), \tag{4}$$

where $\mathbf{M}(\boldsymbol{\theta})$ is a $d \times d$ covariance matrix. We assume

$\mathbf{M}(\boldsymbol{\theta})$ is *continuous in* $\boldsymbol{\theta}$ *and uniformaly bounded below* in the sense that for some constant $\alpha > 0$ we have $\mathbf{M}(\boldsymbol{\theta}) > \alpha \mathbf{I}$ for all $\boldsymbol{\theta} \in \Theta$. (5)

A *minimum* χ^2 *estimate* is a value of $\boldsymbol{\theta}$, depending on $\mathbf{Z}_n$, that minimizes $Q_n(\boldsymbol{\theta})$. With only the above assumptions, a minimum χ^2 estimate may not exist. We avoid the existence question by defining $\boldsymbol{\theta}_n^*(\mathbf{Z}_n)$ to be a *minimum* χ^2 *sequence* if

$$Q_n(\boldsymbol{\theta}_n^*) - \inf_{\boldsymbol{\theta} \in \Theta} Q_n(\boldsymbol{\theta}) \xrightarrow{\text{P}} 0,$$

whatever be the true value of $\boldsymbol{\theta} \in \Theta$.

The main theorem states that every such minimum χ^2 sequence is asymptotically normal, and we find the choice of $\mathbf{M}$ satisfying (5) that gives the minimum asymptotic covariance matrix uniformly for $\boldsymbol{\theta} \in \Theta$. We will also see that when $\mathbf{Z}_n$ is the vector of sufficient statistics from an exponential family (thus including the multinomial distributions), the resulting sequence of estimates is asymptotically equivalent to the maximum-likelihood estimate and is therefore asymptotically efficient.

As an illustrative example, consider Pearson's χ^2. In the notation of Section 9, $d = c$ is the number of cells, $\mathbf{Z}_n = \overline{\mathbf{X}}_n$ is the vector of cell relative frequencies, and $\mathbf{A}(\boldsymbol{\theta}) = \mathbf{p}(\boldsymbol{\theta})$ is the vector of cell probabilities, written as a function of some k-dimensional parameter $\boldsymbol{\theta}$, $k \le c - 1$. Pearson's χ^2 is then exactly $Q_n(\boldsymbol{\theta})$ of (4), where $\mathbf{M}(\boldsymbol{\theta}) = \mathbf{P}^{-1}(\boldsymbol{\theta})$ is the diagonal matrix with the inverse cell probabilities down the diagonal. Moreover, (1) is satisfied with covariance matrix

$$\mathbf{C}(\boldsymbol{\theta}) = \mathbf{M}(\boldsymbol{\theta})^{-1} - \mathbf{A}(\boldsymbol{\theta})\mathbf{A}(\boldsymbol{\theta})^T. \tag{6}$$

The question arises: Can we obtain a better estimate using a matrix, $\mathbf{M}(\boldsymbol{\theta})$, different from $\mathbf{P}^{-1}(\boldsymbol{\theta})$?

To simplify the notation of the main theorem, let $\boldsymbol{\theta}_0$ denote the true value of the parameter, and let $\dot{\mathbf{A}}$, $\mathbf{M}$, and $\mathbf{C}$ denote $\dot{\mathbf{A}}(\boldsymbol{\theta}_0)$, $\mathbf{M}(\boldsymbol{\theta}_0)$, and $\mathbf{C}(\boldsymbol{\theta}_0)$, respectively. The proof is deferred to the end of this section.

Theorem 23. *For any minimum* χ^2 *sequence,* $\sqrt{n}\,(\boldsymbol{\theta}_n^* - \boldsymbol{\theta}_0) \xrightarrow{\mathscr{L}} \mathscr{N}(\mathbf{0}, \boldsymbol{\Sigma})$, *where*

$$\boldsymbol{\Sigma} = (\dot{\mathbf{A}}^T \mathbf{M} \dot{\mathbf{A}})^{-1} \dot{\mathbf{A}}^T \mathbf{M} \mathbf{C} \mathbf{M} \dot{\mathbf{A}} (\dot{\mathbf{A}}^T \mathbf{M} \dot{\mathbf{A}})^{-1}. \tag{7}$$

The problem now is to choose $\mathbf{M}$ to get the smallest asymptotic covariance matrix for $\sqrt{n}\,(\boldsymbol{\theta}_n^* - \boldsymbol{\theta}_0)$. Let $\boldsymbol{\Sigma}(\mathbf{M})$ denote this matrix as a function of $\mathbf{M}$.

Corollary. *If there is a nonsingular* $d \times d$ *matrix* $\mathbf{M}_0$ *such that* $\mathbf{C}\mathbf{M}_0\dot{\mathbf{A}} = \dot{\mathbf{A}}$, *then* $\boldsymbol{\Sigma}(\mathbf{M}_0) = (\dot{\mathbf{A}}^T \mathbf{M}_0 \dot{\mathbf{A}})^{-1}$. *Moreover,*

$$\boldsymbol{\Sigma}(\mathbf{M}_0) \le \boldsymbol{\Sigma}(\mathbf{M}), \qquad \text{for all } \mathbf{M}.$$

Proof.

$$\mathbf{\Sigma}(\mathbf{M}_0) = \left(\dot{\mathbf{A}}^T\mathbf{M}_0\dot{\mathbf{A}}\right)^{-1}\dot{\mathbf{A}}^T\mathbf{M}_0\mathbf{C}\mathbf{M}_0\dot{\mathbf{A}}\left(\dot{\mathbf{A}}^T\mathbf{M}_0\dot{\mathbf{A}}\right)^{-1} = \left(\dot{\mathbf{A}}^T\mathbf{M}_0\dot{\mathbf{A}}\right)^{-1}.$$

Moreover,

$$\mathbf{0} \le \left(\mathbf{M}\dot{\mathbf{A}}(\dot{\mathbf{A}}^T\mathbf{M}\dot{\mathbf{A}})^{-1} - \mathbf{M}_0\dot{\mathbf{A}}\left(\dot{\mathbf{A}}^T\mathbf{M}_0\dot{\mathbf{A}}\right)^{-1}\right)^T$$

$$\times\mathbf{C}\left(\mathbf{M}\dot{\mathbf{A}}(\dot{\mathbf{A}}^T\mathbf{M}\dot{\mathbf{A}})^{-1} - \mathbf{M}_0\dot{\mathbf{A}}\left(\dot{\mathbf{A}}^T\mathbf{M}_0\dot{\mathbf{A}}\right)^{-1}\right)$$

$$= (\dot{\mathbf{A}}^T\mathbf{M}\dot{\mathbf{A}})^{-1}\dot{\mathbf{A}}^T\mathbf{M}\mathbf{C}\mathbf{M}\dot{\mathbf{A}}(\dot{\mathbf{A}}^T\mathbf{M}\dot{\mathbf{A}})^{-1} - \left(\dot{\mathbf{A}}^T\mathbf{M}_0\dot{\mathbf{A}}\right)^{-1} = \mathbf{\Sigma}(\mathbf{M}) - \mathbf{\Sigma}(\mathbf{M}_0). \quad \blacksquare$$

Note: If $\mathbf{C}$ is nonsingular, then one may choose $\mathbf{M}_0 = \mathbf{C}^{-1}$ to obtain the best asymptotic covariance. More generally, the condition $\mathbf{C}\mathbf{M}_0\dot{\mathbf{A}} = \dot{\mathbf{A}}$ implies that the columns of $\dot{\mathbf{A}}$ are in the range space of $\mathbf{C}$. Conversely, if there exists a matrix $\mathbf{X}$ such that $\mathbf{C}\mathbf{X} = \dot{\mathbf{A}}$ then $\mathbf{M}_0$ may be chosen as any generalized inverse of $\mathbf{C}$. [A *generalized inverse* of a matrix $\mathbf{C}$ is a matrix $\mathbf{C}^-$ such that $\mathbf{C}\mathbf{C}^-\mathbf{C} = \mathbf{C}$. Such inverses exist and one may construct them to be nonsingular; see the Rao (1973) Section 1b.5).] For if $\mathbf{M}_0$ is a generalized inverse of $\mathbf{C}$ and if $\mathbf{C}\mathbf{X} = \dot{\mathbf{A}}$ then $\mathbf{C}\mathbf{M}_0\dot{\mathbf{A}} = \mathbf{C}\mathbf{M}_0\mathbf{C}\mathbf{X} = \mathbf{C}\mathbf{X} = \dot{\mathbf{A}}$. Thus, the assumption of the existence of a matrix $\mathbf{M}_0$ such that $\mathbf{C}\mathbf{M}_0\dot{\mathbf{A}} = \dot{\mathbf{A}}$ is equivalent to the assumption that the columns of $\dot{\mathbf{A}}$ are in the range of $\mathbf{C}$, and then $\mathbf{M}_0$ may be taken as any generalized inverse of $\mathbf{C}$.

Pearson's χ^2 provides an example where $\mathbf{C}$ is not invertible. We have $\mathbf{C} = \mathbf{P} - \mathbf{p}\mathbf{p}^T$ and $\dot{\mathbf{A}} = (\partial/\partial\boldsymbol{\theta})\mathbf{p}$. If we take $\mathbf{M}_0 = \mathbf{P}^{-1}$, then

$$\mathbf{C}\mathbf{M}_0\dot{\mathbf{A}} = (\mathbf{I} - \mathbf{p}\mathbf{p}^T\mathbf{P}^{-1})\dot{\mathbf{A}} = (\mathbf{I} - \mathbf{p}\mathbf{1}^T)\dot{\mathbf{A}},$$

where $\mathbf{1}$ is the vector of all 1's. But

$$\mathbf{1}^T\dot{\mathbf{A}} = \sum_1^d \frac{\partial}{\partial\boldsymbol{\theta}}\mathbf{p}_j(\boldsymbol{\theta}) = \frac{\partial}{\partial\boldsymbol{\theta}}\sum_1^d p_j(\boldsymbol{\theta}) = \frac{\partial}{\partial\boldsymbol{\theta}}1 = \mathbf{0},$$

so that $\mathbf{C}\mathbf{M}_0\dot{\mathbf{A}} = \dot{\mathbf{A}}$. Thus, Pearson's choice of $\mathbf{M}_0 = \mathbf{P}^{-1}$ leads to the smallest asymptotic covariance matrix for $\sqrt{n}\,(\boldsymbol{\theta}_n^* - \boldsymbol{\theta}_0)$.

EXAMPLE 1. *The Exponential Family.* Let $X_1, \ldots, X_n$ be i.i.d. with density

$$f(x|\boldsymbol{\pi}) = h(x)\exp\{\boldsymbol{\pi}^T\mathbf{T}(x) - \varphi(\boldsymbol{\pi})\}$$

with respect to $d\nu(x)$ where $\mathbf{T}(x)$ and $\boldsymbol{\pi}$ are d-dimensional vectors, and

$$\varphi(\boldsymbol{\pi}) = \log \int h(x) \exp\{\boldsymbol{\pi}^T \mathbf{T}(x)\}\, d\nu(x)$$

is assumed to exist in an open set in $\mathbb{R}^d$. Then, $E_{\boldsymbol{\pi}}\mathbf{T}(X) = \dot{\varphi}(\boldsymbol{\pi})^T$ and $\mathrm{var}_{\boldsymbol{\pi}}\mathbf{T}(X) = \ddot{\varphi}(\boldsymbol{\pi})$. Let $\mathbf{Z}_n = (1/n)\sum_1^n \mathbf{T}(X_i)$ so that from the Central Limit Theorem, $\sqrt{n}\,(\mathbf{Z}_n - \dot{\varphi}(\boldsymbol{\pi})^T) \xrightarrow{\mathscr{L}} \mathscr{N}(\mathbf{0}, \ddot{\varphi}(\boldsymbol{\pi}))$. Since the parameter space contains an open set in $\mathbb{R}^d$, $\ddot{\varphi}$ is nonsingular and we choose

$$Q_n(\boldsymbol{\pi}) = n\left(\mathbf{Z}_n - \dot{\varphi}(\boldsymbol{\pi})^T\right)^T \ddot{\varphi}(\boldsymbol{\pi})^{-1}\left(\mathbf{Z}_n - \dot{\varphi}(\boldsymbol{\pi})^T\right)$$

If $\boldsymbol{\pi}$ is allowed to range over the entire natural parameter space, then $Q_n(\boldsymbol{\pi})$ has minimum value zero at $\mathbf{Z}_n = \dot{\varphi}(\boldsymbol{\pi})$, so that the minimum χ^2 estimates are identical to the maximum-likelihood estimates. This is essentially the class of distributions for which the minimum χ^2 estimates are the same as the maximum-likelihood estimates. It contains the Pearson's χ^2 since the multinomial distribution is an exponential family.

If $\boldsymbol{\pi}$ is restricted, say to be a function of $\boldsymbol{\theta}$, then the MLE and minimum χ^2 estimates may not be equal. However, they have the same asymptotic covariance matrix. (See Exercise 1.)

Generalized χ^2's

A. Modified χ^2. If the matrix $\mathbf{M}$ is allowed to depend on $\mathbf{Z}_n$, the resulting quadratic form,

$$Q_n(\boldsymbol{\theta}) = n(\mathbf{Z}_n - \mathbf{A}(\boldsymbol{\theta}))^T \mathbf{M}(\mathbf{Z}_n, \boldsymbol{\theta})(\mathbf{Z}_n - \mathbf{A}(\boldsymbol{\theta})),$$

is known as modified χ^2, and the value that minimizes $Q_n(\boldsymbol{\theta})$ is a minimum modified χ^2 estimate. Neyman's $\chi^2 = \Sigma[(\text{obs} - \text{exp})^2/\text{obs}]$ is an example. If condition (5) is replaced by the condition that $\mathbf{M}(\mathbf{z}, \boldsymbol{\theta})$ be jointly continuous in $(\mathbf{z}, \boldsymbol{\theta})$ and uniformly bounded below, then the minimum modified χ^2 estimates are asymptotically equivalent to the minimum χ^2 estimates obtained from the above quadratic form with $\mathbf{M}(\mathbf{Z}_n, \boldsymbol{\theta})$, replaced by its limit $\mathbf{M}(\mathbf{A}(\boldsymbol{\theta}), \boldsymbol{\theta})$. When $\mathbf{M}(\mathbf{Z}_n, \boldsymbol{\theta})$ is chosen independent of $\boldsymbol{\theta}$, it is usually easier to compute the estimates.

Example 2. Consider Pearson's χ^2 with three cells and probabilities depending on a real parameter θ linearly, say, $p_1(\theta) = \frac{1}{3} - \theta$, $p_2(\theta) = \frac{2}{3} - \theta$, and $p_3(\theta) = 2\theta$, where $0 < \theta < \frac{1}{3}$,

$$\chi^2 = \frac{\left(n_1 - n(\frac{1}{3} - \theta)\right)^2}{n(\frac{1}{3} - \theta)} + \frac{\left(n_2 - n(\frac{2}{3} - \theta)\right)^2}{n(\frac{2}{3} - \theta)} + \frac{(n_3 - 2n\theta)^2}{2n\theta}.$$

Taking a derivative with respect to θ and setting it to 0 leads to a sixth-degree polynomial equation in θ. With a Neyman χ^2,

$$\chi^2 = \frac{\left(p_1 - n\left(\frac{1}{3} - \theta\right)\right)^2}{n_1} + \frac{\left(n_2 - n\left(\frac{2}{3} - \theta\right)\right)^2}{n_2} - \frac{(n_3 - 2n\theta)^2}{n_3}.$$

the same operation results in a linear equation for θ.

B. Transformed χ^2. Let $\mathbf{g}: \mathbb{R}^d \to \mathbb{R}^d$ have continuous first derivative $\dot{\mathbf{g}}$ of full rank. Then, by Cramér's Theorem,

$$\sqrt{n}\,(\mathbf{g}(\mathbf{Z}_n) - \mathbf{g}(\mathbf{A}(\boldsymbol{\theta}))) \xrightarrow{\mathscr{L}} \mathscr{N}\left(\mathbf{0}, \dot{\mathbf{g}}(\mathbf{A}(\boldsymbol{\theta}))\mathbf{C}(\boldsymbol{\theta})\dot{\mathbf{g}}(\mathbf{A}(\boldsymbol{\theta}))^T\right)$$

and

$$Q_n(\boldsymbol{\theta}) = n(\mathbf{g}(\mathbf{Z}_n) - \mathbf{g}(\mathbf{A}(\boldsymbol{\theta})))^T[\dot{\mathbf{g}}(\mathbf{A}(\boldsymbol{\theta}))^{T-1}\mathbf{M}(\boldsymbol{\theta})\dot{\mathbf{g}}(\mathbf{A}(\boldsymbol{\theta}))^{-1}](\mathbf{g}(\mathbf{Z}_n) - \mathbf{g}(\mathbf{A}(\boldsymbol{\theta})))$$

leads to minimum χ^2 estimates with the same asymptotic distribution as that for the untransformed χ^2 found in Theorem 23, and is optimized by the same choice of $\mathbf{M}$. One may combine modification and transformation by replacing the matrix in brackets by an estimate. Sometimes the function $\mathbf{g}$ may be chosen so that $\mathbf{g}(\mathbf{A}(\boldsymbol{\theta}))$ is linear in $\boldsymbol{\theta}$.

Example 3. Consider a bioassay problem with response curve $F(x|\boldsymbol{\theta})$, with n samples at each of the levels $x_1, \ldots, x_d$. Let $n_1, \ldots, n_d$ denote the number of responses at these levels, respectively. We form the χ^2:

$$\chi^2 = \sum_1^d \left[\frac{\left(n_1 - nF(x_1|\boldsymbol{\theta})\right)^2}{nF\left(x_j|\boldsymbol{\theta}\right)} + \frac{\left((n - n_j) - n\left(1 - F\left(x_j|\boldsymbol{\theta}\right)\right)\right)^2}{n\left(1 - F\left(x_j|\boldsymbol{\theta}\right)\right)}\right]$$

$$= \sum_1^d \frac{\left(n_i - nF(x_i|\boldsymbol{\theta})\right)^2}{nF\left(x_j|\boldsymbol{\theta}\right)\left(1 - F\left(x_j|\boldsymbol{\theta}\right)\right)} = n\sum_1^d \frac{\left((n_i/n) - F(x_i|\boldsymbol{\theta})\right)^2}{F\left(x_i|\boldsymbol{\theta}\right)\left(1 - F\left(x_j|\boldsymbol{\theta}\right)\right)}.$$

Note the way a Pearson's χ^2 of two cells reduces to a single term.

If $F(x|\boldsymbol{\theta})$ is logistic, $F(x|\boldsymbol{\theta}) = (1 + \exp\{-(\alpha + \beta x)\})^{-1}$ where $\boldsymbol{\theta} = (\alpha, \beta)$, it becomes a tedious task to compute the minimum χ^2 estimates of α and β. However, the transformation $\operatorname{logit}(p) = \log(p/(1-p))$ makes $g(F(x|\boldsymbol{\theta}))$ linear: $\operatorname{logit}(F(x|\boldsymbol{\theta})) = \alpha + \beta x$. Because

$$\frac{d}{dp}\operatorname{logit}(p) = \frac{1}{p(1-p)},$$

the transformed χ^2 becomes

$$\chi^2 = n\sum_1^d F(x_j|\theta)(1 - F(x_j|\theta))\left(\text{logit}\left(\frac{n_j}{n}\right) - \text{logit}(F(x_j|\theta))\right)^2.$$

Using the process of modification, we obtain Berkson's logit χ^2:

$$\text{logit } \chi^2 = n\sum_1^d \frac{n_j}{n}\left(1 - \frac{n_j}{n}\right)\left(\text{logit}\left(\frac{n_j}{n}\right) - (\alpha + \beta x_j)\right)^2.$$

C. Expansion of χ^2 about subefficient estimates. As in the computation of the MLE, one may improve easily computable but subefficient estimates by an application of Newton's method. To find minimum χ^2 estimates, one ordinarily seeks a solution of $d/d\boldsymbol{\theta}(Q_n(\boldsymbol{\theta})) = 0$. In applying Newton's method, several simplifications may be made. First in taking the derivative of $Q_n(\boldsymbol{\theta})$, one may pretend that $M(\boldsymbol{\theta})$ does not depend on $\boldsymbol{\theta}$. This is equivalent to using modified χ^2 by replacing $\mathbf{M}(\boldsymbol{\theta})$ by an estimate, taking a derivative, and then replacing the estimate by $\mathbf{M}(\boldsymbol{\theta})$. Thus we may work with the equation

$$\dot{\mathbf{A}}(\boldsymbol{\theta})^T\mathbf{M}(\boldsymbol{\theta})(\mathbf{Z}_n - \mathbf{A}(\boldsymbol{\theta})) = \mathbf{0}.$$

Second, the equation may be modified by replacing $\dot{\mathbf{A}}(\boldsymbol{\theta})^T\mathbf{M}(\boldsymbol{\theta})$ by an estimate.

Example 4. In estimating the bacterial density of a liquid, the usual experiment shows whether a given cubic centimeter of the liquid contains no bacteria or at least one bacterium. If θ denotes the bacterial density, the number of bacteria in a cubic centimeter is assumed to have a Poisson distribution with parameter θ. The probability of success (no bacteria) in a single trial is then $e^{-\theta}$. In estimating bacterial density by the dilution method, the liquid is successively diluted to several dilution levels, $x_1, \ldots, x_d$, and n trials are carried out at each level. At dilution x_i, the probability of success is $\exp\{-\theta x_i\}$. This leads to a χ^2 of the form of Example 3 with $F(x|\theta) = \exp\{-\theta x\}$,

$$\chi^2 = n\sum_1^d \frac{((n_j/n) - \exp\{-\theta x_j\})^2}{\exp\{-\theta x_j\}(1 - \exp\{-\theta x_j\})},$$

where n_i = the number out of n samples that show no bacteria at level x_i. Pretending the denominator does not depend on θ and taking derivatives, we obtain the equations

$$2n\sum_1^d \frac{((n_j/n) - \exp\{-\theta x_j\})x_j}{(1 - \exp\{-\theta x_j\})} = 0.$$

Provided $n_j \neq n$, we may replace the denominator by $(1 - (n_j/n))$.

D. Linearization of the side conditions. [Neyman (1949)]. In minimizing Q_n, $\mathbf{A}^T = (a_1, \ldots, a_d)$ may be considered as a vector of parameters subject to restrictions, called side conditions, due to the dependence of **A** on $\boldsymbol{\theta}$. If there are k independent parameters, there are $d - k$ side conditions on the a's: $f_j(a_1, \ldots, a_d) = 0$ for $j = 1, \ldots, d - k$. One may then minimize Q_n subject to these side conditions by the method of Lagrange multipliers. A simpler procedure is to minimize Q_n subject to the linearized constraints, that is, the first two terms of the Taylor-series expansion of the f_j about $\mathbf{Z}_n$. The problem then only requires solution of linear equations.

Example 5. In *the log-linear model* with multinomial sampling of sample size n and c cells, the cell probabilities $p_1, \ldots, p_c$ are assumed to be of the form

$$p_i = \exp\left\{\theta_0 + \sum_{j=1}^k x_{ij}\theta_j\right\}, \qquad \text{for } i = 1, \ldots, c,$$

where the x_{ij} are known numbers. It is simpler to work with transformed χ^2 with each cell transformed by $g(z) = \log z$, $g'(z) = 1/z$, and modified so that

$$Q_n = n\sum_1^c (\log(n_i/n) - \log(p_i))^2 (n_i/n) = \sum_1^c (z_i - a_i)^2 n_i,$$

where $a_i = \log p_i = \theta_0 + \sum x_{ij}\theta_j$ and $z_i = \log(n_i/n)$. Although Q_n is quadratic in the θ's, the constraint $1 = \sum_1^c p_i = \sum_1^c \exp\{a_i\}$ makes the problem nonlinear. The expansion of this constraint about **z** gives

$$1 = \sum_1^c \exp\{a_i\} \sim \sum \exp\{z_i\} + \sum \exp\{z_i\}(a - z_i).$$

Because $\sum \exp\{z_i\} = \sum(n_i/n) = 1$, the constraint is $\sum n_i a_i = \sum n_i z_i$, which can be solved for

$$\theta_0 = \frac{1}{n}\sum_i n_i z_i - \frac{1}{n}\sum_{j=1}^{k}\sum_{i=1}^{c} n_i x_{ij}\theta_j.$$

Therefore,

$$a_i = \frac{1}{n}\sum_1^c n_i z_i + \sum_{j=1}^{k}\left(x_{ij} - \sum_{m=1}^{c}\frac{n_m}{n}x_{mj}\right)\theta_j$$

and the minimum transformed χ^2 estimates may be found by solving the linear equations,

$$\frac{\partial}{\partial\theta_j}Q_n = -2\sum_{i=1}^{c} n_i(z_i - a_i)\left(x_{ij} - \sum_{m=1}^{c}\frac{n_m}{n}x_{mj}\right) = 0, \qquad \text{for } j = 1,\ldots,k.$$

Unfortunately, the resulting a_i do not quite satisfy the original constraint, $\Sigma_1^c \exp\{a_i\} = 1$. If it is desired to have this equation satisfied exactly, we may modify the estimates as follows. Find δ so that $\Sigma_1^c \exp\{a_j\} = \exp(\delta\}$, and replace θ_0 by $\theta_0 - \delta$. The resulting estimate satisfies $\Sigma_1^c p_i = 1$, and is still asymptotically efficient.

Proof of the Main Result. We precede the proof of Theorem 23 by some lemmas. With $\boldsymbol{\theta}_0$ denoting the true value of $\boldsymbol{\theta}$, we have $\sqrt{n}(\mathbf{Z}_n - \mathbf{A}(\boldsymbol{\theta}_0)) \xrightarrow{\mathscr{L}} \mathscr{N}(\mathbf{0}, \mathbf{C})$, where $\mathbf{C} = \mathbf{C}(\boldsymbol{\theta}_0)$. We use the metric $\|\mathbf{x}\|$ in $\mathbb{R}^d$ given by

$$\|\mathbf{x}\|^2 = \mathbf{x}^T\mathbf{M}(\boldsymbol{\theta}_0)\mathbf{x} = \mathbf{x}^T\mathbf{M}\mathbf{x}.$$

We say a sequence of random vectors, $\mathbf{V}_n$, is *tight* if for every $\varepsilon > 0$ there exists r_ε such that $P\{\|\mathbf{V}_n\| < r_\varepsilon\} > 1 - \varepsilon$ for all n sufficiently large.

LEMMA 1. $\sqrt{n}(\mathbf{Z}_n - \mathbf{A}(\boldsymbol{\theta}_n^*))$ *is tight.*

Proof. Let $\varepsilon > 0$. Find $r > 0$ such that $P\{\sqrt{n}\|\mathbf{Z}_n - \mathbf{A}(\boldsymbol{\theta}_0)\| < r\} > 1 - \varepsilon/2$ for n sufficiently large. Since

$$P\left\{Q_n(\boldsymbol{\theta}_n^*) - \inf_{\boldsymbol{\theta}\in\Theta} Q_n(\boldsymbol{\theta}) \le \varepsilon\right\} > 1 - \varepsilon/2$$

for n sufficiently large, we also have for n sufficiently large,

$$P\left\{\sqrt{n}\,\|\mathbf{Z}_n - \mathbf{A}(\boldsymbol{\theta}_0)\| < r, \qquad Q_n(\boldsymbol{\theta}_n^*) - \inf_{\boldsymbol{\theta}\in\Theta} Q_n(\boldsymbol{\theta}) \le \varepsilon\right\} > 1 - \varepsilon.$$

Because $\mathbf{M}(\boldsymbol{\theta})$ is uniformly bounded below, we can find $\delta > 0$ such that $\mathbf{M}(\boldsymbol{\theta}) > \delta\mathbf{M}(\boldsymbol{\theta}_0)$ for all $\boldsymbol{\theta} \in \Theta$. The lemma then follows from the implication

$$n\|\mathbf{Z}_n - \mathbf{A}(\boldsymbol{\theta}_0)\|^2 < r^2 \quad \text{and} \quad Q_n(\boldsymbol{\theta}_n^*) - \inf_{\boldsymbol{\theta}\in\Theta} Q_n(\boldsymbol{\theta}) \le \varepsilon$$

$$\Rightarrow n\|\mathbf{Z}_n - \mathbf{A}(\boldsymbol{\theta}_n^*)\|^2 \le (1/\delta)Q_n(\boldsymbol{\theta}_n^*) \qquad [\text{since } \delta\mathbf{M}(\boldsymbol{\theta}_0) > \mathbf{M}(\boldsymbol{\theta})]$$

$$\le (1/\delta)\Big(\inf_{\boldsymbol{\theta}\in\Theta} Q_n(\boldsymbol{\theta}) + \varepsilon\Big) \le (1/\alpha)\big(Q(\boldsymbol{\theta}_0) + \varepsilon\big)$$

$$= (1/\delta)\big(n\|\mathbf{Z}_n - \mathbf{A}(\boldsymbol{\theta}_0)\|^2 + \varepsilon\big)$$

$$\le (1/\delta)(r^2 + \varepsilon) = r_\varepsilon^2$$ ■

Corollary 1. *$\sqrt{n}\,(\mathbf{A}(\boldsymbol{\theta}_n^*) - \mathbf{A}(\boldsymbol{\theta}_0))$ is tight.*

Proof. $\sqrt{n}\,(\mathbf{A}(\boldsymbol{\theta}_n^*) - \mathbf{A}(\boldsymbol{\theta}_0)) = \sqrt{n}\,(\mathbf{Z}_n - \mathbf{A}(\boldsymbol{\theta}_0)) - \sqrt{n}\,(\mathbf{Z}_n - \mathbf{A}(\boldsymbol{\theta}_n^*))$. ■

Corollary 2. $\boldsymbol{\theta}_n^* \xrightarrow{P} \boldsymbol{\theta}_0$.

Proof. This follows since $\mathbf{A}(\boldsymbol{\theta}_n^*) \xrightarrow{P} \mathbf{A}(\boldsymbol{\theta}_0)$ and $\mathbf{A}$ is bicontinuous. ■

Let $\boldsymbol{\Pi}$ denote the projection onto the range space of $\dot{\mathbf{A}}$ using the metric, $\|\mathbf{x}\|^2 = \mathbf{x}^T\mathbf{M}\mathbf{x}$. In other words, $\boldsymbol{\Pi}\mathbf{x} = \dot{\mathbf{A}}\mathbf{y}$ where $\mathbf{y}$ minimizes $\|\mathbf{x} - \dot{\mathbf{A}}\mathbf{y}\|^2$ for $\mathbf{y} \in \mathbb{R}^k$. We find $\boldsymbol{\Pi}$ as follows.

$$\frac{\partial}{\partial\mathbf{y}}\|\mathbf{x} - \dot{\mathbf{A}}\mathbf{y}\|^2 = \frac{\partial}{\partial\mathbf{y}}\big(\mathbf{x} - \dot{\mathbf{A}}\mathbf{y}\big)^T\mathbf{M}\big(\mathbf{x} - \dot{\mathbf{A}}\mathbf{y}\big) = -2\dot{\mathbf{A}}^T\mathbf{M}\big(\mathbf{x} - \dot{\mathbf{A}}\mathbf{y}\big) = 0$$

$$\Rightarrow \dot{\mathbf{A}}^T\mathbf{M}\dot{\mathbf{A}}\mathbf{y} = \dot{\mathbf{A}}^T\mathbf{M}\mathbf{x}.$$

Since $\dot{\mathbf{A}}$ has full rank and $\mathbf{M}$ is nonsingular, $\dot{\mathbf{A}}^T\mathbf{M}\dot{\mathbf{A}}$ is nonsingular so that $\mathbf{y} = (\dot{\mathbf{A}}^T\mathbf{M}\dot{\mathbf{A}})^{-1}\dot{\mathbf{A}}^T\mathbf{M}\mathbf{x}$. Hence

$$\boldsymbol{\Pi} = \dot{\mathbf{A}}\big(\dot{\mathbf{A}}^T\mathbf{M}\dot{\mathbf{A}}\big)^{-1}\dot{\mathbf{A}}^T\mathbf{M}.$$

Lemma 2. $\sqrt{n}\,(\boldsymbol{\Pi}\mathbf{Z}_n - \mathbf{A}(\boldsymbol{\theta}_n^*)) \xrightarrow{P} 0$.

Proof. *Picture*:

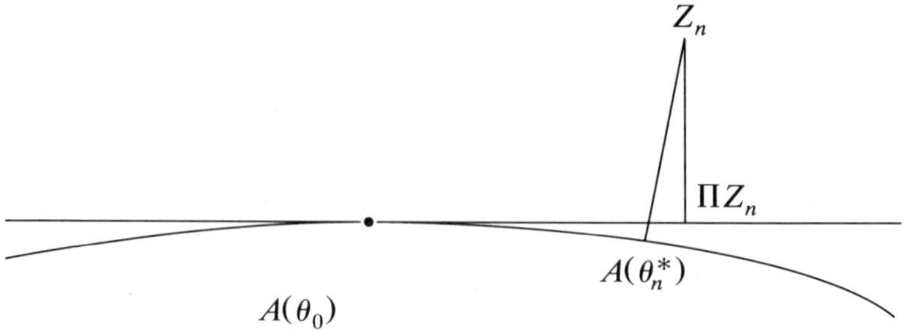

Let $\varepsilon > 0$. Using continuous differentiability and bicontinuity of $\mathbf{A}(\boldsymbol{\theta})$, we may find $\delta > 0$ such that

$$\left\| \mathbf{A}(\boldsymbol{\theta}) - \mathbf{A}(\boldsymbol{\theta}_0) - \dot{\mathbf{A}}^T(\boldsymbol{\theta} - \boldsymbol{\theta}_0) \right\| < \varepsilon \left\| \mathbf{A}(\boldsymbol{\theta}) - \mathbf{A}(\boldsymbol{\theta}_0) \right\|$$

provided $\|\mathbf{A}(\boldsymbol{\theta}) - \mathbf{A}(\boldsymbol{\theta}_0)\| < \delta$. Since $\boldsymbol{\theta}_n^* \xrightarrow{\text{P}} \boldsymbol{\theta}_0$, $Q_n(\boldsymbol{\theta}_n^*)$ comes arbitrarily close to $\|\mathbf{Z}_n - \mathbf{A}(\boldsymbol{\theta}_n^*)\|^2$ with high probability for n large. From this we may conclude that

$$\left\| \mathbf{A}(\boldsymbol{\theta}_n^*) - \mathbf{A}(\boldsymbol{\theta}_0) - \dot{\mathbf{A}}^T(\boldsymbol{\theta}_n^* - \boldsymbol{\theta}_0) \right\| < \varepsilon \left\| \mathbf{A}(\boldsymbol{\theta}_n^*) - \mathbf{A}(\boldsymbol{\theta}_0) \right\|$$

whenever $\|\mathbf{Z}_n - \mathbf{A}(\boldsymbol{\theta}_0)\| < \delta/3$, say, with high probability for n large. Let $d_n = \|\mathbf{Z}_n - \boldsymbol{\Pi}\mathbf{Z}_n\|$ and $\varepsilon_n = \varepsilon\|\mathbf{A}(\boldsymbol{\theta}_n^*) - \mathbf{A}(\boldsymbol{\theta}_0)\|$. Then $\|\mathbf{Z}_n - \mathbf{A}(\boldsymbol{\theta}_n^*)\| \le d_n + \varepsilon_n$ because there is at least one point $\mathbf{A}(\boldsymbol{\theta})$ this close to $\mathbf{Z}_n$. Moreover,

$$\left\| \boldsymbol{\Pi}\mathbf{Z}_n - \boldsymbol{\Pi}\mathbf{A}(\boldsymbol{\theta}_n^*) \right\|^2 \le (d_n + \varepsilon_n)^2 = (d_n + \varepsilon_n)^2 = 4d_n\varepsilon_n,$$

and hence

$$\left\| \boldsymbol{\Pi}\mathbf{Z}_n - \mathbf{A}(\boldsymbol{\theta}_n^*) \right\| \le \varepsilon_n + (4d_n\varepsilon_n)^{1/2}.$$

Now since both $\sqrt{n}\,\|\mathbf{A}(\boldsymbol{\theta}_n^*) - \mathbf{A}(\boldsymbol{\theta}_0)\|$ and $\sqrt{n}\,\|\mathbf{Z}_n - \boldsymbol{\Pi}\mathbf{Z}_n\|$ are tight, we have that $\sqrt{n}\,\|\boldsymbol{\Pi}\mathbf{Z}_n - \mathbf{A}(\boldsymbol{\theta}_n^*)\|$ is bounded by $\sqrt{\varepsilon}$ times something tight. ■

Proof of Theorem 23. Expand $\mathbf{A}(\boldsymbol{\theta}_n^*)$ about $\boldsymbol{\theta}_0$:

$$\begin{aligned}
\mathbf{A}(\boldsymbol{\theta}_n^*) - \mathbf{A}(\boldsymbol{\theta}_0) &= \int_0^1 \dot{\mathbf{A}}(\boldsymbol{\theta}_0 + \lambda(\boldsymbol{\theta}_n^* - \boldsymbol{\theta}_0))\, d\lambda(\boldsymbol{\theta}_n^* - \boldsymbol{\theta}_0) \\
&= \mathbf{A}^*(\boldsymbol{\theta}_n^*)(\boldsymbol{\theta}_n^* - \boldsymbol{\theta}_0).
\end{aligned}$$

Since $\boldsymbol{\theta}_n^* \xrightarrow{\text{P}} \boldsymbol{\theta}_0$ and $\dot{\mathbf{A}}(\boldsymbol{\theta})$ is continuous, $\mathbf{A}^*(\boldsymbol{\theta}_n^*) \xrightarrow{\text{P}} \dot{\mathbf{A}}$. Therefore, for n

sufficiently large, $\mathbf{A}^*(\boldsymbol{\theta}_n^*)$ has full rank k, so that

$$\sqrt{n}\,(\boldsymbol{\theta}_n^* - \boldsymbol{\theta}_0) = \left(\mathbf{A}^*(\boldsymbol{\theta}_0^*)^T \mathbf{M}\mathbf{A}^*(\boldsymbol{\theta}_n^*)\right)^{-1} \mathbf{A}^*(\boldsymbol{\theta}_n^*)^T \mathbf{M}\sqrt{n}\,(\mathbf{A}(\boldsymbol{\theta}_n^*) - \mathbf{A}(\boldsymbol{\theta}_0)).$$

From Lemma 2,

$$\sqrt{n}\,(\mathbf{A}(\boldsymbol{\theta}_n^*) - \mathbf{A}(\boldsymbol{\theta}_0)) \sim \sqrt{n}\,\boldsymbol{\Pi}(\mathbf{Z}_n - \mathbf{A}(\boldsymbol{\theta}_0)),$$

and since

$$\sqrt{n}\,(\mathbf{Z}_n - \mathbf{A}(\boldsymbol{\theta}_0)) \xrightarrow{\mathscr{L}} \mathscr{N}(\mathbf{0}, \mathbf{C}),$$

we have

$$\sqrt{n}\,(\mathbf{A}(\boldsymbol{\theta}_n^*) - \mathbf{A}(\boldsymbol{\theta}_0)) \xrightarrow{\mathscr{L}} \mathscr{N}(\mathbf{0}, \boldsymbol{\Pi}\mathbf{C}\boldsymbol{\Pi}^T).$$

Hence

$$\sqrt{n}\,(\boldsymbol{\theta}_n^* - \boldsymbol{\theta}_0) \xrightarrow{\mathscr{L}} \mathscr{N}\!\left(\mathbf{0}, (\dot{\mathbf{A}}^T\mathbf{M}\dot{\mathbf{A}})^{-1}\dot{\mathbf{A}}^T\mathbf{M}\boldsymbol{\Pi}\mathbf{C}\boldsymbol{\Pi}^T\mathbf{M}\dot{\mathbf{A}}(\dot{\mathbf{A}}^T\mathbf{M}\dot{\mathbf{A}})^{-1}\right).$$

Writing $\boldsymbol{\Pi} = \dot{\mathbf{A}}(\dot{\mathbf{A}}^T\mathbf{M}\dot{\mathbf{A}})^{-1}\dot{\mathbf{A}}^T\mathbf{M}$ and simplifying gives the $\boldsymbol{\Sigma}$ of the theorem. ■

EXERCISES

1. Prove the last statement of Example 1 when θ is a one-dimensional parameter such that $\boldsymbol{\pi}(\theta)$ has continuous derivatives.
2. In Example 2 assume $n = 100$, $n_1 = 20$, $n_2 = 50$, $n_3 = 30$, and find
   (a) the minimum χ^2 estimate,
   (b) the minimum modified χ^2 estimate, and
   (c) the MLE.
3. (a) For the response curve $F(x|\boldsymbol{\theta}) = \Phi(\alpha + \beta x)$, where $\Phi(x)$ is the distribution function of the standard normal distribution, find the linearizing transformation, call it probit (p), and find the resulting modified transformed χ^2.
   (b) For the Cauchy response curve $F(x|\theta) = (1/\pi)(\arctan(\alpha + \beta x) + \pi/2)$, find the linearizing transformation, give it a nice catchy name, and find the resulting modified transformed χ^2.
4. As a given instance of estimating bacterial density by the dilution method, suppose there are three dilution levels, $x_1 = 1$, $x_2 = \frac{1}{2}$, and $x_3 = \frac{1}{4}$, and suppose we have a sample of size $n = 10$ at each level. Given the data $n_1 = 0$, $n_2 = 4$, and $n_3 = 8$, find the minimum χ^2 estimate of θ as indicated in Example 4.

5. In Example 5, suppose $c = 3$ and $k = 1$, with $a_1 = \theta_0$, $a_2 = \theta_0 + \theta_1$, $a_3 = \theta_0 - \theta_1$. If $n_1 = 30$, $n_2 = 20$, and $n_3 = 50$, find the resulting estimate adjusted so that $\Sigma\, p_i = 1$.
6. Let $\mathbf{Y}_1, \ldots, \mathbf{Y}_n$ be i.i.d. d-dimensional random vectors with mean $\mathbf{A}(\boldsymbol{\theta})$ and covariance matrix $\mathbf{C}(\boldsymbol{\theta})$. The parameter space is the open square $\Theta = \{(\theta_1, \theta_2)\colon\ 0 < \theta_1 < \pi/2, 0 < \theta_2 < \pi/2\}$. Write $\mathbf{A}(\boldsymbol{\theta}) = (\mu_1(\boldsymbol{\theta}), \ldots, \mu_d(\boldsymbol{\theta}))^T$ and

$$\mathbf{C}(\boldsymbol{\theta}) = \begin{bmatrix} \sigma_1^2(\boldsymbol{\theta}) & 0 & \cdots & 0 \\ 0 & \sigma_2^2(\boldsymbol{\theta}) & \cdots & 0 \\ \vdots & \vdots & \ddots & \vdots \\ 0 & 0 & \cdots & \sigma_d^2(\boldsymbol{\theta}) \end{bmatrix},$$

where for some numbers $0 \le x_i \le 1$, $\mu_i(\boldsymbol{\theta}) = \sin(\theta_1 x_i - \theta_2)$ and $\sigma_i^2(\boldsymbol{\theta}) = \cos^2(\theta_1 x_i - \theta_2)$.

(a) Find some asymptotically optimal minimum χ^2 estimates $\hat{\theta}_1$, $\hat{\theta}_2$ as explicit functions of the x_i and $\mathbf{Y}_i$.

(b) What is the asymptotic joint distribution of $(\hat{\theta}_1, \hat{\theta}_2)$?

(c) If $x_1, \ldots, x_d$ may be chosen by the experimenter, how should they be chosen subject to $0 \le x_i \le 1$?

24

General Chi-Square Tests

We treat the general theory of χ^2 tests, give applications to the treatment of contingency tables, and consider the more general problem of testing against restricted alternatives. We make the general assumptions of Section 23, and we choose $\mathbf{M}(\boldsymbol{\theta})$ to be a nonsingular generalized inverse of $\mathbf{C}(\boldsymbol{\theta})$. Therefore, our assumptions are

(1) $\sqrt{n}\,(\mathbf{Z}_n - \mathbf{A}(\boldsymbol{\theta}_0)) \xrightarrow{\mathscr{L}} \mathscr{N}(\mathbf{0}, \mathbf{C}(\boldsymbol{\theta}_0))$, $\mathbf{Z} \in \mathbb{R}^d$, $\boldsymbol{\theta}_0 \in \Theta$ open $\subset \mathbb{R}^k$.
(2) $\mathbf{A}(\boldsymbol{\theta})$ is bicontinuous; $\dot{\mathbf{A}}(\boldsymbol{\theta})$ is continuous and has full rank $k \le d$.
(3) $\mathbf{M}(\boldsymbol{\theta})$ is continuous nonsingular and there exists $\alpha > 0$ such that $\mathbf{M}(\boldsymbol{\theta}) > \alpha\mathbf{I}$ for all $\boldsymbol{\theta} \in \Theta$.
(4) $\mathbf{C}(\boldsymbol{\theta})\mathbf{M}(\boldsymbol{\theta})\mathbf{C}(\boldsymbol{\theta}) = \mathbf{C}(\boldsymbol{\theta})$ and $\mathbf{C}(\boldsymbol{\theta})\mathbf{M}(\boldsymbol{\theta})\dot{\mathbf{A}}(\boldsymbol{\theta}) = \dot{\mathbf{A}}(\boldsymbol{\theta})$.

Our main objective is to find the asymptotic distribution of $Q_n(\boldsymbol{\theta}_n^*)$, where Q_n is the quadratic form

$$Q_n(\boldsymbol{\theta}) = n(\mathbf{Z}_n - \mathbf{A}(\boldsymbol{\theta}))^T\mathbf{M}(\boldsymbol{\theta})(\mathbf{Z}_n - \mathbf{A}(\boldsymbol{\theta})),$$

and $\boldsymbol{\theta}_n^*$ is a minimum χ^2 sequence. Under the above assumptions, the results of the previous section show that any minimum χ^2 sequence satisfies $\sqrt{n}\,(\boldsymbol{\theta}_n^* - \boldsymbol{\theta}_0) \xrightarrow{\mathscr{L}} \mathscr{N}(\mathbf{0}, (\dot{\mathbf{A}}^T\mathbf{M}\dot{\mathbf{A}})^{-1})$, where $\dot{\mathbf{A}} = \dot{\mathbf{A}}(\boldsymbol{\theta}_0)$ and $\mathbf{M} = \mathbf{M}(\boldsymbol{\theta}_0)$. The statistic $Q_n(\boldsymbol{\theta}_n^*)$ may be used as a goodness-of-fit test of the model by rejecting the model when $Q_n(\boldsymbol{\theta}_n^*)$ is too large.

Theorem 24. *Under assumptions* (1)–(4), $Q_n(\boldsymbol{\theta}_n^*) \xrightarrow{\mathscr{L}} \chi^2_{\nu-k}$, *where* ν *is the rank of the matrix* $\mathbf{C}(\boldsymbol{\theta}_0)$.

Proof. From Lemma 2 of Section 23, $\sqrt{n}(\mathbf{A}(\boldsymbol{\theta}_n^*) - \mathbf{A}(\boldsymbol{\theta}_0)) \sim \sqrt{n}\,\boldsymbol{\Pi}(\mathbf{Z}_n - \mathbf{A}(\boldsymbol{\theta}_0))$, where $\boldsymbol{\Pi} = \dot{\mathbf{A}}(\dot{\mathbf{A}}^T\mathbf{M}\dot{\mathbf{A}})^{-1}\dot{\mathbf{A}}^T\mathbf{M}$. Hence,

$$\sqrt{n}(\mathbf{Z}_n - \mathbf{A}(\boldsymbol{\theta}_n^*)) = \sqrt{n}(\mathbf{Z}_n - \mathbf{A}(\boldsymbol{\theta}_0)) - \sqrt{n}(\mathbf{A}(\boldsymbol{\theta}_n^*) - \mathbf{A}(\boldsymbol{\theta}_0))$$
$$\sim \sqrt{n}(\mathbf{I} - \boldsymbol{\Pi})(\mathbf{Z}_n - \mathbf{A}(\boldsymbol{\theta}_0)).$$

Since $\sqrt{n}(\mathbf{Z}_n - \mathbf{A}(\boldsymbol{\theta}_0)) \xrightarrow{\mathscr{L}} \mathbf{Y} \in \mathscr{N}(\mathbf{0}, \mathbf{C})$ where $\mathbf{C} = \mathbf{C}(\boldsymbol{\theta}_0)$, and since $\mathbf{M}(\boldsymbol{\theta}_n^*) \to \mathbf{M}$, we may conclude

$$Q_n(\boldsymbol{\theta}_n^*) \xrightarrow{\mathscr{L}} \mathbf{Y}^T(\mathbf{I} - \boldsymbol{\Pi})^T\mathbf{M}(\mathbf{I} - \boldsymbol{\Pi})\mathbf{Y} = \mathbf{W}^T\mathbf{W}$$

where $\mathbf{W} = \mathbf{M}^{1/2}(\mathbf{I}\text{-}\boldsymbol{\Pi})\mathbf{Y} \in \mathscr{N}(\mathbf{0}, \boldsymbol{\Sigma})$ and $\boldsymbol{\Sigma} = \mathbf{M}^{1/2}(\mathbf{I} - \boldsymbol{\Pi})\mathbf{C}(\mathbf{I} - \boldsymbol{\Pi})^T\mathbf{M}^{1/2}$. From Lemma 3 of Section 8, it is sufficient to show that $\boldsymbol{\Sigma}$ is a projection of rank $\nu - k$. To show $\boldsymbol{\Sigma}^2 = \boldsymbol{\Sigma}$, first note that $\mathbf{C}\mathbf{M}\dot{\mathbf{A}} = \dot{\mathbf{A}}$ implies $\mathbf{C}\boldsymbol{\Pi}^T\mathbf{M} = \boldsymbol{\Pi}$, so that $\mathbf{C}(\mathbf{I} - \boldsymbol{\Pi})^T\mathbf{M} = \mathbf{C}\mathbf{M} - \boldsymbol{\Pi}$, and $(\mathbf{I} - \boldsymbol{\Pi})\mathbf{C}(\mathbf{I} - \boldsymbol{\Pi})^T\mathbf{M} = (\mathbf{I} - \boldsymbol{\Pi})\mathbf{C}\mathbf{M}$. Similarly, $\mathbf{M}(\mathbf{I} - \boldsymbol{\Pi})\mathbf{C}(\mathbf{I} - \boldsymbol{\Pi})^T = \mathbf{M}\mathbf{C}(\mathbf{I} - \boldsymbol{\Pi})^T$. Hence using $\mathbf{C}\mathbf{M}\mathbf{C} = \mathbf{C}$,

$$\begin{aligned}\boldsymbol{\Sigma}^2 &= \mathbf{M}^{1/2}(\mathbf{I} - \boldsymbol{\Pi})\mathbf{C}(\mathbf{I} - \boldsymbol{\Pi})^T\mathbf{M}(\mathbf{I} - \boldsymbol{\Pi})\mathbf{C}(\mathbf{I} - \boldsymbol{\Pi})^T\mathbf{M}^{1/2}\\ &= \mathbf{M}^{1/2}(\mathbf{I} - \boldsymbol{\Pi})\mathbf{C}\mathbf{M}\mathbf{C}(\mathbf{I} - \boldsymbol{\Pi})^T\mathbf{M}^{1/2} = \mathbf{M}^{1/2}(\mathbf{I} - \boldsymbol{\Pi})\mathbf{C}(\mathbf{I} - \boldsymbol{\Pi})^T\mathbf{M}^{1/2}\\ &= \boldsymbol{\Sigma}.\end{aligned}$$

Finally, noting that $\mathbf{C}\mathbf{M}$ is a projection so that $\operatorname{rank}(\mathbf{C}\mathbf{M}) = \operatorname{trace}(\mathbf{C}\mathbf{M})$,

$$\begin{aligned}\operatorname{rank}\boldsymbol{\Sigma} &= \operatorname{trace}\boldsymbol{\Sigma} = \operatorname{trace}\left(\mathbf{M}^{1/2}(\mathbf{I} - \boldsymbol{\Pi})\mathbf{C}(\mathbf{I} - \boldsymbol{\Pi})^T\mathbf{M}^{1/2}\right)\\ &= \operatorname{trace}\left((\mathbf{I} - \boldsymbol{\Pi})\mathbf{C}(\mathbf{I} - \boldsymbol{\Pi})^T\mathbf{M}\right) = \operatorname{trace}((\mathbf{I} - \boldsymbol{\Pi})\mathbf{C}\mathbf{M})\\ &= \operatorname{trace}(\mathbf{C}\mathbf{M}) - \operatorname{trace}(\boldsymbol{\Pi}\mathbf{C}\mathbf{M}) = \operatorname{rank}(\mathbf{C}\mathbf{M}) - \operatorname{trace}(\boldsymbol{\Pi})\\ &= \operatorname{rank}(\mathbf{C}) - \operatorname{rank}(\boldsymbol{\Pi}) = \nu - k. \quad \blacksquare\end{aligned}$$

Power. We may use this result to test the model given by assumption (1) by rejecting if $Q_n(\boldsymbol{\theta}_n^*)$ is too large. We may find an approximation to the power of this test by finding the asymptotic distribution of $Q_n(\boldsymbol{\theta}_n^*)$ when assumption (1) is changed to

(1′) $\sqrt{n}(\mathbf{Z}_n - \mathbf{A}(\boldsymbol{\theta}_0)) \xrightarrow{\mathscr{L}} \mathbf{Y} \in \mathscr{N}(\boldsymbol{\delta}, \mathbf{C}(\boldsymbol{\theta}_0))$.

Then Lemmas 1 and 2 of Section 23 are still valid, and in Theorem 24 one can conclude

$$Q_n(\boldsymbol{\theta}_n^*) \xrightarrow{\mathscr{L}} \mathbf{Y}^T(\mathbf{I} - \boldsymbol{\Pi})^T\mathbf{M}(\mathbf{I} - \boldsymbol{\Pi})\mathbf{Y} = \mathbf{W}^T\mathbf{W},$$

where $\mathbf{W} = \mathbf{M}^{1/2}(\mathbf{I} - \mathbf{\Pi})\mathbf{Y} \in \mathcal{N}(\mathbf{M}^{1/2}(\mathbf{I} - \mathbf{\Pi})\boldsymbol{\delta}, \boldsymbol{\Sigma})$. Thus from the lemma of Section 10, $Q_n(\boldsymbol{\theta}_0^*)$ has asymptotically a noncentral χ^2 distribution, $Q_n(\boldsymbol{\theta}_n^*) \xrightarrow{\mathscr{L}} \chi^2_{\nu-k}(\lambda)$, with noncentrality parameter $\lambda = \boldsymbol{\delta}^T(\mathbf{I} - \mathbf{\Pi})^T\mathbf{M}(\mathbf{I} - \mathbf{\Pi})\boldsymbol{\delta}$.

Note: These results are valid for an arbitrary minimum χ^2 sequence, $\boldsymbol{\theta}_n^*$. This may be any of the minimum modified, transformed, et cetera χ^2's —they are all asymptotically equivalent. When sampling from an exponential family of distributions (like the multinomial), these estimates are also asymptotically equivalent to maximum-likelihood estimates.

To be able to apply Theorem 24 to Pearson's χ^2, we should check that $\mathbf{M} = \mathbf{P}^{-1}$ is a generalized inverse of $\mathbf{C} = \mathbf{P} - \mathbf{p}\mathbf{p}^T$. (We have not needed this before.) This follows from

$$\begin{aligned} \mathbf{CMC} &= (\mathbf{I} - \mathbf{p}\mathbf{p}^T\mathbf{P}^{-1})\mathbf{C} = (\mathbf{I} - \mathbf{p}\mathbf{1}^T)(\mathbf{P} - \mathbf{p}\mathbf{p}^T) \\ &= \mathbf{P} - \mathbf{p}\mathbf{1}^T\mathbf{P} - \mathbf{p}\mathbf{p}^T + \mathbf{p}(\mathbf{1}^T\mathbf{p})\mathbf{p}^T \\ &= \mathbf{P} - \mathbf{p}\mathbf{p}^T - \mathbf{p}\mathbf{p}^T + \mathbf{p}\mathbf{p}^T = \mathbf{C}. \end{aligned}$$

Example 1. *A contingency table.* Samples of size n are chosen from each of r populations, each observation resulting in one of c possible outcomes or cells. Let p_{ij} represent the probability that an observation from the ith population results in the jth outcome, and let n_{ij} be the total number of such observations. We have

$$\sum_{j=1}^{c} p_{ij} = 1 \quad \text{and} \quad \sum_{j=1}^{c} n_{ij} = n, \qquad \text{for all } i = 1, \ldots, r.$$

To test the hypothesis of homogeneity of the populations

$$H_0\colon p_{ij} = \pi_j, \qquad \text{for all } i \text{ and } j,$$

where the π_j are unknown numbers such that $\sum_1^c \pi_j = 1$, we form the χ^2,

$$Q_n(\boldsymbol{\pi}) = \sum_{i=1}^{r}\sum_{j=1}^{c} \frac{(n_{ij} - n\pi_j)^2}{n\pi_j}.$$

When H_0 is true, $Q_n(\boldsymbol{\pi}_n^*)$ will have, for large n, an approximate χ^2 distribution. The degrees of freedom may be calculated as follows. For each i, $\sum_{j=1}^{c}(n_{ij} - n\pi_j)^2/n\pi_j$ is an ordinary χ^2 with $(c-1)$ d.f. The sum of r independent χ^2's of this type gives a χ^2 with $r(c-1)$ d.f. There are $c-1$ independent π_j. When we estimate them, we lose $c-1$ d.f. ending with $r(c-1) - (c-1) = (r-1)(c-1)$ d.f.

To find a minimum χ^2 sequence, we may use Lagrange multipliers. Taking derivatives of $Q_n(\boldsymbol{\pi}) + \lambda(\sum_1^c \pi_j - 1)$ pretending the denominators in $Q_n(\boldsymbol{\pi})$ do not depend on $\boldsymbol{\pi}$, we obtain

$$\frac{\partial}{\partial \pi_j}\left(Q_n(\boldsymbol{\pi}) + \lambda\left(\sum_1^c \pi_j - 1\right)\right)$$

$$= \sum_{i=1}^r \frac{-2n(n_{ij} - n\pi_j)}{n\pi_j} + \lambda = 0, \qquad \text{for } j = 1, \ldots, c.$$

This leads to

$$\frac{1}{n\pi_j}\sum_{i=1}^r n_{ij} = \frac{\lambda}{2n} + r \quad \text{or} \quad \pi_j^* = \frac{2}{\lambda + 2nr} n_{\cdot j}.$$

The constraint $\sum_1^c \pi_j^* = 1$ then gives $\pi_j^* = (1/nr)n_{\cdot j}$ = average relative frequency of cell j. These are, in fact, the maximum-likelihood estimates for this problem. We reject H_0 if

$$Q_n(\boldsymbol{\pi}^*) = n\sum_i \sum_j \frac{\left(n_{ij}/n - (1/nr)n_{\cdot j}\right)^2}{(1/nr)n_{\cdot j}} > \chi^2_{(r-1)(c-1);\,\alpha}.$$

To find the power at an arbitrary point (p_{ij}), we must compute the noncentrality parameter. This is done by replacing n_{ij}/n whenever it occurs in $Q_n(\boldsymbol{\pi}^*)$ by p_{ij}:

$$\lambda = n\sum_i \sum_j \frac{\left(p_{ij} - (1/r)p_{\cdot j}\right)^2}{(1/r)p_{\cdot j}}.$$

If (p_{ij}) are the true values of the parameters, then the distribution of $Q_n(\boldsymbol{\pi}^*)$ is approximately the $\chi^2_{(r-1)(c-1)}(\lambda)$ distribution.

Testing Against Restricted Alternatives. The tests discussed above are designed to be good against all alternatives. One can obtain a more sensitive test when it is known that the alternatives lie in some restricted class. Suppose that $\boldsymbol{\theta}$ is known to lie in Θ, an open set in $\mathbb{R}^k$, and that it is desired to test H_0: $\boldsymbol{\theta} \in \Theta_0$, an open smooth submanifold of Θ of dimension $k - r$ (r represents the number of restrictions under H_0). It is reasonable to reject H_0 if Θ is much better at explaining the data than is Θ_0, where the minimum χ^2 value may be used as a measure of how good the explanation is. This test rejects H_0 if

$$\inf_{\boldsymbol{\theta} \in \Theta_0} Q_n(\boldsymbol{\theta}) - \inf_{\boldsymbol{\theta} \in \Theta} Q_n(\boldsymbol{\theta})$$

is too large, or, equivalently, if $Q_n(\boldsymbol{\theta}_n^*) - Q_n(\hat{\boldsymbol{\theta}}_n)$ is too large, where $\boldsymbol{\theta}_n^*$ and $\hat{\boldsymbol{\theta}}_n$ are minimum χ^2 sequences under Θ_0 and Θ, respectively.

Let $\boldsymbol{\theta}_0$ denote the true value of $\boldsymbol{\theta}$, and suppose $\boldsymbol{\theta}_0 \in \Theta_0$. Let T_0 and T denote the tangent planes to $\mathbf{A}(\boldsymbol{\theta})$ for $\boldsymbol{\theta} \in \Theta_0$ and $\boldsymbol{\theta} \in \Theta$, respectively, and let $\boldsymbol{\Pi}_0$ and $\boldsymbol{\Pi}$ denote the projections along the metric $\|\mathbf{x}\|^2 = \mathbf{x}^T\mathbf{M}\mathbf{x}$ to the planes T_0 and T, respectively. Then

$$\begin{aligned} Q_n(\boldsymbol{\theta}_n^*) - Q(\hat{\boldsymbol{\theta}}_n) &\sim n\|\mathbf{Z}_n - \mathbf{A}(\boldsymbol{\theta}_n^*)\|^2 - n\|\mathbf{Z}_n - \mathbf{A}(\hat{\boldsymbol{\theta}}_n)\|^2 \\ &\sim n\|(\mathbf{I} - \boldsymbol{\Pi}_0)(Z_n - \mathbf{A}(\boldsymbol{\theta}_0))\|^2 - n\|(\mathbf{I} - \boldsymbol{\Pi})(\mathbf{Z}_n - \mathbf{A}(\boldsymbol{\theta}_0))\|^2 \\ &= n\|(\boldsymbol{\Pi} - \boldsymbol{\Pi}_0)(\mathbf{Z}_n - \mathbf{A}(\boldsymbol{\theta}_0))\|^2. \end{aligned}$$

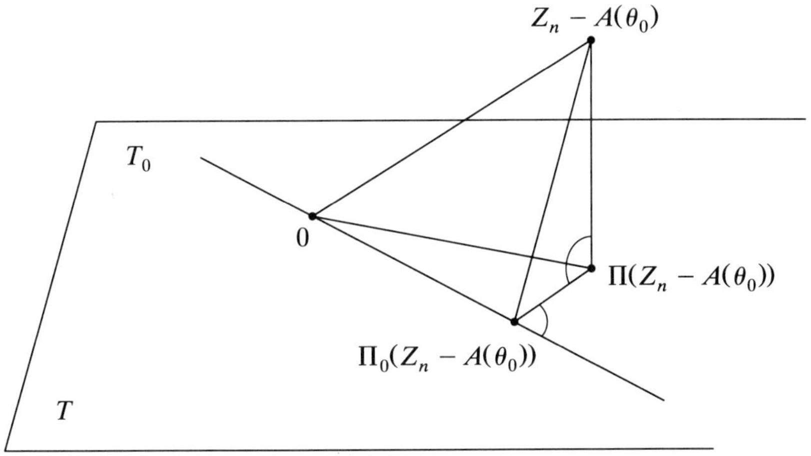

Since $\mathbf{\Pi}$ and $\mathbf{\Pi}_0$ are projections and $\mathbf{\Pi}\mathbf{\Pi}_0 = \mathbf{\Pi}_0\mathbf{\Pi} = \mathbf{\Pi}_0$, it follows that $(\mathbf{\Pi} - \mathbf{\Pi}_0)$ is a projection and that

$$\begin{aligned}\operatorname{rank}(\mathbf{\Pi} - \mathbf{\Pi}_0) &= \operatorname{trace}(\mathbf{\Pi} - \mathbf{\Pi}_0) = \operatorname{trace}\mathbf{\Pi} - \operatorname{trace}\mathbf{\Pi}_0 \\ &= k - (k - r) = r.\end{aligned}$$

Hence $Q_n(\boldsymbol{\theta}_n^*) - Q_n(\hat{\boldsymbol{\theta}}_n) \xrightarrow{\mathscr{L}} \chi_r^2$. Note that $Q_n(\boldsymbol{\theta}_n^*) - Q_n(\hat{\boldsymbol{\theta}}_n)$ and $Q_n(\hat{\boldsymbol{\theta}}_n)$ are asymptotically independent. Thus, $Q_n(\hat{\boldsymbol{\theta}}_n)$ provides an independent check on the validity of the model.

Example 2. Humans may be classified into one of four blood phenotypes: O, A, B, and AB. Inheritance into these groups is controlled through three alleles; O, A, and B, at one locus, with O recessive to both A and B. The general theory predicts that the four blood phenotypes, O: A: B: AB, occur in the proportions p^2: $q^2 + 2pq$: $r^2 + 2pr$: $2qr$, where p, q, and r are the relative frequencies of the alleles O, A, and B, respectively, in the whole population, and $p + q + r = 1$. It is desired to test the hypothesis that $p = \frac{1}{2}$, $q = \frac{1}{3}$, and $r = \frac{1}{6}$, based on a sample of size 770 with the observed frequencies: 180, 360, 132, 98, of the four blood types; O, A, B, AB, respectively.

The null hypothesis is simple, so if we were testing against all alternatives, we would reject if $\chi^2 > \chi^2_{3;\,0.05}$, where

$$\begin{aligned}\chi^2 &= \frac{(180 - 770(0.25))^2}{770(0.25)} + \frac{(360 - 770(0.444))^2}{770(0.444)} \\ &\quad + \frac{(132 - 770(0.194))^2}{770(0.194)} + \frac{(98 - 770(0.111))^2}{770(0.111)} \\ &= \frac{(180 - 193)^2}{193} + \frac{(360 - 342)^2}{342} \\ &\quad + \frac{(132 - 149)^2}{149} + \frac{(98 - 85)^2}{85} = 5.73.\end{aligned}$$

Since $\chi^2_{3;\,0.05} = 7.815$, we accept H_0 at the 5% level.

However, we should be testing against the restricted alternative that the four cell probabilities are $p^2: q^2 + 2pq: r^2 + 2pr: 2qr$ for some p, q, and r that sum to 1. Hence we should first subtract $Q_n(\hat{\boldsymbol{\theta}}_n)$ where $\hat{\boldsymbol{\theta}}_n$ represents minimum χ^2 estimates of p, q, r. These estimates may be computed by numerical methods. They turn out to be about $\hat{p} = 0.47$, $\hat{q} = 0.36$, $\hat{r} = 0.17$, and

$$Q_n(\hat{\boldsymbol{\theta}}_n) = \frac{(180-170)^2}{170} + \frac{(360-361)^2}{361} + \frac{(132-146)^2}{146} + \frac{(98-94)^2}{94} = 2.10.$$

We reject at the 5% level if the difference, $\chi^2 - Q_n(\hat{\boldsymbol{\theta}}_n)$, is greater than $\chi^2_{2;\,0.05}$. In this case, $5.73 - 2.10 = 3.63 < \chi^2_{2;\,0.05} = 5.99$, so we do not reject. Note that $Q_n(\hat{\boldsymbol{\theta}}_n)$ is exactly the χ^2 we would use to test the hypothesis that the blood types have the given relative frequencies for some p, q, r. It provides an independent check on the validity of the general theory for this population. It has 1 degree of freedom.

EXERCISES

1. Consider three hypotheses about a given die with probabilities p_j that side j comes up for $j = 1, \ldots, 6$.

   H_0: The die is fair; that is, $p_j = \frac{1}{6}$ for all j.
   H_1: The die has been shaved slightly so that opposite faces come up with equal probability; that is, H_1: $p_1 = p_6$, $p_2 = p_5$, $p_3 = p_4$.
   H: The probabilities p_j are completely arbitrary.
   The die was tossed 120 times with the following results: $n_1 = 10$, $n_2 = 24$, $n_3 = 20$, $n_4 = 26$, $n_5 = 24$, $n_6 = 16$, where n_j is the number of times side j came up.
   (a) Test H_0 vs H at the 5% level.
   (b) Test H_1 vs H at the 5% level.
   (c) Test H_0 vs H_1 at the 5% level.
   (d) Find the power for each of the above tests at the alternative $p_1 = p_2 = p_3 = p_4 = \frac{1}{8}$, $p_5 = p_6 = \frac{1}{4}$.
2. A sample of 200 married couples was taken from a certain population. Husbands and wives were interviewed separately to determine whether

their main source of news was from the newspapers, radio, or television. The results may be found in the following table.

		Husband		
		Papers	Radio	TV
	Papers	15	6	10
Wife	Radio	11	10	20
	TV	23	15	90

Let p_{ij} denote the probability that a randomly selected couple will fall in cell (i, j). Perform the following tests at the 5% level.

(a) Test H_1: $p_{ij} = p_{ji}$ for all i and j (symmetry).

(b) Test H_0: $p_{ij} = p_i p_j$ for some $p_1 + p_2 + p_3 = 1$ (symmetry and independence).

(c) Test H_0 against H_1.

3. N balls are distributed at random in to $I \times J$ cells, where cell (i, j) has probability $p_{ij} \geq 0$, $i = 1, \ldots, I$, $j = 1, \ldots, J$, $\Sigma_i \Sigma_j p_{ij} = 1$. Let n_{ij} represent the number of balls that fall in cell (i, j), $\Sigma_i \Sigma_j n_{ij} = N$.
   (a) Find the χ^2 test of the hypothesis H: $\Sigma_j p_{ij} = 1/I$, for $i = 1, \ldots, I$. How many degrees of freedom?
   (b) Find the χ^2 test of the hypothesis H_0: p_{ij} is independent of i (that is, $p_{1j} = p_{2j} = \cdots = p_{Ij}$ for $j = 1, \ldots, J$). How many degrees of freedom?
   (c) Find the χ^2 test of H_0 against $H - H_0$. How many degrees of freedom?
4. Consider a three-factor contingency table with probabilities p_{ijk}, for cell (i, j, k) for $i = 1, \ldots, I$, $j = 1, \ldots, J$, and $k = 1, \ldots, K$, such that $\Sigma_i \Sigma_j \Sigma_k p_{ijk} = 1$. Suppose a sample of size N is taken and let n_{ijk} denote the number of observations that fall in cell (i, j, k). Find the χ^2 tests of the following hypotheses. Find the maximum-likelihood estimates and the degrees of freedom.

(a) H_0: $p_{ijk} = p_i q_j r_k$	(three-way independence)
(b) H_0: $p_{ijk} = p_i q_{jk}$	(independence of the first factor from the other two)
(c) H_0: $p_{ijk} = \pi_i q_{jk}$,	where the π_i are known (the first factor has a given probability vector and is independent of the other two)
(d) H_0: $p_{ijk} = p_{i\mid k} q_{j\mid k} r_k$	(conditional independence of the first two factors given the third)
(e) H_0: $p_{ijk} = p_i q_j r_{k\mid ij}$	(marginal independence of the first two factors)

5. To test the effectiveness of five different insecticide treatments, $T1$, $T2$, $T3$, $T4$, $T5$, for the control of two species of ticks, $S1$, $S2$, cattle were chosen at random and randomly assigned treatments. After treatment, the hides were inspected for the presence of living and dead ticks. The data are as follows.

	$S1$		$S2$	
	killed	not killed	killed	not killed
$T1$	30	20	42	35
$T2$	42	11	41	20
$T3$	63	51	22	18
$T4$	20	41	12	31
$T5$	11	17	21	31

(a) Test the hypothesis at the 5% level that there is no difference between the species with regard to these treatments; that is, test H_0: $p_i = \pi_i$ for $i = 1, \ldots, 5$, where $p_1, \ldots, p_5$ are the probabilities of death for species $S1$, and $\pi_1, \ldots, \pi_5$ are the probabilities of death for species $S2$. (Use modified χ^2.)

(b) Find the approximate power of this test at the alternative $p_i = \pi_i + 0.1$, $i = 1, 2, 3, 4, 5$.

Appendix

SOLUTIONS TO THE EXERCISES OF SECTION 1

1. Since $\Gamma(1 + 1/n) = (1/n)\Gamma(1/n)$, we have $\Gamma(1/n) \sim n$. If $f_n(x)$ represents the density of $\mathscr{B}e(1/n, 1/n)$, then $f_n(x) \sim x^{-1}(1-x)^{-1}/(2n)$. Hence, for any small $\varepsilon > 0$, $P(\varepsilon < X_n < 1 - \varepsilon) \to 0$. Since by symmetry, $P(X_n \le \varepsilon) = P(X_n \ge 1 - \varepsilon)$, we have that $P(X_n \le \varepsilon) \to \frac{1}{2}$ for all $0 < \varepsilon < 1$. Thus, $F_n(x)$ converges to the distribution function of X for all $x \neq 0$, $x \neq 1$ showing that X_n converges in law to X.

   For $\alpha \neq \beta$, the symmetry argument does not work, so instead we compute

$$\begin{aligned} P(X_n \le \varepsilon) &= \int_0^\varepsilon f_n(x)\,dx \\ &\sim \frac{\alpha\beta}{n(\alpha+\beta)} \int_0^\varepsilon x^{(\alpha/n)-1}(1-x)^{(\beta/n)-1}\,dx \\ &\ge \frac{\alpha\beta}{n(\alpha+\beta)} \int_0^\varepsilon x^{(\alpha/n)-1}\,dx \\ &= (\beta/(\alpha+\beta))\varepsilon^{\alpha/n} \to \beta/(\alpha+\beta). \end{aligned}$$

   Similarly, $P(X_n \ge 1 - \varepsilon) \ge (\alpha/(\alpha+\beta))\varepsilon^{\beta/n} \to \alpha/(\alpha+\beta)$, and because the sum of these two pieces is no greater than 1, we must have $P(X_n \le \varepsilon) \to \beta/(\alpha+\beta)$. This implies that X_n converges in law to $\mathscr{B}(1, \beta/(\alpha+\beta))$.

2. $P(X_n \le x) = k/n$ where $k/n \le x < (k+1)/n$. Then, since $|k/n - x| < 1/n$, we have $P(X_n \le x) \to x$, showing that X_n converges in law to X where X is $\mathscr{U}(0, 1)$.

   From the information given, one cannot tell whether X_n converges in probability to X because the joint distribution of X_n and X has not been defined.

3. (a) Suppose that $0 < r < s$ and $E|X|^s < \infty$. By Hölder's inequality, $EZ^p \le (EZ)^p$ for any random variable $Z > 0$ and any $0 < p < 1$. Replace Z by $|X_n - X|^s$ and p by r/s, and find

$$E|X_n - X|^r \le \left(E|X_n - X|^s\right)^{r/s}.$$

Thus, $E|X_n - X|^s < \infty$ implies $E|X_n - X|^r < \infty$.

(b) The same inequality shows that $E|X_n - X|^s \to 0$ implies $E|X_n - X|^r \to 0$.

4. If $X_n = n$ with probability $1/n^2$ and $X_n = 0$ otherwise, then $E|X_n| = 1/n \to 0$ and $E|X_n|^2 = 1$ for all n.

5. In one dimension, $E(X_n - \mu)^2 = \text{var}(X_n) + (EX_n - \mu)^2$. So if $EX_n \to \mu$ and $\text{var}(X_n) \to 0$, then $E(X_n - \mu)^2 \to 0$. Conversely, if $E(X_n - \mu)^2 \to 0$, then $\text{var}(X_n) \le E(X_n - \mu)^2 \to 0$ and $(EX_n - \mu)^2 \le E(X_n - \mu)^2 \to 0$.

In d dimensions, the same proof works treating each summand of $(X_n - \mu)^T(X_n - \mu) = \sum_{i=1}^d (X_{ni} - \mu_i)^2$ separately.

6. Let $\varepsilon > 0$, and find an integer k such that $1/k < \varepsilon/2$. Since F is continuous, we can find numbers x_j such that $F(x_j) = j/k$, for $j = 1, \ldots, k-1$. Since $F_n(x_j) \to F(x_j)$ as $n \to \infty$, we can find N_j such that for $n > N_j$ we have $|F_n(x_j) - F(x_j)| < 1/k$. Let $N = \max\{N_1, \ldots, N_{k-1}\}$. If $n > N$ and $x_j \le x \le x_{j+1}$, then

$$F_n(x) \le F_n(x_{j+1}) \le F(x_{j+1}) + 1/k \le F(x) + 2/k.$$

Similarly,

$$F_n(x) \ge F_n(x_j) \ge F(x_j) - 1/k \ge F(x) - 2/k.$$

Hence, if $n > N$, $|F_n(x) - F(x)| \le 2/k < \varepsilon$ for all x.

7. (a) Note that $0 \le X_1 \le X_2 \le \cdots \le \lim_{n\to\infty} X_n = X$. This shows that $EX_n \le EX$, so that $\limsup EX_n \le EX$. From the Fatou–Lebesgue Lemma with $Y \equiv 0$, we have $\liminf EX_n \ge EX$. Combining these two inequalities gives $\lim EX_n = EX$.

(b) If $|X_n| \le Y$, then we have $-Y \le -X_n$. So, assuming $X_n \xrightarrow{\text{a.s.}} X$, the Fatou–Lebesgue Lemma gives $\liminf E(-X_n) \ge E(-X)$ or, equivalently, $\limsup EX_n \le EX$. We also have $-Y \le X_n$, so again from the Fatou–Lebesgue Lemma, $\liminf EX_n \ge EX$. Combining these two inequalities gives $\lim EX_n = EX$.

SOLUTIONS TO THE EXERCISES OF SECTION 2

1. (a) $E|X_n|^r < \infty$ if and only if $r < \alpha$. Therefore $E|X_n/n|^r = E|X_n|^r/n^r \to 0$ if and only if $r < \alpha$.

(b) We are to show that $P(|X_n/n| > \varepsilon \text{ i.o.}) = 0$ for every $\varepsilon > 0$. By the Borel–Cantelli Lemma, this holds provided $\Sigma_n P(|X_n/n| > \varepsilon) < \infty$ for every $\varepsilon > 0$. Now $P(X_n > n\varepsilon) = 1$ for $n\varepsilon \leq 1$, while for $n > 1/\varepsilon$,

$$P(X_n > n\varepsilon) = \int_{n\varepsilon}^{\infty} \alpha x^{-(\alpha+1)}\, dx = (n\varepsilon)^{-\alpha}.$$

Thus, the series $\Sigma_n P(X_n > n\varepsilon)$ converges for all $\varepsilon > 0$ if and only if $\alpha > 1$. Hence X_n/n converges almost surely to 0 if [and only if, using Exercise 4(b) and the independence of the X_n] $\alpha > 1$.

2. If $\Sigma E|\mathbf{X}_n - \mathbf{X}|^r < \infty$, then $E|\mathbf{X}_n - \mathbf{X}|^r \to 0$, so that $\mathbf{X}_n$ converges to $\mathbf{X}$ in the rth mean. Moreover, from Chebyshev's inequality, $\Sigma P(|\mathbf{X}_n - \mathbf{X}| > \varepsilon) \leq \Sigma E|\mathbf{X}_n - \mathbf{X}|^r/\varepsilon^r < \infty$ for arbitrary $\varepsilon > 0$, which implies $P(|\mathbf{X}_n - \mathbf{X}| > \varepsilon \text{ i.o.}) = 0$ using the Borel–Cantelli Lemma. Thus, $\mathbf{X}_n$ converges to $\mathbf{X}$ almost surely.
3. If $\mathbf{X}_n$ does not converge in the rth mean to $\mathbf{X}$, then there exists an $\varepsilon > 0$ such that

$$E|\mathbf{X}_{n'} - \mathbf{X}|^r > \varepsilon \text{ for some subsequence } n'. \qquad (*)$$

Since $\mathbf{X}_n \xrightarrow{\text{P}} \mathbf{X}$, one can apply Theorem 2(d) and find a subsubsequence n'' of the subsequence n' such that $\mathbf{X}_{n''} \xrightarrow{\text{a.s.}} \mathbf{X}$. But from Theorem 2(b), $\mathbf{X}_{n''} \xrightarrow{r} \mathbf{X}$, which contradicts $(*)$. Similarly, from Theorem 2(c), $\mathbf{X}_{n''} \xrightarrow{r} \mathbf{X}$ for $r = 1$, contradicting $(*)$ for $r = 1$.
4. (a) Let $Z \in \mathscr{U}(0,1)$, and let $A_n = \{Z < 1/n\}$. Then $P(A_n \text{ i.o.}) = 0$, but $\Sigma P(A_n) = \Sigma(1/n) = \infty$.

(b) We will show $P(A_n$ finitely often$) = 0$.

$$\begin{aligned}
P(A_n \text{ f.o.}) &= P\Big(\bigcup_n \bigcap_{j>n} A_j^c\Big) \\
&= \lim_{n\to\infty} P\Big(\bigcap_{j>n} A_j^c\Big), \quad \text{because } \bigcap_{j>n} A_j^c \text{ are nondecreasing} \\
&= \lim_{n\to\infty} \prod_{j>n} P(A_j^c), \quad \text{because the } A_n^c \text{ are independent} \\
&= \lim_{n\to\infty} \prod_{j>n} \big(1 - P(A_j)\big) \\
&\leq \lim_{n\to\infty} \prod_{j>n} \exp\{-P(A_j)\}, \quad \text{because } 1 - x \leq \exp\{-x\} \\
&= \lim_{n\to\infty} \exp\Big\{-\sum_{j>n} P(A_j)\Big\} = 0,
\end{aligned}$$

since $\Sigma_{j>n} P(A_j) = \infty$ for all n.

5. (a) For $\varepsilon > 0$, $P(|X_n| > \varepsilon) \le P(X_n \ne 0) = 1/n \to 0$. Hence, X_n converges in probability to zero for all α.
   (b) X_n converges to 0 almost surely if and only if $P(|X_n| > \varepsilon \text{ i.o.}) = 0$ for all $\varepsilon > 0$. Since the X_n are independent, the Borel–Cantelli Lemma and its converse, 4(b), implies that this is equivalent to $\Sigma P(|X_n| > \varepsilon) < \infty$ for all $\varepsilon > 0$. Since $\Sigma 1/n = \infty$, we have that X_n converges to zero almost surely if and only if $\alpha < 0$.
   (c) $E|X_n|^r = n^{\alpha r}(1/n) \to 0$ if and only if $\alpha < 1/r$.
6. (a) $|f_n(x) - g(x)| = f_n(x) - g(x) + 2(g(x) - f_n(x))^+$. Hence,

$$\int |f_n(x) - g(x)|\,d\nu(x)$$

$$= \int (f_n(x) - g(x))\,d\nu(x) + 2\int (g(x) - f_n(x))^+\,d\nu(x).$$

   The first integral is zero since $\int f_n(x)\,d\nu(x) = \int g(x)\,d\nu(x) = 1$. The second term converges to zero by the Lebesgue Dominated Convergence Theorem, since $(g(x) - f_n(x))^+ \le g(x)$.
   (b)

$$\begin{aligned}\sup_A |P(X_n \in A) - P(X \in A)| &= \sup_A \left| \int_A (f_n(x) - g(x))\,d\nu(x) \right| \\ &\le \sup_A \int_A |f_n(x) - g(x)|\,d\nu(x) \\ &= \int |f_n(x) - g(x)|\,d\nu(x) \\ &\to 0.\end{aligned}$$

7. Write $|X_n| = X_n^+ + X_n^-$, where $X_n^+ = \max\{X_n, 0\}$ and $X_n^- = (-X_n)^+$. From $X_n \xrightarrow{\text{a.s.}} X$ we may conclude that $X_n^+ \xrightarrow{\text{a.s.}} X^+$ and $X_n^- \xrightarrow{\text{a.s.}} X^-$. By Fatou's Lemma, we have $\liminf EX_n^+ \ge EX^+$ and $\liminf EX_n^- \ge EX^-$. Therefore,

$$E|X| = \lim E|X_n| \ge \liminf EX^+ + \liminf EX_n^- \ge EX^+ + EX^- = E|X|.$$

   Since we have equality throughout, we must have $\lim EX_n^+ = EX^+$ and $\lim EX_n^- = EX^-$. We may now apply Scheffé's Theorem to the positive and negative parts and conclude $E|X_n^+ - X^+| \to 0$ and $E|X_n^- - X^-| \to 0$. The result then follows from $E|X_n - X| = E|(X_n^+ - X^+) - (X_n^- - X^-)| \le E|X_n^+ - X^+| + E|X_n^- - X^-| \to 0$.
8. From the Schwartz inequality, $E|X_nX| \le \sqrt{EX_n^2 EX^2}$. From $EX_n^2 \to EX^2$, it follows that $\limsup_{n\to\infty} E|X_nX| \le EX^2$. Hence, the Fatou–Lebesgue Lemma implies $E|X_nX| \to EX^2$. From Exercise 7, $E|X_nX -$

$X^2| \to 0$, and in particular, $EX_nX \to EX^2$. The result now follows from $E(X_n - X)^2 = EX_n^2 - 2EX_nX + EX^2 \to 0$.

SOLUTIONS TO THE EXERCISES OF SECTION 3

1. (a) Let $X_n = X + (1/n)$. Then $X_n \to X$ in law, yet $Eg(X_n) = P(0 \le X \le 9)$ does not converge to $Eg(X) = P(1 \le X \le 9)$.
   (b) $g(x) = \exp\{-x^2\}$ is continuous and bounded so that $Eg(X_n) \to Eg(X)$.
   (c) $g(x) = \text{sgn}(\cos(x))$ is continuous at all points except $\pm\pi/2, \pm 3\pi/2, \pm 5\pi/2, \ldots$. None of these points is an integer; hence $P(X \in C(g)) = 1$, and $Eg(X_n) \to Eg(X)$.
   (d) Let $X_n = X$ with probability $(n-1)/n$ and $X_n = n$ with probability $1/n$. Then $X_n \to X$ in probability and hence in law; yet $EX_n = ((n-1)/n)EX + n/n \to EX + 1$.
2. Use characteristic functions. Since $\mathbf{a}'\mathbf{X}_n \xrightarrow{\mathscr{L}} \mathbf{a}'\mathbf{X}$ for every $\mathbf{a}$,

$$\Phi_{\mathbf{a}'\mathbf{X}_n}(t) \to \Phi_{\mathbf{a}'\mathbf{X}}(t), \qquad \text{for all } \mathbf{a} \text{ and } t.$$

   The result then follows from

$$\Phi_{\mathbf{X}_n}(\mathbf{a}) = E\exp\{i\mathbf{a}'\mathbf{X}_n\} = \Phi_{\mathbf{a}'\mathbf{X}_n}(1) \to \Phi_{\mathbf{a}'\mathbf{X}}(1) = \Phi_{\mathbf{X}}(\mathbf{a})$$

   for all $\mathbf{a}$.
3. By Scheffé's Useful Convergence Theorem, we have $\int|f_n(x) - f(x)|\,d\nu(x) \to 0$ as $n \to \infty$. Hence,

$$\begin{aligned} |E(g(X_n) - g(X))| &= \left|\int g(x)(f_n(x) - f(x))\,d\nu(x)\right| \\ &\le \int |g(x)||f_n(x) - f(x)|\,d\nu(x) \\ &\le B\int |f_n(x) - f(x)|\,d\nu(x) \to 0, \end{aligned}$$

   where B is a bound for $|g(x)|$.
4. (a) The characteristic function of $\mathscr{B}(n, p_n)$ is

$$\begin{aligned} E\exp\{itS_n\} &= \sum_{j=0}^{n} e^{itj}\binom{n}{j} p_n^j (1-p_n)^{n-j} \\ &= \sum_{j=0}^{n}\binom{n}{j}(p_n e^{it})^j (1-p_n)^{n-j} = (p_n e^{it} + 1 - p_n)^n \end{aligned}$$

from the binomial theorem. The characteristic function of $\mathscr{P}(\lambda)$ is

$$Ee^{itZ} = \sum_{j=0}^{\infty} e^{itj} e^{-\lambda}\lambda^j/j! = e^{-\lambda} \sum_{j=0}^{\infty} (e^{it}\lambda)^j/j! = e^{-\lambda+\lambda e^{it}} = \exp\{\lambda(e^{it}-1)\}.$$

Let $\lambda_n = np_n$. Then $\lambda_n \to \lambda$ and

$$E\exp\{itS_n\} = \left(\frac{\lambda_n}{n}e^{it} + 1 - \frac{\lambda_n}{n}\right)^n$$

$$= \left(1 + \frac{\lambda_n(e^{it}-1)}{n}\right)^n \to \exp\{\lambda(e^{it}-1)\},$$

so $S_n \xrightarrow{\mathscr{L}} Z$ from the Continuity Theorem.

(b) The same method may be used. The log of the characteristic function of S_n is

$$\log E\exp\{itS_n\} = \log \prod_{j=1}^{n} \left(1 + p_{jn}(e^{it}-1)\right) = \sum_{j=1}^{n} \log\left(1 + p_{jn}(e^{it}-1)\right).$$

The Taylor expansion of $\log(1+z)$ for z in a neighborhood of 0 gives $\log(1+z) = z + zg(z)$, where $g(z)$ is a continuous function such that $g(0) = 0$. Since $\max_{j\le n} p_{jn} \to 0$, we have $g(p_{jn}(e^{it}-1)) \to 0$ uniformly in j. Hence, for all t as $n \to \infty$,

$$\log E\exp\{itS_n\} = \sum_{j=1}^{n} \left(p_{jn}(e^{it}-1) + p_{jn}(e^{it}-1)g\left(p_{jn}(e^{it}-1)\right)\right)$$

$$= (e^{it}-1)\left(\sum_{j=1}^{n} p_{jn}\right) + (e^{it}-1)\sum_{j=1}^{n} p_{jn}g\left(p_{jn}(e^{it}-1)\right)$$

$$\to \lambda(e^{it}-1),$$

the log of the characteristic function of $\mathscr{P}(\lambda)$.

5. Let U_i be iid $\mathscr{U}(0,1)$ random variables, and let $X_i = I(U_i > 1 - p_i)$. Then, $X_1, \ldots, X_n$ are independent Bernoulli trials with $P(X_i = 1) = p_i$ for $i = 1, \ldots, n$. Now define Y_i to have a $\mathscr{P}(p_i)$ distribution: let $Y_i = 0$ if $U_i < F(0)$ and for $k = 1, 2, \ldots$ let $Y_i = k$ if $F(k-1) < U_i < F(k)$, where F represents the distribution function of $\mathscr{P}(p_i)$. Since $P(X_i = 0) = 1 - p_i \le \exp(-p_i) = P(Y_i = 0)$, we have that $Y_i = 0$ whenever $X_i = 0$. Let $Z = \Sigma_1^n Y_i$.

(1) To show $|P(S_n \in A) - P(Z \in A)| \le P(S_n \ne Z)$, suppose without loss of generality that $P(S_n \in A) \ge P(Z \in A)$. Then,

$$P(S_n \in A) - P(Z \in A) \le P(S_n \in A) - P(S_n \in A \text{ and } Z \in A)$$
$$= P(S_n \in A \text{ and } Z \notin A) \le P(S_n \ne Z).$$

(2) If $S_n \ne Z$, then for at least one i, we have $X_i \ne Y_i$. Hence,

$$P(S_n \ne Z) \le P\left(\bigcup_1^n \{X_i \ne Y_i\}\right) \le \sum_1^n P(X_i \ne Y_i).$$

(3) $P(X_i \ne Y_i) = 1 - P(X_i = 0) - P(Y_i = 1) = 1 - (1 - p_i') - p_i \exp(-p_i) = p_i(1 - \exp(-p_i)) \le p_i^2$. Combining these, we have

$$|P(S_n \in A) - P(Z \in A)| \le P(S_n \ne Z) \le \sum_1^n P(X_i \ne Y_i) \le \sum_1^n p_i^2.$$

SOLUTIONS TO THE EXERCISES OF SECTION 4

1. (a) $E\hat{\beta}_n = [\Sigma(\alpha + \beta z_j)(z_j - \bar{z}_n)]/[\Sigma(z_j - \bar{z}_n)^2] = \beta$. (In fact, the Gauss–Markov Theorem states that least-squares estimates are best linear unbiased estimates.)

$$\operatorname{Var}(\hat{\beta}_n) = \frac{\Sigma\sigma^2(z_j - \bar{z}_n)^2}{\left(\Sigma(z_j - \bar{z}_n)^2\right)^2} = \frac{\sigma^2}{\Sigma(z_j - \bar{z}_n)^2}.$$

Thus, $\hat{\beta}_n$ converges in quadratic mean to β, if and only if $\Sigma_{j=1}^n (z_j - \bar{z}_n)^2 \to \infty$.

(b) $E\hat{\alpha}_n = E\bar{X}_n - E\hat{\beta}_n\bar{z}_n = (\alpha + \beta\bar{z}_n) - \beta\bar{z}_n = \alpha$. We may write

$$\hat{\alpha}_n = \sum X_j\left(\frac{1}{n} - \frac{(z_j - \bar{z}_n)\bar{z}_n}{\Sigma(z_i - \bar{z}_n)^2}\right)$$

and compute $\operatorname{var}(\hat{\alpha}_n) = \sigma^2(1/n + \bar{z}_n^2/\Sigma(z_j - \bar{z}_n)^2)$. Hence, $\hat{\alpha}_n$ is consistent in quadratic mean if and only if,

$$\frac{\bar{z}_n^2}{\sum_{j=1}^n (z_j - \bar{z}_n)^2} \to 0.$$

2. $X_1 = \varepsilon_1$, $X_2 = \beta\varepsilon_1 + \varepsilon_2$, $X_3 = \beta^2\varepsilon_1 + \beta\varepsilon_2 + \varepsilon_3$, et cetera. In general, $X_n = \sum_1^n \varepsilon_j \beta^{n-j}$, and

$$\bar{X}_n = (1/n) \sum_{i=1}^{n} \sum_{j=1}^{i} \varepsilon_j \beta^{i-j} = (1/n) \sum_{j=1}^{n} \varepsilon_j (1 - \beta^{n-j+1})/(1-\beta).$$

Hence

$$\begin{aligned} E\bar{X}_n &= (1/n)(\mu/(1-\beta)) \sum_1^n (1-\beta^j) \\ &= (1/n)(\mu/(1-\beta))(n - \beta(1-\beta^n)/(1-\beta)) \\ &= \mu/(1-\beta) - (\beta\mu/n)\left((1-\beta^n)/(1-\beta)^2\right) \to \mu/(1-\beta), \end{aligned}$$

$$\operatorname{var}\left(\bar{X}_n\right) = (1/n^2) \sum_1^n \sigma^2 \left(1 - \beta^{n-j+1}\right)^2 / (1-\beta)^2 \le \sigma^2/n \to 0,$$

and $E(\bar{X}_n - \mu/(1-\beta))^2 = \operatorname{var}(\bar{X}_n) + (E\bar{X}_n - \mu/(1-\beta))^2 \to 0$.

3. It is sufficient to show that $\operatorname{var}(\bar{X}_n) \to 0$ as $n \to \infty$:

$$\operatorname{var}\left(\bar{X}_n\right) = \frac{1}{n^2} \sum_{i=1}^{n} \sum_{j=1}^{n} \operatorname{cov}(X_i, X_j) \le \frac{c}{n^2} \sum_{i=1}^{n} \sum_{j=1}^{n} |\rho_{ij}|.$$

Let $\varepsilon > 0$ be arbitrary and find N so that $|\rho_{ij}| < \varepsilon$ for all i and j such that $|i-j| > N$. Then in the double summation with n very large, $(n-N)^2$ of the $|\rho_{ij}|$ are less than ε and the rest may be bounded by 1. We obtain

$$\operatorname{var}\left(\bar{X}_n\right) \le \frac{1}{n^2}\left[(n-N)^2\varepsilon + \left(n^2 - (n-N)^2\right)\right] \le \varepsilon + \frac{1}{n}[N^2 + 2N].$$

Thus for n sufficiently large, we have $\operatorname{var}(\bar{X}_n) \le 2\varepsilon$, say, and since ε is arbitrary, the proof is complete.

4. The integral I is defined as

$$I = \lim_{z \to \infty} \int_1^z (1/x) \sin(2\pi x)\, dx = 0.153 \cdots.$$

For $\hat{I}_n$ to converge almost surely to I, we need $|(1/Y)\sin(2\pi/Y)|$ to have finite expectation when Y has a uniform distribution on $[0, 1]$. But

$$E|(1/Y)\sin(2\pi/Y)| = \int_0^1 \frac{1}{y}\left|\sin\left(\frac{2\pi}{y}\right)\right| dy = \int_1^\infty \frac{1}{x}|\sin(2\pi x)|\, dx = \infty,$$

so $\hat{I}_n$ does not converge almost surely to I. One cannot tell from the theorem of this section whether or not $\hat{I}_n$ converges to I in probability.

5. (a) For $0 < p < 1$,

$$\begin{aligned} H(px_1 + (1-p)x_2) &= \sup_\theta(\theta(px_1 + (1-p)x_2) - \log M(\theta)) \\ &= \sup_\theta(p[\theta x_1 - \log M(\theta)] + (1-p)[\theta x_2 - \log M(\theta)]) \\ &\le \sup_\theta(p[\theta x_1 - \log M(\theta)]) \\ &\quad + \sup_\theta((1-p)[\theta x_2 - \log M(\theta)]) = pH(x_1) + (1-p)H(x_2). \end{aligned}$$

(b) First note that at $\theta = 0$, $\theta x - \log M(\theta) = 0$, so $H(x) \ge 0$ for all x. Now, from Jensen's inequality, since $\exp\{\theta x\}$ is convex in x for all θ, we have $M(\theta) \ge \exp\{\theta\mu\}$, or $\theta\mu - \log M(\theta) \le 0$ for all θ. Thus, $H(\mu) = 0$.

(c) For the normal distribution, $\mathscr{N}(\mu, \sigma^2)$ with $\sigma^2 > 0$, $M(\theta) = Ee^{\theta X} = e^{\theta\mu + \sigma^2\theta^2/2}$, so that $\log M(\theta) = \theta\mu + \sigma^2\theta^2/2$. If $\varphi(\theta) = \theta z - \theta\mu - \sigma^2\theta^2/2$, then $\varphi'(\theta) = z - \mu - \sigma^2\theta = 0$ shows that φ has a maximum at $\theta = (z-\mu)/\sigma^2$. Therefore,

$$H(z) = \frac{(z-\mu)^2}{\sigma^2} - \frac{(z-\mu)^2}{2\sigma^2} = \frac{(z-\mu)^2}{2\sigma^2}.$$

For the Poisson distribution, $\mathscr{P}(\lambda)$, $\lambda > 0$, we have $M(\theta) = \exp\{-\lambda + \lambda e^\theta\}$. If $\varphi(\theta) = \theta z + \lambda - \lambda e^\theta$, then $\varphi(\theta)$ has its maximum at $\theta = \log(z/\lambda)$ if $z > 0$, and at $\theta = -\infty$ if $z \le 0$. Hence,

$$H(z) = \begin{cases} z\log(z/\lambda) + \lambda - z, & \text{if } z \ge 0, \\ +\infty, & \text{if } z < 0. \end{cases}$$

with the convention that $0 \log 0 = 0$.

For the Bernoulli distribution, $P(x = 1) = p$ and $P(X = 0) = q = 1 - p$, $0 < p < 1$, we have $M(\theta) = pe^\theta + q$. If $\varphi(\theta) = \theta z - \log(pe^\theta + q)$, then $\varphi(\theta)$ has its maximum at $\theta = \log(zq/((1 - z)p)$ if $0 < z < 1$, at $\theta = -\infty$ if $z \le 0$, and at $\theta = +\infty$ if $z \ge 1$. Hence

$$H(z) = \begin{cases} z\log\dfrac{z}{p} + (1-z)\log\dfrac{1-z}{q}, & \text{for } 0 \le z \le 1, \\ +\infty, & \text{otherwise}. \end{cases}$$

6. As in the proof of Chebyshev's inequality,

$$\begin{aligned} E\exp\{\theta\overline{X}_n\} &\ge E\exp\{\theta\overline{X}_n\}I(\overline{X}_n \ge \mu + \varepsilon \\ &\ge \exp\{\theta(\mu + \varepsilon)\}P(\overline{X}_n \ge \mu + \varepsilon), \end{aligned}$$

for all n and θ. Hence

$$\begin{aligned} P(\overline{X}_n \geq \mu + \varepsilon) &\leq \exp\{-\theta(\mu + \varepsilon) E \exp\{\theta \overline{X}_n\} \\ &= \exp\{-\theta(\mu + \varepsilon)\} M(\theta/n)^n \\ &= \exp\left\{-n\left(\frac{\theta}{n}(\mu + \varepsilon) - \log M\left(\frac{\theta}{n}\right)\right)\right\} \\ &\leq \exp\{-nH(\mu + \varepsilon)\}. \end{aligned}$$

7. (a) Since $y > \mu$, we have $\theta' > 0$. Hence,

$$\begin{aligned} P_{\theta'}(|\overline{X}_n - y| < \delta) &= \int \cdots \int I(|\bar{x}_n - y| < \delta) e^{\theta'(x_1 + \cdots + x_n)} f(x_1) \\ &\qquad \times \cdots f(x_n)\, dx_1 \cdots dx_n / M(\theta)^n \\ &\leq e^{\theta' n(y+\delta)} P_0(|\overline{X}_n - y| < \delta)/M(\theta)^n \\ &= \exp\{n(\theta(y + \delta) - \log M(\theta)\} P_0(|\overline{X}_n - y| < \delta) \\ &\leq \exp\{nH(y + \delta)\} P_0(|\overline{X}_n - y| < \delta). \end{aligned}$$

(b) The left side of this inequality tends to 1 by the weak Law of Large Numbers. Hence

$$\begin{aligned} P(\overline{X}_n > \mu + \varepsilon) &\geq P(|\overline{X}_n - y| < \delta) \\ &\geq \exp\{-nH(y + \delta)\} P_{\theta'}(|\overline{X}_n - y| < \delta). \end{aligned}$$

Hence

$$\liminf_{n \to \infty} \frac{1}{n} \log P(\overline{X}_n > \mu + \varepsilon) \geq -H(y + \delta)$$

Since δ is an arbitrary positive number, this inequality holds in the limit as $\delta \to 0$. Since we are assuming $H(\mathbf{x})$ to be continuous at $x = \mu + \varepsilon$, the result follows.

8. $P(\overline{X}_n > 1) = 0$ for all n, so $P(\overline{X}_n > 1) = \exp\{-nH(1^+)\}$, because $H(1^+) = \infty$. $P(\overline{X}_n \geq 1) = P(n \text{ successes}) = p^n = \exp\{n \log p\} = \exp\{-nH(1)\}$.

SOLUTIONS TO THE EXERCISES OF SECTION 5

1. (a)

$$\boldsymbol{\mu} = \begin{pmatrix} \theta_1 \\ \theta_2 \end{pmatrix} \quad \text{and} \quad \mathrm{E}\mathbf{XX}' = \begin{pmatrix} \theta_1 & 0 \\ 0 & \theta_2 \end{pmatrix},$$

so

$$\boldsymbol{\Sigma} = \begin{pmatrix} \theta_1(1-\theta_1) & -\theta_1\theta_2 \\ -\theta_1\theta_2 & \theta_2(1-\theta_2) \end{pmatrix}$$

The central limit theorem gives $\sqrt{n}(\overline{\mathbf{X}}_n - \boldsymbol{\mu}) \xrightarrow{\mathscr{L}} \mathscr{N}(\mathbf{0}, \boldsymbol{\Sigma})$.

(b) $EX = \theta$, $EI(X = 0) = e^{-\theta}$, $\operatorname{var} X = \theta$, $\operatorname{var}(I(X = 0)) = e^{-\theta}(1 - e^{-\theta})$, and $EXI(X = 0) = 0$ so $\operatorname{cov}(X, I(X = 0)) = -\theta e^{-\theta}$. Hence, $\sqrt{n}((\overline{X}_n, Z_n) - (\theta, e^{-\theta})) \xrightarrow{\mathscr{L}} \mathscr{N}(0, \boldsymbol{\Sigma})$, where

$$\boldsymbol{\Sigma} = \begin{pmatrix} \theta & -\theta e^{-\theta} \\ -\theta e^{-\theta} & e^{-\theta}(1 - e^{-\theta}) \end{pmatrix}.$$

2. $EX_j = 0$ and $\operatorname{var}(X_j) = j$, so $B_n^2 = \Sigma_1^n j = n(n+1)/2$. Since $|X_j| = \sqrt{j}$ with probability 1,

$$E\{X_j^2 I(|X_j| > \varepsilon B_n)\} = jI\{\sqrt{j} > \varepsilon B_n\} = jI\{j > \varepsilon^2 n(n+1)/2\}.$$

This is equal to zero for all $1 \le j \le n$ when $n + 1 > 2/\varepsilon^2$. Hence, for all $\varepsilon > 0$,

$$\frac{1}{B_n^2} \sum_1^n E\{X_j^2 I(|X_j| > \varepsilon B_n)\} = 0,$$

for $n > 2/\varepsilon^2$. Thus, the Lindeberg condition is satisfied and $(1/B_n)\Sigma_1^n X_j \xrightarrow{\mathscr{L}} \mathscr{N}(0, 1)$, which in turn implies that

$$\overline{X}_n \xrightarrow{\mathscr{L}} \mathscr{N}(0, \tfrac{1}{2}).$$

3. Since $\operatorname{var}(X_n) = \sigma^2$, we have $B_n^2 = n\sigma^2$. The Central Limit Theorem now follows, because the Lindeberg Condition is satisfied: For every $\varepsilon > 0$,

$$\frac{1}{n\sigma^2} \sum_1^n E\{X_j^2 I(|X_j| > \varepsilon\sigma\sqrt{n})\}$$

$$= \frac{1}{\sigma^2} E\{X_1^2 I(|X_1| > \varepsilon\sigma\sqrt{n})\} \to 0 \text{ as } n \to \infty.$$

4. If for all j, $X_j = \pm v_j$ with probability $p_j/2$ each, and $X_j = 0$ otherwise, then $EX_j = 0$, and $\operatorname{var}(X_j) = 1$ if $p_j v_j^2 = 1$. We want to choose v_j and $p_j = 1/v_j^2$ so that the Lindeberg Condition is not satisfied.

Here $B_n^2 = n$, so that we compute

$$\frac{1}{n}\sum_1^n EX_j^2 I\left(|X_j| > \varepsilon\sqrt{n}\right) = \frac{1}{n}\sum_1^n v_j^2 p_j I\left(v_j > \varepsilon\sqrt{n}\right) = \frac{1}{n}\sum_1^n I\left(v_j^2 > \varepsilon^2 n\right).$$

If we choose $v_j^2 = j$ (so $p_j = 1/j$), then this becomes approximately $(1/n)(n - \varepsilon^2 n) \to (1 - \varepsilon^2) \neq 0$. Thus the Lindeberg Condition is not satisfied. But since $\max_{j \le n} \sigma_{nj}^2/B_n^2 = 1/n \to 0$ as $n \to \infty$, the Lindeberg Condition is necessary and sufficient for asymptotic normality of $Z_n/B_n = \sqrt{n}\,\overline{X}_n$, so that $\sqrt{n}\,\overline{X}_n$ does not converge in law to $\mathcal{N}(0, 1)$.

5. The mean and variance of T_n are

$$\mu_n = ET_n = \sum_{j=1}^n Ez_{nj}X_j = \mu \sum_{j=1}^n z_{nj},$$

$$\sigma_n^2 = \operatorname{var}(T_n) = \sum_{j=1}^n \operatorname{var}\left(z_{nj}X_j\right) = \sigma^2 \sum_{j=1}^n z_{nj}^2.$$

Since $T_n - \mu_n = \sum_{j=1}^n z_{nj}(X_j - \mu)$, we use the Lindeberg–Feller Theorem with $X_{nj} = z_{nj}(X_j - \mu)$. Thus, we have $EX_{nj} = 0$, $\operatorname{var}(X_{nj}) = \sigma_{nj}^2 = \sigma^2 z_{nj}^2$, $Z_n = T_n - \mu_n$, and $B_n^2 = \sigma_n^2 = \sigma^2 \sum_{j=1}^n z_{nj}^2$ using the notation of the theorem. Therefore $Z_n/B_n = (T_n - \mu_n)/\sigma_n \xrightarrow{\mathcal{L}} \mathcal{N}(0, 1)$ provided the Lindeberg Condition is satisfied. Let $\varepsilon > 0$. Then,

$$\frac{1}{B_n^2}\sum_{j=1}^n E\left\{X_{nj}^2 I\left(|X_{nj}| \ge \varepsilon B_n\right)\right\}$$

$$= \frac{1}{B_n^2}\sum_{j=1}^n z_{nj}^2 E\left\{(X_j - \mu)^2 I\left(|X_j - \mu| \ge \frac{\varepsilon B_n}{|z_{nj}|}\right)\right\}$$

$$\le \frac{1}{B_n^2}\sum_{j=1}^n z_{nj}^2 E\left\{(X_j - \mu)^2 I\left(|X_j - \mu| \ge \frac{\varepsilon B_n}{\max_{j \le n}|z_{nj}|}\right)\right\}.$$

Since the X_j are identically distributed, the expectation does not depend on j and so may be factored outside the summation sign. Then the summation of z_{nj}^2 may be canceled by the same term in B_n^2, giving

$$\frac{1}{B_n^2}\sum_{j=1}^{n} E\{X_{nj}^2 I(|X_{nj}| \geq \varepsilon B_n)\}$$

$$\leq \frac{1}{\sigma^2} E\left\{(X_1-\mu)^2 I\left(|X_1-\mu| \geq \frac{\varepsilon B_n}{\max\limits_{j\leq n}|z_{nj}|}\right)\right\}.$$

We are given that $\max_{j\leq n} z_{nj}^2/B_n^2 \to 0$, and since the variance of X_1 is finite, this last expectation converges to zero. Thus the Lindeberg Condition is satisfied.

6. The mean and variance of S_n are $ES_n = \Sigma_{k=1}^n ER_k = \Sigma_1^n 1/k$, and $\text{var}(S_n) = \Sigma_1^n \text{var}(R_k) = \Sigma_1^n(1/k)(1-(1/k))$. If we let X_{nj} in the Lindeberg–Feller Theorem denote $R_j - (1/j)$, then $EX_{nj} = 0$ and $B_n^2 = \text{var}(S_n)$. We must check the Lindeberg Conditions. We use the fact that $|X_{nj}| = |R_j - (1/j)| < 1$ to deduce that

$$\frac{1}{B_n^2}\sum_1^n E\{X_{nj}^2 I(|X_{nj}| > \varepsilon B_n)\} \leq \frac{1}{B_n^2}\sum_1^n E\{X_{nj}^2 I(1 > \varepsilon B_n)\} = I(1 > \varepsilon B_n).$$

For fixed $\varepsilon > 0$, this is equal to zero for n sufficiently large, since B_n converges to infinity. Thus the Lindeberg Condition is satisfied.

7. Since

$$EX_k = (1/k)\sum_1^{k-1} i = (1/k)(k(k-1)/2) = (k-1)/2,$$

and

$$\text{var}\, X_k = (1/k)\sum_1^{k-1} i^2 - ((k-1)/2)^2 = (k^2-1)/12,$$

we have

$$ET_n = \sum_1^n \frac{k-1}{2} = \frac{n(n-1)}{4}$$

and

$$\text{var}\, T_n = \sum_1^n \frac{k^2-1}{12} = \frac{1}{12}\left[\frac{n(n+1)(2n+1)}{6} - n\right]$$

$$= \frac{n(n-1)(2n+5)}{72}.$$

To show asymptotic normality of $(T_n - ET_n)/\sqrt{\text{var } T_n}$, we check the Lindeberg Condition. We use $X_{nj} = X_j - ((j-1)/2)$ so that $EX_{nj} = 0$, and $B_n^2 = \text{var } T_n$. Because X_j is bounded between 0 and $j-1$, we have that $|X_{nj}| \le (j-1)/2 \le (n-1)/2$ for $j \le n$. Hence,

$$\frac{1}{B_n^2}\sum_{j=1}^{n} E\{X_{nj}^2 I(|X_{nj}| \ge \varepsilon B_n)\} \le \frac{1}{B_n^2}\sum_{j=1}^{n} E\{X_{nj}^2 I((n-1)/2 \ge \varepsilon B_n)\}$$

$$= I((n-1)/2 \ge \varepsilon B_n).$$

For fixed $\varepsilon > 0$, this is equal to zero for n sufficiently large, since B_n is of the order $n^{3/2}$. Thus the Lindeberg Condition is satisfied and the normalized versions of T_n and τ_n are asymptotically normal.

8. For this distribution, $\mu = 0$, $\sigma^2 = 1$, and $\rho = 1$. Hence,

$$c_n = \sqrt{n}\,\sup_x |F_n(x) - \Phi(x)|. \qquad (*)$$

If $n = 1$, then $F_1(x) = 0$ for $x < -1$, $F_1(x) = \frac{1}{2}$ for $-1 \le x < 1$, and $F_1(x) = 1$ for $x \ge 1$; so the supremum in $(*)$ occurs at x close to ± 1, and $c_1 = \max\{1 - \Phi(1), \Phi(1) - 1/2\} = \Phi(1) - 1/2 = 0.3413\cdots$. For $n = 2$, $F_2(x) = 0$ for $x < -\sqrt{2}$, $F_2(x) = \frac{1}{4}$ for $-\sqrt{2} \le x < 0$, $F_2(x) = \frac{3}{4}$ for $0 \le x < \sqrt{2}$, and $F_2(x) = 1$ for $x \ge \sqrt{2}$; so the supremum in $(*)$ occurs for x close to 0, and $c_2 = \sqrt{2}\,\frac{1}{4} = 0.3536\cdots$. For arbitrary $n \ge 2$, we expect the supremum in $(*)$ to occur for x close to zero where the largest jump in $F_n(x)$ occurs. So take n even, $n = 2k$, and evaluate

$$c_n = \sqrt{n}\,|F_n(0) - \Phi(0)| = \sqrt{n}\,q/2,$$

where q represents the size of the jump in $F_n(x)$ at $x = 0$. Thus, q is the probability that a binomial random variable of sample size $2k$ and probability of success $\frac{1}{2}$ is equal to k. Using Stirling's approximation to $k!$, we find

$$c_n = \sqrt{n}\binom{n}{k}\left(\tfrac{1}{2}\right)^n/2 = \sqrt{n}\,(2k!)/(k!^2 2^{2k+1})$$

$$\sim \sqrt{n}\left[(2k/e)^{2k}(\pi 2k)^{1/2}\right]/\left[(k/e)^{2k}(\pi k)2^{2k+1}\right]$$

$$= 1/\sqrt{2\pi} = 0.3989\cdots.$$

This shows that the constant c in the Berry–Esseen Theorem is at least $0.3989\cdots$.

9. Since the coefficients of skewness and kurtosis are independent of location and scale, we may assume that the underlying distribution has mean 0 and variance 1. Then,

$$ES_n^2 = nEX^2 = n,$$

$$ES_n^3 = E\sum\sum\sum X_i X_j X_k = nEX^3 = n\beta_1,$$

$$ES_n^4 = E\sum\sum\sum\sum X_i X_j X_k X_l = nEX^4 + 3n(n-1)(EX^2)^2$$
$$= n(\beta_2 + 3) + 3n(n-1).$$

From this, we may compute

$$\beta_{1n} = ES_n^3/(ES_n^2)^{3/2} = \beta_1/\sqrt{n},$$

$$\beta_{2n} = ES_n^4/(ES_n^2)^2 - 3 = (n(\beta_2+3) + 3n(n-1))/n^2 - 3 = \beta_2/n.$$

The Edgeworth Expansion (12) is independent of scale change, and since the exponential distribution with mean 1 is just a scale change from the χ_2^2 distribution, Table 1 represents the normal and Edgeworth approximations for a sample of size 5 from χ_2^2. But from the above, it is also valid for a sample of size 10 from the χ_1^2 distribution or a sample of size 1 from the χ_{10}^2 distribution.

10. The mean of the uniform distribution on $(0,1)$ is $\mu = \frac{1}{2}$ and the variance is $\sigma^2 = \frac{1}{12}$. The coefficient of skewness is $\beta_1 = 0$, since the distribution is symmetric about $\frac{1}{2}$. The fourth moment about the mean is

$$E\left(X - \tfrac{1}{2}\right)^4 = \int_0^1 (x - 1/2)^4\,dx = 2\int_0^{1/2} y^4\,dy = 2\left(\tfrac{1}{2}\right)^5/5 = \tfrac{1}{80},$$

so the coefficient of kurtosis is $\beta_2 = (\frac{1}{80})/(\frac{1}{12})^2 - 3 = 1.8 - 3 = -1.2$. With $n = 3$, we have $P(S_n \le 6) = P(\sqrt{n}(\bar{X}_n - \frac{1}{2})/\sigma \le 1)$. The normal approximation to this probability is $\Phi(1) = 0.8413$ from Table 1. The Edgeworth Expansion is $\Phi(1) - \beta_2(1-3)/(24n)\varphi(1) = 0.8413 - 0.0081 = 0.8332$. The exact probability is

$$P(X_1 + X_2 + X_3 \le 2) = 1 - P(X_1 + X_2 + X_3 \ge 2)$$
$$= 1 - P(X_1 + X_2 + X_3 \le 1) = 1 - \tfrac{1}{6} = 0.8333,$$

since $P(X_1 + X_2 + X_3 \le 1) = \frac{1}{6}$ is the volume of the unit tetrahedron.

SOLUTIONS TO THE EXERCISES OF SECTION 6

1. (a) Let n' be a subsequence; we are to show there exists a subsubsequence n'' such that $\mathbf{f}(X_{n''}) \to \mathbf{f}(\mathbf{X})$ almost surely. Since $\mathbf{X}_{n'} \to \mathbf{X}$ in probability, there exists a subsubsequence n'' such that $\mathbf{X}_{n''} \to \mathbf{X}$ almost surely. Hence for $\mathbf{X} \in C(\mathbf{f})$, we have $\mathbf{f}(\mathbf{X}_{n''}) \to \mathbf{f}(\mathbf{X})$ and since $P\{\mathbf{X} \in C(\mathbf{f})\} = 1$, this implies $\mathbf{f}(\mathbf{X}_{n''}) \to \mathbf{f}(\mathbf{X})$ almost surely.

   (b) Since $|\mathbf{Y}_n - \mathbf{X}| \le |\mathbf{Y}_n - \mathbf{X}_n| + |\mathbf{X}_n - \mathbf{X}|$, we have for all $\varepsilon > 0$,

$$\{|\mathbf{Y}_n - \mathbf{X}| > \varepsilon\} \subset \{|\mathbf{Y}_n - \mathbf{X}_n| > \varepsilon/2\} \cup \{|\mathbf{X}_n - \mathbf{X}| > \varepsilon/2\}.$$

   Hence,

$$P\{|\mathbf{Y}_n - \mathbf{X}| > \varepsilon\} \le P\{|\mathbf{Y}_n - \mathbf{X}_n| > \varepsilon/2\} + P\{|\mathbf{X}_n - \mathbf{X}| > \varepsilon/2\} \to 0.$$

   (c)

$$P\left\{\left|\begin{pmatrix}\mathbf{X}_n\\ \mathbf{Y}_n\end{pmatrix} - \begin{pmatrix}\mathbf{X}\\ \mathbf{Y}\end{pmatrix}\right| > \varepsilon\right\} \le P\left\{|\mathbf{X}_n - \mathbf{X}| > \frac{\varepsilon}{\sqrt{2}}\right\} + P\left\{|\mathbf{Y}_n - \mathbf{Y}| > \frac{\varepsilon}{\sqrt{2}}\right\} \to 0.$$

2.

$$\begin{aligned}\Phi_{X_n, Y_n}(u, v) &= \Phi_{X_n}(u)\Phi_{Y_n}(v), \qquad \text{because of independence}\\ &\to \Phi_X(u)\Phi_Y(v)\\ &= \Phi_{X,Y}(u, v), \qquad \text{if } X \text{ and } Y \text{ are independent}.\end{aligned}$$

3. Let $-1 < \beta < 1$. Since $X_0 = 0$ and $X_j = \beta X_{j-1} + e_j$, we have $\Sigma_1^n X_j = \beta \Sigma_1^{n-1} X_j + \Sigma_1^n e_j$. This implies that $(1 - \beta)\Sigma_1^n X_j = \Sigma_1^n e_j - \beta X_n$, or

$$\sqrt{n}\left((1 - \beta)\bar{X}_n - \mu\right) = \sqrt{n}\,(\bar{e}_n - \mu) - \beta X_n/\sqrt{n}\,.$$

By the Central Limit Theorem, $\sqrt{n}\,(\bar{e}_n - \mu) \xrightarrow{\mathscr{L}} \mathscr{N}(0, \sigma^2)$. We now show that $\sqrt{n}\,((1 - \beta)\bar{X}_n - \mu)$ and $\sqrt{n}\,(\bar{e}_n - \mu)$ are asymptotically equivalent by showing that the difference, $\beta X_n/\sqrt{n}$ converges to 0 in probability. Since $X_n = \Sigma_1^n e_j \beta^{n-j}$ (see the solution to Exercise 2 of Section 4), we have $E(X_n/\sqrt{n}) = \mu\, \Sigma_1^n \beta^{n-j}/\sqrt{n} \to 0$, and $\operatorname{var}(X_n/\sqrt{n}) = \sigma^2 \Sigma_1^n \beta^{2(n-j)}/n \to 0$. This implies that $X_n/\sqrt{n}$ converges to 0 in quadratic mean (Exercise 5 of Section 1), and hence in probability. An application of Theorem 6(b) now gives that $\sqrt{n}\,((1 - \beta)\bar{X}_n - \mu) \xrightarrow{\mathscr{L}} \mathscr{N}(0, \sigma^2)$, or

$$\sqrt{n}\left(\bar{X}_n - \frac{\mu}{1 - \beta}\right) \xrightarrow{\mathscr{L}} \mathscr{N}\left(0, \frac{\sigma^2}{(1 - \beta)^2}\right).$$

For $\beta = -1$, $\bar{X}_n = (1/n)(e_2 + e_4 + \cdots + e_n)$ for even n, and $\bar{X}_n = (1/n)(e_1 + e_3 + \cdots + e_n)$ for n odd. In either case, $\sqrt{n}(\bar{X}_n - \mu/2)$ is approximately $\mathcal{N}(0, \sigma^2/2)$ for large n. For $\beta = +1$, we have $X_n = \sum_1^n e_j$ and $\bar{X}_n = (1/n)\sum_1^n(n+1-j)e_j$. If $\mu > 0$ for example, this converges to infinity in probability. In spite of this, we can show that $\bar{X}_n$, properly normalized, converges in law to a normal distribution. $\bar{X}_n$ is equivalent in distribution to $Z_n = \sum_1^n je_j$, so consider $Z_n - EZ_n = \sum_1^n j(e_j - \mu)$. We check the Lindeberg Conditions with $X_{nj} = j(e_j - \mu)$. We have $EX_{nj} = 0$ and $\mathrm{var}(X_{nj}) = j^2\sigma^2$, so $B_n^2 = \sum_1^n j^2\sigma^2 = \sigma^2 n(n+1)(2n+1)/6$. Then,

$$\frac{1}{B_n^2}\sum_{j=1}^n E\{X_{nj}^2 I(|X_{nj}| \geq \varepsilon B_n)\}$$

$$= \frac{1}{B_n^2}\sum_{j=1}^n j^2 E\left\{(e_j - \mu)^2 I\left((e_j - \mu)^2 \geq \frac{\varepsilon B_n^2}{j^2}\right)\right\}$$

$$\leq \frac{1}{B_n^2}\sum_{j=1}^n j^2 E\left\{(e_j - \mu)^2 I\left((e_j - \mu)^2 \geq \frac{\varepsilon B_n^2}{n^2}\right)\right\}$$

$$= \frac{1}{\sigma^2}E\left\{(e_1 - \mu)^2 I\left((e_1 - \mu)^2 \geq \frac{\varepsilon B_n^2}{n^2}\right)\right\} \to 0,$$

because $B_n^2/n^2 \to \infty$. Hence $(Z_n - EZ_n)/B_n \xrightarrow{\mathscr{L}} \mathcal{N}(0,1)$, which is equivalent to

$$\frac{1}{\sqrt{n}}\left(\bar{X}_n - n\frac{\mu}{2}\right) \xrightarrow{\mathscr{L}} \mathcal{N}(0, \sigma^2/3).$$

4. (a) Let U_n and V_n be sequences of mean 0, variance 1 random variables such that $\mathrm{corr}(U_n, V_n) \to 1$. Then, $E(U_n - V_n)^2 = 2(1 - \mathrm{corr}(U_n, V_n)) \to 0$, so that $U_n - V_n$ converges to zero in quadratic mean. This implies convergence in probability, so U_n and V_n are asymptotically equivalent and from Theorem 6(b), they have the same limit laws. This observation may be applied directly to the sequences $U_n = (X_n - EX_n)/\sqrt{\mathrm{var}(X_n)}$ and $V_n = (Y_n - EY_n)/\sqrt{\mathrm{var}(Y_n)}$ of normalized variables with $\mathrm{corr}(X_n, Y_n) \to 1$, since $\mathrm{corr}(U_n, V_n) = \mathrm{corr}(X_n, Y_n)$.
   (b) The variables X_n and Y_n themselves may not be asymptotically equivalent. Here is a counterexample. Let U and V be distinct independent mean 0 random variables on $[-1, 1]$ such that $\mathrm{var}(U) = \mathrm{var}(V)$, and let W be independent with $P(W = -1) =$

$P(W = +1) = \frac{1}{2}$. Let $(X_n, Y_n) = (nW, nW)$ with probability $1/n$, and $= (U, V)$ with probability $(n-1)/n$. Then $X_n \to U$ in law and $Y_n \to V$ in law, yet $\text{var}(X_n) = n + ((n-1)/n)\text{var}(U)$, $\text{Var}(Y_n) = n + ((n-1)/n)\text{var}(V)$, and $\text{cov}(X_n, Y_n) = n$, so that $\text{corr}(X_n, Y_n) \to 1$.

5.

$$E(X_n - Y_n)^2 \geq \text{var}(X_n - Y_n)$$

$$= \text{var}(X_n) - 2\,\text{cov}(X_n, Y_n) + \text{var}(Y_n) \geq 0.$$

Since $\text{cov}(X_n, Y_n) \leq \sqrt{\text{var}(X_n)}\sqrt{\text{var}(Y_n)}$, we have $E(X_n - Y_n)^2 \geq (\sqrt{\text{var}(X_n)} - \sqrt{\text{var}(Y_n)})^2$. Dividing both sides by $\text{var}(X_n)$ and noting that the left side tends to zero shows that $(1 - \sqrt{\text{var}(Y_n)}/\sqrt{\text{var}(X_n)})^2 \to 0$, or equivalently, $\text{var}(Y_n)/\text{var}(X_n) \to 1$. Now, dividing both sides of the original inequality by $\sqrt{\text{var}(X_n)}\sqrt{\text{var}(Y_n)}$ gives

$$\sqrt{\text{var}(X_n)}/\sqrt{\text{var}(Y_n)} - 2\,\text{corr}(X_n, Y_n) + \sqrt{\text{var}(Y_n)}/\sqrt{\text{var}(X_n)}$$

$$\leq E(X_n - Y_n)^2/\left(\sqrt{\text{var}(X_n)}\sqrt{\text{var}(Y_n)}\right) \to 0.$$

Hence, $\text{corr}(X_n, Y_n) \to 1$. The last line follows directly from Exercise 4.

6. (a) By Slutsky's Theorem part (a), we have $\log X_n \xrightarrow{\mathscr{L}} \log X$, since log is continuous on $(0, \infty)$. Also by part (a), $\log Y_n - \log X_n \xrightarrow{\mathscr{L}} 0$. Then by part (b) of Slutsky's Theorem, $\log Y_n \xrightarrow{\mathscr{L}} \log X$, and again by part (a), $Y_n \xrightarrow{\mathscr{L}} X$.
   (b) If $(X_{1n}, \ldots, X_{kn}) \xrightarrow{\mathscr{L}} (X_1, \ldots, X_k) > (0, \ldots, 0)$, and if $(X_{1n}/Y_{1n}, \ldots, X_{kn}/Y_{kn}) \xrightarrow{\text{P}} (1, \ldots, 1)$ as $n \to \infty$, then $(Y_{1n}, \ldots, Y_{kn}) \xrightarrow{\mathscr{L}} (X_1, \ldots, X_k)$. The proof is essentially the same as in part (a).

SOLUTIONS TO THE EXERCISES OF SECTION 7

1. $\sqrt{n}(s_x^2 - \sigma^2) \xrightarrow{\mathscr{L}} \mathscr{N}(0, \mu_4 - \sigma^4)$, $g(x) = \log(x)$, $g'(x) = 1/x$, and $g'(\sigma^2) = 1/\sigma^2$. Hence from Theorem 7,

$$\sqrt{n}\left(\log(s_x^2) - \log(\sigma^2)\right) \xrightarrow{\mathscr{L}} \mathscr{N}(0, \mu_4/\sigma^4 - 1) = \mathscr{N}(0, \beta_2 - 1)$$

where $\beta_2 = \mu_4/\sigma^4$.

2. Taking $m_1' = (1/n)\Sigma(X_j - \mu)$ and $m_2' = (1/n)\Sigma(X_j - \mu)^2$ allows us to use central moments in the computation of the covariance matrix.

Then, $\sqrt{n}\,((m_1', m_2') - (0, \sigma^2)) \xrightarrow{\mathscr{L}} \mathscr{N}((0,0),\boldsymbol{\Sigma})$, where

$$\boldsymbol{\Sigma} = \begin{pmatrix} \operatorname{var}(X-\mu) & \operatorname{cov}((X-\mu)^2, X-\mu) \\ \operatorname{cov}((X-\mu)^2, X-\mu) & \operatorname{var}((X-\mu)^2) \end{pmatrix}$$

$$= \begin{pmatrix} \sigma^2 & \mu_3 \\ \mu_3 & \mu_4 - \sigma^4 \end{pmatrix}.$$

Take

$$g(x,y) = \begin{pmatrix} x \\ y - x^2 \end{pmatrix}, \qquad \dot{g}(x,y) = \begin{pmatrix} 1 & 0 \\ -2x & 1 \end{pmatrix}, \qquad \dot{g}(0,\sigma^2) = I.$$

Then, by Theorem 7,

$$\sqrt{n}\begin{pmatrix} \overline{X}_n - \mu \\ s_x^2 - \sigma^2 \end{pmatrix} \xrightarrow{\mathscr{L}} \mathscr{N}\left(\begin{pmatrix} 0 \\ 0 \end{pmatrix}, \begin{pmatrix} \sigma^2 & \mu_3 \\ \mu_3 & \mu_4 - \sigma^4 \end{pmatrix}\right).$$

3. (a) $g(u,v) = \sqrt{v}/u$, $\dot{g}(\mu, \sigma^2) = (-\sigma/\mu^2, 1/(2\mu\sigma))$.

$$\sqrt{n}\left(\frac{s_x}{\overline{X}_n} - \frac{\sigma}{\mu}\right) \xrightarrow{\mathscr{L}} \mathscr{N}(0, \dot{g}\boldsymbol{\Sigma}\dot{g}^T) = \mathscr{N}\left(0, \frac{\mu_4 - \sigma^4}{4\mu^2\sigma^2} - \frac{\mu_3}{\mu^3} + \frac{\sigma^4}{\mu^4}\right).$$

If the parent distribution is normal, then $\mu_3 = 0$ and $\mu_4 = 3\sigma^4$, so that the limiting distribution is $\mathscr{N}(0, \sigma^2(1/2 + \sigma^2/\mu^2)/\mu^2)$.

(b) Without loss of generality, take $\mu = 0$; then $\sqrt{n}\,((m_1', m_2', m_3') - (0, \sigma^2, \mu_3)) \to \mathscr{N}((0,0,0), \boldsymbol{\Sigma})$, where

$$\boldsymbol{\Sigma} = \begin{pmatrix} \sigma^2 & \mu_3 & \mu_4 \\ \mu_3 & \mu_4 - \sigma^4 & \mu_5 - \sigma^2\mu_3 \\ \mu_4 & \mu_5 - \sigma^2\mu_3 & \mu_6 - \mu_3^2 \end{pmatrix}.$$

Since $m_3 = m_3' - 3m_2'm_1' + 2(m_1')^2$, we let $g(u,v,w) = w - 3uv + 2u^3$ and find that $\dot{g}(0,\sigma^2,\mu_3) = (-3\sigma^2, 0, 1)$, so that

$$\sqrt{n}\,(m_3 - \mu_3) \xrightarrow{\mathscr{L}} \mathscr{N}(0, \dot{g}\boldsymbol{\Sigma}\dot{g}^T) = \mathscr{N}(0, \mu_6 - \mu_3^2 - 6\sigma^2\mu_4 + 9\sigma^6).$$

4. $E(X) = \alpha/(\alpha+\beta) = \theta/(\theta+1)$ and $\operatorname{var}(X) = \alpha\beta/((\alpha+\beta)^2(\alpha+\beta+1)) = \theta/((\theta+1)^2(\theta+2))$. Hence,

$$\sqrt{n}\left(\overline{X}_n - \frac{\theta}{\theta+1}\right) \xrightarrow{\mathscr{L}} \mathscr{N}\left(0, \frac{\theta}{(\theta+1)^2(\theta+2)}\right).$$

Let $g(x) = x/(1-x)$ so that $g'(x) = 1/(1-x)^2$ and $g'(\theta/(\theta+1)) = (\theta+1)^2$. Then we find

$$\sqrt{n}\left(\hat{\theta}_n - \theta\right) \xrightarrow{\mathscr{L}} \mathscr{N}\left(0, \frac{\theta(\theta+1)^2}{(\theta+2)}\right).$$

5. (a) Using $g(x, y) = y/x$ in Cramér's Theorem applied to the result of Exercise 2, we find $\dot{g}(\mu, \sigma^2) = (-\sigma^2/\mu^2, 1/\mu)$ and

$$\sqrt{n}\left(\frac{s^2}{\overline{X}_n} - \frac{\sigma^2}{\mu}\right) \xrightarrow{\mathscr{L}} \mathscr{N}(0, \dot{g}\boldsymbol{\Sigma}\dot{g}^T)$$

$$= \mathscr{N}\left(0, \frac{1}{\mu^4}\left(\sigma^6 - 2\mu\sigma^2\mu_3 + \mu^2\mu_4 - \mu^2\sigma^4\right)\right).$$

(b) The first four moments of the Poisson distribution, $\mathscr{P}(\lambda)$, are $\mu = \lambda$, $\mu_2 = \sigma^2 = \lambda$, $\mu_3 = \lambda$, and $\mu_4 = 3\lambda^2 + \lambda$. Substituting these values into the result of part (a), we find

$$\sqrt{n}\left(\frac{s^2}{\overline{X}_n} - 1\right) \xrightarrow{\mathscr{L}} \mathscr{N}(0, 2),$$

independent of λ.

6. (a) Since $g'(p) = 1 - 2p$ and $\sqrt{n}(X_n - p) \xrightarrow{\mathscr{L}} \mathscr{N}(0, p(1-p))$, we have, by Theorem 7,

$$\sqrt{n}\left(g(X_n) - g(p)\right) \xrightarrow{\mathscr{L}} \mathscr{N}\left(0, (1-2p)^2 p(1-p)\right).$$

If $p = 1/2$, this gives $\sqrt{n}(X_n(1 - X_n) - 0.25) \xrightarrow{\mathscr{L}} \mathscr{N}(0, 0)$. This just says $\sqrt{n}X_n(1 - X_n) \xrightarrow{\mathscr{L}} 0.25$.

(b) Since $g''(p) = -2$, (11) gives

$$n\left(X_n(1-X_n) - p(1-p)\right) \sim -p(1-p)\left[\chi_1^2(\gamma_n^2) - \gamma_n^2\right],$$

where $\gamma_n^2 = n(1-2p)^2/(4p(1-p))$. When $p = \frac{1}{2}$, this gives $n(X_n(1 - X_n) - 0.25) \xrightarrow{\mathscr{L}} -0.25\chi_1^2$ or, equivalently, $4n(0.25 - X_n(1 - X_n)) \xrightarrow{\mathscr{L}} \chi_1^2$. Since g is quadratic, the expansion (9) is exact, so if X_n were exactly normal, the above noncentral χ^2 approximation would be exact.

(c) When $p = 0.6$ and $n = 100$, (a) becomes $(X_n(1 - X_n) - 0.24) \sim \mathscr{N}(0, 0.96)$, and (b) becomes $(X_n(1 - X_n) - 0.24) \sim -0.0024[\chi_1^2(\gamma^2) - \gamma^2]$, where $\gamma^2 = 4.1667$. At $y = 0.25$, (a) gives $P(X_n(1 - X_n) \le y) \sim \Phi(1.021) = 0.8463$, whereas (b) gives $P(X_n(1 - X_n) \le y) = 1.0$, obviously the correct answer. At $y = 0.24$, (a) gives $P(X_n(1 - X_n) \le y) \sim 0.5000$ and (b) gives

$$P(X_n(1 - X_n) \le y) \sim P(\chi_1^2(\gamma^2) - \gamma^2 \ge 0)$$
$$= P\big((\mathscr{N}(0,1) + \gamma)^2 \ge \gamma^2\big)$$
$$= \Phi(0) + \Phi(-2|\gamma|) \simeq 0.5000.$$

At $y = 0.23$, (a) gives $P(X_n(1 - X_n) \le y) \sim \Phi(-1.021) = 0.1537$, and (b) gives

$$P(X_n(1 - X_n) \le y) \sim P(\chi_1^2(\gamma^2) \ge 2\gamma^2)$$
$$\simeq 1 - \Phi(\sqrt{8.3333} - \sqrt{4.1667}) = 0.1990.$$

We see that the normal approximation, (a), is rather poor.

SOLUTIONS TO THE EXERCISES OF SECTION 8

1. We use the notation μ_{jk} to represent $E\{(X - EX)^j(Y - EY)^k\}$. From Theorem 8, $\sqrt{n}((s_x^2, s_{xy}) - (\sigma_x^2, \sigma_{xy}) \to \mathscr{N}((0,0), \mathbf{\Sigma})$, where

$$\mathbf{\Sigma} = \begin{pmatrix} \mu_{40} - \mu_{20}^2 & \mu_{31} - \mu_{20}\mu_{11} \\ \mu_{31} - \mu_{20}\mu_{11} & \mu_{22} - \mu_{11}^2 \end{pmatrix}.$$

Take $g(u, v) = v/u$. Then $\dot{g}(u, v) = (-v/u^2, 1/u)$, and so

$$\sqrt{n}(\hat{\beta} - \beta) \to \mathscr{N}(0, \dot{g}(\mu_{20}, \mu_{11})\mathbf{\Sigma}\dot{g}(\mu_{20}, \mu_{11})')$$
$$= \mathscr{N}\big(0, [\mu_{40}\mu_{11}^2 - 2\mu_{31}\mu_{20}\mu_{11} + \mu_{22}\mu_{20}^2]/\mu_{20}^4\big).$$

For the bivariate normal distribution, $\mu_{40} = 3\sigma_x^4$, $\mu_{31} = 3\rho\sigma_x^3\sigma_y$, $\mu_{22} = (1 + 2\rho^2)\sigma_x^2\sigma_y^2$, and $\mu_{11} = \rho\sigma_x\sigma_y$. Hence the asymptotic variance is

$$[3\rho^2\sigma_x^6\sigma_y^2 - 6\rho^2\sigma_x^6\sigma_y^2 + (1 + 2\rho^2)\sigma_x^6\sigma_y^2]/\sigma_x^8 = (1 - \rho^2)\sigma_y^2/\sigma_x^2.$$

2. Because from Theorem 8, $\sqrt{n}(s_{xy} - \sigma_{xy}) \to \mathscr{N}(0, \mu_{22} - \mu_{11}^2)$, we have

$$\frac{\sqrt{n}(s_{xy} - \sigma_{xy})}{(\mu_{22} - \mu_{11}^2)^{1/2}} \to \mathscr{N}(0,1).$$

Hence,

$$\frac{\sqrt{n}\,(s_{xy} - \sigma_{xy})}{\left(m_{22} - s_{xy}^2\right)^{1/2}} \to \mathcal{N}(0,1),$$

where m_{22} is the sample estimate of μ_{22}, namely

$$m_{22} = (1/n)\sum_1^n \left(X_j - \overline{X}_n\right)^2\left(Y_j - \overline{Y}_n\right)^2.$$

3. (a) Because the mean and variance of $\mathcal{P}(\lambda)$ are both λ, we have $\sqrt{n}\,(\overline{X}_n - \lambda) \to \mathcal{N}(0, \lambda)$. We seek a transformation g such that $g'(\lambda)^2\lambda = 1$. Solving the differential equation $g'(\lambda) = \pm 1/\sqrt{\lambda}$ gives, say, $g(\lambda) = 2\sqrt{\lambda}$. Hence,

$$\sqrt{n}\left(\sqrt{\overline{X}_n} - \sqrt{\lambda}\right) \to \mathcal{N}(0, \tfrac{1}{4}).$$

(b) If X is binomial, $\mathcal{B}(n, p)$, then the mean of X/n is p and the variance of X/n is $p(1-p)$. We seek a transformation g such that $g'(p)^2 \cdot p(1-p) = 1$. Solving $g'(p) = (p(1-p))^{-1/2}$ gives, say, $g(p) = \arcsin(2p - 1)$, or, alternatively, $g(p) = \frac{1}{2}\arcsin(\sqrt{p})$. Hence,

$$\sqrt{n}\,(\arcsin(2X/n - 1) - \arcsin(2p - 1)) \to \mathcal{N}(0,1).$$

4. Let s_x^2 and s_y^2 be the sample variances from independent samples of size n from distributions with finite variances and fourth moments about the mean (σ_x^2, μ_{4x}) and (σ_y^2, μ_{4y}), respectively. Then, $\sqrt{n}\,(s_x^2 - \sigma_x^2)$ and $\sqrt{n}\,(s_y^2 - \sigma_y^2)$ converge in law jointly to independent normal distributions with means 0 and variances $\mu_{4x} - \sigma_x^4$ and $\mu_{4y} - \sigma_y^4$, respectively. Then applying the transformation $g(x, y) = x/y$ with gradient $g'(x, y) = (1/y, -x/y^2)$ to (s_x^2, s_y^2), we find that

$$\sqrt{n}\left(s_x^2/s_y^2 - \sigma_x^2/\sigma_y^2\right) \xrightarrow{\mathcal{L}} \mathcal{N}(0, \gamma^2),$$

where

$$\begin{aligned}\gamma^2 &= \left(\mu_{4x} - \sigma_x^4\right)/\sigma_y^4 + \left(\mu_{4y} - \sigma_y^4\right)\sigma_x^4/\sigma_y^8 \\ &= \left(\beta_{2x} + \beta_{2y} - 2\right)\sigma_x^4/\sigma_y^4,\end{aligned}$$

where β_{2x} and β_{2y} are the coefficients of kurtosis for the distributions. For sampling from normal distributions, we have $\gamma^2 = 4\sigma_x^4/\sigma_y^4$.

SOLUTIONS TO THE EXERCISES OF SECTION 9

1. Neyman's modified χ^2 may be written in the form

$$\chi_N^2 = n\left(\overline{\mathbf{X}}_n - \mathbf{p}\right)^T \hat{\mathbf{P}}_n^{-1}\left(\overline{\mathbf{X}}_n - \mathbf{p}\right),$$

where $\hat{\mathbf{P}}_n$ is the matrix $\mathbf{P}$ with each p_j replaced by its estimate, n_j/n. By the Law of Large Numbers, $\hat{\mathbf{P}}_n \to \mathbf{P}$ in probability, and by the central Limit Theorem, $\sqrt{n}\,(\overline{\mathbf{X}}_n - \mathbf{p}) \to \mathbf{Y} \in \mathscr{N}(0, \boldsymbol{\Sigma})$. Hence as in the proof of Theorem 9, $n(\overline{\mathbf{X}}_n - \mathbf{p})^T \hat{\mathbf{P}}_n^{-1}(\overline{\mathbf{X}}_n - \mathbf{p}) \to \mathbf{Y}^T\mathbf{P}^{-1}\mathbf{Y} \in \chi_{c-1}^2$.

2. Find Q orthogonal such that $\mathbf{QPQ}^T = \mathbf{D}$, diagonal. Let $\mathbf{Y} = \mathbf{QX}$ so that $\mathbf{Y} \in \mathscr{N}(0, \mathbf{QQ}^T) = \mathscr{N}(0, \mathbf{I})$ and $\mathbf{X}^T\mathbf{PX} = \mathbf{X}^T\mathbf{Q}^T\mathbf{DQX} = \mathbf{Y}^T\mathbf{DY}$. Then,

$$\mathbf{Y}^T\mathbf{DY} \in \chi_{c-1}^2, \qquad \text{iff } r \text{ of the } d_j \text{ are 1 and the rest are zero}$$

$$\text{iff } \mathbf{P} \text{ is a projection of rank } r$$

as in the proof of Lemma 3.

3. First note that $\Phi = \mathbf{Q} - \mathbf{qq}^T$, $\mathbf{Q}^{-1}\mathbf{q} = \mathbf{1}$ and $\mathbf{1}^T\mathbf{q} = 1 - p_c$. From this it follows that

$$\begin{aligned}(\mathbf{Q}^{-1} + \mathbf{11}^T/p_c)(\mathbf{Q} - \mathbf{qq}^T) &= \mathbf{I} - \mathbf{Q}^{-1}\mathbf{qq}^T + \mathbf{11}^T\mathbf{Q}/p_c - \mathbf{11}^T\mathbf{qq}^T/p_c \\ &= \mathbf{I} - \mathbf{1q}^T + \mathbf{1q}^T/p_c - (1 - p_c)\mathbf{1q}^T/p_c \\ &= \mathbf{I},\end{aligned}$$

so that $\boldsymbol{\Phi}^{-1} = (\mathbf{Q} - \mathbf{qq}^T)^{-1} = \mathbf{Q}^{-1} + \mathbf{11}^T/p_c$.

From the Central Limit Theorem, $\sqrt{n}\,(\mathbf{Y}_n - \mathbf{q}) \to \mathscr{N}(\mathbf{0}, \boldsymbol{\Phi})$. Hence, $Z = n(\overline{\mathbf{Y}}_n - \mathbf{q})^T\boldsymbol{\Phi}^{-1}(\overline{\mathbf{Y}}_n - \mathbf{q}) \to \chi_{c-1}^2$ from Lemma 1. It must be shown that Z is identical to Pearson's χ^2.

$$\begin{aligned}&n\left(\overline{\mathbf{Y}}_n - \mathbf{q}\right)^T \boldsymbol{\Phi}^{-1}\left(\overline{\mathbf{Y}}_n - \mathbf{q}\right) \\ &\quad = \mathbf{n}\left(\overline{\mathbf{Y}}_n - \mathbf{q}\right)^T \mathbf{Q}^{-1}\left(\overline{\mathbf{Y}}_n - \mathbf{q}\right) \\ &\qquad + n\left(\overline{\mathbf{Y}}_n - \mathbf{q}\right)^T \mathbf{11}^T\left(\overline{\mathbf{Y}}_n - \mathbf{q}\right)/p_c \\ &\quad = n\left(\overline{\mathbf{Y}}_n - \mathbf{q}\right)^T \mathbf{Q}^{-1}\left(\overline{\mathbf{Y}}_n - \mathbf{q}\right) + n(n_c/n - p_c)^2/p_c \\ &\quad = n\left(\overline{\mathbf{X}}_n - \mathbf{p}\right)^T \mathbf{P}^{-1}\left(\overline{\mathbf{X}}_n - \mathbf{p}\right),\end{aligned}$$

exactly Pearson's χ^2.

4. With $g(x) = \log(x_1)$, we have $g'(x) = 1/x$, and

$$\chi_g^2 = n \sum \frac{\left(\log(n_j/n) - \log(p_j)\right)^2}{(1/p_j)^2 p_j}$$

$$= n \sum \left(\log(n_j/n) - \log(p_j)\right)^2 p_j.$$

The modified transformed χ^2 is

$$\sum \left(\log(n_j/n) - \log(p_j)\right)^2 n_j.$$

SOLUTIONS TO THE EXERCISES OF SECTION 10

1. The noncentrality parameter is

$$\lambda = 100\left[\frac{(0.25 - 0.2)^2}{0.25} + \frac{(0.5 - 0.6)^2}{0.5} + \frac{(0.25 - 0.2)^2}{0.25}\right] = 4.$$

There are two degrees of freedom, so from the Fix Tables (Table 3) for $\alpha = 0.05$, we obtain $\beta = 0.42\cdots$, and for $\alpha = 0.01$, we obtain $\beta = 0.20\cdots$. To find n to achieve a power of 0.9 at $\alpha = 0.05$, we solve $(n/100)4 = 12.655$ to find that $n = 317$. For a power of 0.9 at $\alpha = 0.01$, we solve $(n/100)4 = 17.427$, to find $n = 436$.

2. (a) If $X \in \chi_r^2(\lambda)$, then X may be written in the form $X = (Y_1 + \sqrt{\lambda})^2 + Y_2^2 + \cdots + Y_r^2$, where $Y_1, \ldots, Y_r$ are i.i.d. normal mean 0 variance 1 random variables. Hence,

$$EX = E\left(Y_1 + \sqrt{\lambda}\right)^2 + EY_2^2 + \cdots + EY_r^2$$

$$= (1 + \lambda) + 1 + \cdots + 1 = r + \lambda.$$

To find var(X), first compute for $Y \in \mathcal{N}(0, 1)$,

$$\operatorname{var}\left\{\left(Y + \sqrt{\lambda}\right)^2\right\} = E\left(Y + \sqrt{\lambda}\right)^4 - \left(E\left(Y + \sqrt{\lambda}\right)^2\right)^2$$

$$= \left[EY^4 + 6\lambda EY^2 + \lambda^2\right] - (1 + \lambda)^2$$

$$= \left[3 + 6\lambda + \lambda^2\right] - (1 + 2\lambda + \lambda^2) = 2 + 4\lambda.$$

Hence,

$$\operatorname{var}(X) = (2 + 4\lambda) + 2 + \cdots + 2 = 2r + 4\lambda.$$

(b) We show that the moment-generating function of $(X - (r + \lambda))/(2 + 4\lambda)^{1/2}$ converges to $\exp\{+t^2/2\}$, the moment-generating function of $\mathcal{N}(0, 1)$, as $\max(r, \lambda) \to \infty$. The moment-generating function of X is $\varphi_X(t) = (1 - 2t)^{-r/2} \exp\{\lambda t/(1 - 2t)\}$; hence the moment-generating function of $(X - a)/b$ is

$$\varphi_{(X-a)/b}(t) = \varphi_X(t/b)\exp\{-at/b\}$$
$$= (1 - 2t/b)^{-r/2} \exp\{\lambda t/(b - 2t) - at/b\}.$$

From this, we find

$$\log \varphi_{(X-a)/b}(t)$$
$$= -(r/2)\log(1 - 2t/b) + (t/b)(\lambda/(1 - 2t/b) - a)$$
$$= -(r/2)\left[-2t/b - 4(t/b)^2/2\right]$$
$$+(t/b)[\lambda + 2\lambda t/b - a] + O\left((t/b)^3\right).$$

If $a = \lambda + r$, the linear terms cancel, and if $b = (2r + 4\lambda)^{1/2}$, we are left with $t^2/2 + O((t/b)^3) \to t^2/2$ as $b \to \infty$. When we notice that $b \to \infty$ if and only if $\max(r, \lambda) \to \infty$, we are done.

(c) Since $\chi^2_{20;\,.05} = 31.410$, we want to find λ such that

$$P\left(\chi^2_{20}(\lambda) > 31.410\right) = 0.5.$$

By part (b), this distribution is approximately $\mathcal{N}(20 + \lambda, 40 + 4\lambda)$, so we solve $20 + \lambda = 31.410$ to obtain $\lambda = 11.410$ as the approximation. The true value of λ given by the Fix Tables is $\lambda = 12.262$, rather close. If $\lambda = 11.410$ were used, the actual power found in the Fix Tables is about 0.47.

3. From the Central Limit Theorem, $\sqrt{n}(\overline{\mathbf{X}}_n - \mathbf{p}) \xrightarrow{\mathcal{L}} \mathbf{Z} \in \mathcal{N}(0, \boldsymbol{\Sigma})$, where $\boldsymbol{\Sigma} = \mathbf{P} - \mathbf{p}\mathbf{p}^T$. From Cramér's Theorem, $\sqrt{n}(\mathbf{g}(\overline{\mathbf{X}}_n) - \mathbf{g}(\mathbf{p})) \xrightarrow{\mathcal{L}} \dot{\mathbf{g}}(\mathbf{p})\mathbf{Z}$. Then $\sqrt{n}(\mathbf{g}(\mathbf{p}) - \mathbf{g}(\mathbf{p}_n^0)) \to \dot{\mathbf{g}}(\mathbf{p})\boldsymbol{\delta}$ implies that

$$\sqrt{n}\left(\mathbf{g}(\overline{\mathbf{X}}_n) - \mathbf{g}(\mathbf{p}_n^0)\right) = \sqrt{n}\left(\mathbf{g}(\overline{\mathbf{X}}_n) - \mathbf{g}(\mathbf{p})\right)$$
$$+\sqrt{n}\left(\mathbf{g}(\mathbf{p}) - \mathbf{g}(\mathbf{p}_n^0)\right) \xrightarrow{\mathcal{L}} \dot{\mathbf{g}}(\mathbf{p})\mathbf{Y},$$

where $\mathbf{Y} = \mathbf{Z} + \boldsymbol{\delta} \in \mathcal{N}(\boldsymbol{\delta}, \boldsymbol{\Sigma})$. From this, we have $\sqrt{n}\,\dot{\mathbf{g}}(\mathbf{p}_n^0)^{-1}(\mathbf{g}(\overline{\mathbf{X}}_n) - \mathbf{g}(\mathbf{p}_n^0)) \xrightarrow{\mathcal{L}} \mathbf{Y}$, so that

$$\chi^2_{\mathbf{g}} = n\left(\mathbf{g}(\overline{\mathbf{X}}_n) - \mathbf{g}(\mathbf{p}_n^0)\right)^T \dot{\mathbf{g}}(\mathbf{p}_n^0)^{-1}\left(\mathbf{P}_n^0\right)^{-1}$$
$$\dot{\mathbf{g}}(\mathbf{p}_n^0)^{-1}\left(\mathbf{g}(\overline{\mathbf{X}}_n) - \mathbf{g}(\mathbf{p}_n^0)\right) \xrightarrow{\mathcal{L}} \mathbf{Y}^T\mathbf{P}^{-1}\mathbf{Y}.$$

From the proof of Theorem 10, this has a $\chi^2_{c-1}(\lambda)$ distribution with $\lambda = \boldsymbol{\delta}^T \mathbf{P} \boldsymbol{\delta}$.

SOLUTIONS TO THE EXERCISES OF SECTION 11

1. The Y_j form a stationary 1-dependent Bernoulli sequence. The mean is $\boldsymbol{\mu} = EY_1 = E(1 - X_0)X_1 = E(1 - X_0)EX_1 = qp$. The variance is $\sigma_{00} = qp(1 - qp)$ and the covariance of lag 1 is $\sigma_{01} = \text{cov}(Y_1, Y_2) = EY_1Y_2 - EY_1EY_2 = 0 - (qp)^2$. Hence,
$$\sqrt{n}\left(\overline{Y}_n - qp\right) \xrightarrow{\mathscr{L}} \mathscr{N}(0, \sigma^2),$$
where $\sigma^2 = \sigma_{00} + 2\sigma_{01} = qp - 3(qp)^2$.
2. The Z_j are $(r + 1)$ dependent with $EZ_j = q^2p^r$ (where $q = 1 - p$), and $EZ_j^2 = q^2p^r$, $EZ_jZ_{j+r+1} = q^3p^{2r}$, and $EZ_jZ_{j+k} = 0$ for $1 \le k \le r$. Thus, $\text{var}(Z_j) = q^2p^r - q^4p^{2r}$, $\text{cov}(Z_j, Z_{j+k}) = -q^4p^{2r}$ for $1 \le k \le r$, $\text{cov}(Z_j, Z_{j+r+1} = q^3p^{2r} - q^4p^{2r}$ and $\text{cov}(Z_j, Z_{j+k}) = 0$ otherwise. Because the Z_j are stationary and $(r + 1)$ dependent, $\sqrt{n}(S_n/n - q^2p^r) \xrightarrow{\mathscr{L}} \mathscr{N}(0, \sigma^2)$, where
$$\sigma^2 = q^2p^r + 2q^3p^{2r} - (2r + 3)q^4p^{2r}.$$
3. Here $Y_j = X_{j-1}X_j$ is a stationary 1-dependent Bernoullli sequence with mean $\mu = EX_{j-1}X_j = p^2$, variance $\sigma_{00} = p^2(1 - p^2)$ and covariance of lag 1, $\sigma_{01} = EX_0X_1^2X_2 - (p^2)^2 = p^3(1 - p)$. Hence,
$$\sqrt{n}\left(\overline{Y}_n - p^2\right) \xrightarrow{\mathscr{L}} \mathscr{N}(0, \sigma_{00} + 2\sigma_{01}) = \mathscr{N}(0, p^2(1 - p)(1 + 3p)).$$
4. (a) Because $a\overline{X} + b\overline{Z} = (1/n)\Sigma_1^n X_i(a + bX_{i+1})$, we let $Y_i = X_i(a + bX_{i+1})$. Then $Y_1, Y_2, \cdots$ is a stationary 1-dependent sequence with mean $EY_i = a\mu + b\mu^2$ and variance
$$\begin{aligned}\sigma_{00} &= \text{var}\, Y_1 = EX_1^2E(a + bX_2)^2 - \mu^2(a + b\mu)^2\\ &= (\sigma^2 + \mu^2)(b^2\sigma^2 + b^2\mu^2 + 2ab\mu + a^2) - \mu^2(a^2 + 2ab\mu + b^2\mu^2)\\ &= \sigma^2(a^2 + 2ab\mu + b^2(\sigma^2 + 2\mu^2)).\end{aligned}$$
and covariance at lag 1,
$$\begin{aligned}\sigma_{01} &= \text{cov}(Y_1, Y_2) = EX_1E(a + bX_2)X_2E(a + bX_3) - \mu^2(a + b\mu)^2\\ &= \mu(a\mu + b\sigma^2 + b\mu^2)(a + b\mu) - \mu^2(a + b\mu)^2\\ &= \mu(a + b\mu)b\sigma^2.\end{aligned}$$

Therefore,

$$\sqrt{n}\left(a\overline{X}_n + b\overline{Z}_n - \mu(a + b\mu)\right)$$

$$\xrightarrow{\mathscr{L}} \mathscr{N}(0, \sigma_{00} + 2\sigma_{01})$$

$$= \mathscr{N}\left(0, \sigma^2\left(a^2 + 4ab\mu + b^2(\sigma^2 + 4\mu^2)\right)\right).$$

This is the distribution of $aX + bZ$ when $(X, Z) \in \mathscr{N}(\mathbf{0}, \mathbf{\Sigma})$, where

$$\mathbf{\Sigma} = \begin{pmatrix} \sigma^2 & 2\sigma^2\mu \\ 2\sigma^2\mu & \sigma^4 + 4\sigma^2\mu^2 \end{pmatrix}.$$

Since $a\sqrt{n}(\overline{X}_n - \mu) + b\sqrt{n}(\overline{Z}_n - \mu^2) \xrightarrow{\mathscr{L}} aX + bZ$, we have, from Exercise 2 of Section 3, $\sqrt{n}(\overline{X}_n - \mu, \overline{Z}_n - \mu^2) \xrightarrow{\mathscr{L}} \mathscr{N}(\mathbf{0}, \mathbf{\Sigma})$.

(b) Now we apply Cramér's Theorem using the function $g(x, z) = z - x^2$. We have $\dot{g}(x, z) = (-2x, 1)$, $g(\mu, \mu^2) = 0$, and $\dot{g}(\mu, \mu^2) = (-2\mu, 1)$. Thus we find

$$\sqrt{n}\left(\overline{Z}_n - \overline{X}_n^2\right) \xrightarrow{\mathscr{L}} \mathscr{N}(0, \sigma^4).$$

5. The sequence $Z_1, Z_2, \cdots$ forms a 2-dependent stationary sequence of Bernoulli variables (Z_1 and Z_4 are independent, for example). We have $EZ_1 = P(X_0 > X_1 < X_2) = \frac{1}{3}$, because this is just the probability that of three independent numbers chosen from a distribution, the second one is the smallest. The distribution is continuous, so there are no ties. Because Z_1 is Bernoulli, $\text{var}(Z_1) = \frac{1}{3}\frac{2}{3} = \frac{2}{9}$. And not both Z_1 and Z_2 can be positive, so $EZ_1Z_2 = 0$ and $\text{cov}(Z_1, Z_2) = -\frac{1}{9}$. To compute $\text{cov}(Z_1, Z_3)$, we must evaluate $EZ_1Z_3 = P(X_0 > X_1 < X_2 > X_3 < X_4)$. All $5! = 120$ orderings of X_0, X_1, X_2, X_3, X_4 are equally likely, and we must count the number of orderings such that $X_0 > X_1 < X_2 > X_3 < X_4$. Either X_1 or X_3 must be the smallest, and there are exactly 8 orderings with X_1 the smallest and 8 with X_3 the smallest for a total of 16 orderings. Thus, $\text{cov}(Z_1, Z_3) = \frac{16}{120} - \frac{1}{9} = \frac{1}{45}$. We find $\sigma^2 = \frac{2}{9} + 2(-\frac{1}{9}) + 2\frac{1}{45} = \frac{2}{45}$. Hence,

$$\sqrt{n}\left(\frac{S_n}{n} - \frac{1}{3}\right) \xrightarrow{\mathscr{L}} \mathscr{N}\left(0, \frac{2}{45}\right).$$

6. (a) Let $U_i = X_i^2$ and $V_i = X_i X_{i+1}$. Then $W_i = aX_i + bU_i + cV_i$ is a 1-dependent sequence with mean $EW_i = b\sigma^2$. Then $EW_i^2 = \operatorname{var} W_i = a^2\sigma^2 + 2ab\mu_3 + b^2\mu_4 + c^2\sigma^4$ and $\mathrm{EW_iW_{i+1}} = \mathrm{b}^2\sigma^4$, so that $\sigma_{00} = \operatorname{var} W_i = a^2\sigma^2 + 2ab\mu_3 + b^2\mu_4 + c^2\sigma^4 - b^2\sigma^4$, and $\sigma_{01} = EW_iW_{i+1} - b^2\sigma^4 = 0$. From the theorem of this section,

$$\sqrt{n}\left(a\overline{X}_n + b\overline{U}_n + c\overline{V}_n - b\sigma^2\right)$$

$$\xrightarrow{\mathscr{L}} \mathscr{N}\left(0, a^2\sigma^2 + 2ab\mu_3 + b^2\left(\mu_4 - \sigma^4\right) + c^2\sigma^4\right).$$

This is the distribution of $aX + bU + cV$ when $(X, U, V) \in \mathscr{N}(\mathbf{0}, \mathbf{\Sigma})$, where

$$\mathbf{\Sigma} = \begin{pmatrix} \sigma^2 & \mu_3 & 0 \\ \mu_3 & \mu_4 - \sigma^4 & 0 \\ 0 & 0 & \sigma^4 \end{pmatrix}.$$

Then by Exercise 2 of Section 3 we have $\sqrt{n}(\overline{X}_n, \overline{U}_n - \sigma^2, \overline{V}_n) \xrightarrow{\mathscr{L}} \mathscr{N}(\mathbf{0}, \mathbf{\Sigma})$.

(b) Note $r_n = g(\overline{X}_n, \overline{U}_n, \overline{V}_n)$ where $g(x, u, v) = (v - x^2)/(u - x^2)$. We have $g(0, \sigma^2, 0) = 0$, and because $\dot{g}(x, u, v) = (2x(v - u), -(v - x^2), u - x^2)/(u - x^2)^2$, we have $\dot{g}(0, \sigma^2, 0) = (0, 0, 1/\sigma^2)$. Hence from Cramér's Theorem, $\sqrt{n}(r_n - 0) \xrightarrow{\mathscr{L}} \mathscr{N}(0, \sigma^4/\sigma^4) = \mathscr{N}(0, 1)$.

7. We may assume without loss of generality that $\tau = 1$ and $\xi = 0$ and hence $\mu = 0$. Let $Y_t^{(k)} = \sum_{|j| \le k} z_j X_{t-j}$ and $S_n^{(k)} = \sum_{t=1}^n Y_t^{(k)}$. Then $Y_t^{(k)}$ is a stationary $2k$-dependent sequence with mean 0 and covariances,

$$\sigma_{0t}^{(k)} = \operatorname{cov}\left(Y_0^{(k)}, Y_t^{(k)}\right) = \sum_{|j| \le k} \sum_{|i| \le k} z_j z_i EX_{-j} X_{t-i} = \sum_{j=t-k}^{k} z_j z_{t-j},$$

for $t \ge 0$. Hence by Theorem 11, $S_n^{(k)}/\sqrt{n} \xrightarrow{\mathscr{L}} \mathscr{N}(0, \sigma_k^2)$, where $\sigma_k^2 = \sigma_{00}^{(k)} + 2\sum_{t=1}^{2k} \sigma_{0t}^{(k)}$. Also $\sigma_k^2 \to \sigma^2$, because the latter is absolutely convergent. Thus, by the lemma, we will be finished when we show $(S_n - S_n^{(k)})/\sqrt{n} \to 0$ uniformly in n as $k \to \infty$. Since

$$Y_t - Y_t^{(k)} = \sum_{j<-k} z_j X_{t-j} + \sum_{j>k} z_j X_{t-j},$$

we may break $(S_n - S_n^{(k)})$ into two pieces,

$$S_n - S_n^{(k)} = \sum_{t=1}^{n} \sum_{j<-k} z_j X_{t-j} + \sum_{t=1}^{n} \sum_{j>k} z_j X_{t-j} = U_n^{(k)} + V_n^{(k)},$$

say, and show that $U_n^{(k)}/\sqrt{n}$ and $V_n^{(k)}/\sqrt{n}$ are both uniformly small in n as $k \to \infty$. For this we compute

$$E\left(V_n^{(k)}\right)^2 \le \sum_{i>k} \sum_{j>k} |z_i|\,|z_j| \sum_{s=1}^{n} \sum_{t=1}^{n} EX_{s-i}X_{t-j}$$

$$\le \sum_{i>k} \sum_{j>k} |z_i|\,|z_j| n = n\left(\sum_{j>k} |z_j|\right)^2.$$

Thus, by Chebyshev's inequality,

$$P\left(\left|V_n^{(k)}\right|/\sqrt{n} > \varepsilon\right) \le E\left(V_n^{(k)}/\sqrt{n}\right)^2/\varepsilon^2 \le \left(\sum_{j>k} |z_j|\right)^2/\varepsilon^2 \to 0$$

uniformly in n as $k \to \infty$. Similarly, $U_n^{(k)}/\sqrt{n} \to 0$ uniformly in n as $k \to \infty$. Similarly, $U_n^{(k)}/\sqrt{n} \to 0$ uniformly in n as $k \to \infty$. Finally, the sum converges to zero uniformly in n, since

$$P\left(\left|U_n^{(k)} + V_n^{(k)}\right|\sqrt{n} > 2\varepsilon\right) \le P\left(\left|U_n^{(k)}\right| + \left|V_n^{(k)}\right| > 2\varepsilon\sqrt{n}\right)$$

$$\le P\left(\left|U_n^{(k)}\right| > \varepsilon\sqrt{n}\right) + P\left(\left|V_n^{(k)}\right| > \varepsilon\sqrt{n}\right).$$

This completes the proof.

SOLUTIONS TO THE EXERCISES OF SECTION 12

1. (a) This is a special case of Example 1 with $z_j = j$ and m replacing n. Since $\bar{z}_N = (N+1)/2$,

$$\sum_1^N z_j^2 = N(N+1)(2N+1)/6,$$

$$\sum_1^N \left(z_j - \bar{z}_N\right)^2 = N(N-1)(N+1)/12,$$

and $\max_j(z_j - \bar{z}_N)^2 = (N-1)^2/4$, condition (9) is satisfied if $\min(m, N-m) \to \infty$, because $N \max_j(z_j - \bar{z}_N)^2/\Sigma_1^N(z_j - \bar{z}_N)^2$ is bounded. From Lemma 1,

$$ES_N = N((N+1)/2)(m/N) = m(N+1)/2$$

and

$$\begin{aligned}\operatorname{var}(S_N) &= (N/(N-1))(N(N-1)(N+1)/12)(m(N-m)/N^2)\\ &= m(N-m)(N+1)/12.\end{aligned}$$

Hence we have $(S_N - ES_N)/\sqrt{\operatorname{var}(S_N)} \xrightarrow{\mathcal{L}} \mathcal{N}(0,1)$.

(b) Not necessarily. If $m/N \to r$ as $N \to \infty$, then

$$\sqrt{N}\left(\frac{S_N}{N^2} - \frac{m(N+1)}{2N^2}\right) \xrightarrow{\mathcal{L}} \mathcal{N}\left(0, \frac{r(1-r)}{12}\right).$$

However, for this to imply that $\sqrt{N}(S_N/N^2 - r/2)$ has the same asymptotic distribution, we must have the sequences be asymptotically equivalent; that is, the difference must converge to zero, $\sqrt{N}(m(N+1)/(2N^2) - r/2) \to 0$. This requires a faster rate of convergence; namely, we need $\sqrt{N}(m/N \to r) \to 0$.

2. (a) This is also a special case of the sampling problem, where it was shown that

$$\max_j (a(j) - \bar{a}_N)^2 / \sum_1^N (a(j) - \bar{a}_N)^2 \le N/(n(N-n)).$$

From this we may deduce $\max_j (z_j - \bar{z}_N)^2/\Sigma_1^N (z_j - \bar{z}_N)^2 \le N/(m(N-m))$ also. Thus, condition (9) is satisfied if $N^3/(n(N-n)m(N-m)) \to 0$ or $n(N-n)m(N-m)/N^3 \to \infty$. In particular, if $\min(n, N-n) \to \infty$ and $\min(m, N-m)/N$ is bounded away from 0, then S_N is asymptotically normal. Since the mean of the hypergeometric is mn/N and the variance is $mn(N-m)(N-n)/(N^2(N-1))$, we have that if $\sqrt{N}(m/N - r) \to 0$ and $\sqrt{N}(n/N - s) \to 0$, then

$$\sqrt{N}(S_n/N - rs) \xrightarrow{\mathcal{L}} \mathcal{N}(0, rs(1-r)(1-s)).$$

(b) The probability mass function of the hypergeometric distribution is

$$\begin{aligned}P(S_N = x) &= \frac{\binom{m}{x}\binom{N-m}{n-x}}{\binom{N}{n}}\\ &= \frac{m!n!(N-m)!(N-n)!}{x!(m-x)!(n-x)!N!(N-m-n+x)!}.\end{aligned}$$

We are to show this converges to $e^{-\lambda}\lambda^x/x!$ for all fixed $x = 0, 1, \ldots,$ as $\min(n, m) \to \infty$, and $mn/N \to \lambda$. The $1/x!$ term is already present. Next note that

$$\frac{m!n!}{(m-x)!(n-x)!} \sim m^x n^x \quad \text{and} \quad \frac{(N-n-m)!}{(N-m-n+x)!} \sim N^{-x},$$

so that the product converges to λ^x. We will be finished when we show $(N-m)!(N-n)!/(N!(N-m-n)!) \to e^{-\lambda}$. But

$$\begin{aligned}\frac{(N-m)!(N-n)!}{N!(N-m-n)!} &= \frac{(N-m)\cdots(N-m-n+1)}{N\cdots(N-n+1)}\\ &= \left(1-\frac{m}{N}\right)\cdots\left(1-\frac{m}{N-n+1}\right)\\ &\leq \left(1-\frac{m}{n}\right)^n \to \exp\left\{-\lim_{n\to\infty}\frac{mn}{N}\right\} = e^{-\lambda}.\end{aligned}$$

Similarly,

$$\begin{aligned}\frac{(N-m)!(N-n)!}{N!(N-m-n)!} &\geq \left(1-\frac{m}{N-n+1}\right)^n\\ &\to \exp\left\{-\lim_{n\to\infty}\frac{mn}{N-n+1}\right\} = e^{-\lambda},\end{aligned}$$

completing the proof.

3. (a) Given $U_1 = u$, the rank of U_1 is one more than the number of U_j's less than u. Thus the conditional distribution of $R_1 - 1$ given $U_1 = u$ is binomial with sample size $N - 1$ and probability u. Hence,

$$\begin{aligned}ER_1U_1 &= E\left[U_1E\{R_1|U_1\}\right] = E\left[U_1((N-1)U_1+1)\right]\\ &= (N-1)EU_1^2 + EU_1\\ &= (N-1)/3 + \tfrac{1}{2} = (2N+1)/6.\end{aligned}$$

Then $ER_1^2 = (N+1)(2N+1)/6$ and $EU_1^2 = \frac{1}{3}$ gives

$$E(R_1 - NU_1)^2 = ER_1^2 - 2NER_1U_1 + N^2EU_1^2 = (N+1)/6.$$

From $\mathrm{var}(R_1) = (N+1)(N-1)/12$, we conclude $E(R_1 - NU_1)^2/\mathrm{var}(R_1) = 2/(N-1) \to 0$.

(b) Since $0 \le \lceil NU_1 \rceil - NU_1 < 1$, we have $E(\lceil NU_1 \rceil - NU_1)^2 < 1$ so that $E(\lceil NU_1 \rceil - NU_1)^2/\text{var}(R_1) \to 0$.

(c)

$$(x+y)^2 = x^2 + 2xy + y^2$$
$$= 2x^2 + 2y^2 - (x^2 - 2xy + y^2) \le 2x^2 + 2y^2.$$

Hence,

$$E(R_1 - \lceil NU_1 \rceil)^2/\text{var}(R_1)$$
$$\le 2\left[E(R_1 - NU_1)^2 + E(NU_1 - \lceil NU_1 \rceil)^2\right]/\text{var}(R_1) \to 0.$$

This implies $\text{corr}(R_1, \lceil NU_1 \rceil) \to 1$ so condition (10) is satisfied.

(d) For $a(j) = j$, we have $\bar{a}_N = (N+1)/2$, $\max_j (a(j) - \bar{a}_N)^2 = (N-1)^2/4$, and $\sum_1^N (a(j) - \bar{a}_N)^2 = N(N+1)(N-1)/12$, so that

$$N \max_j (a(j) - \bar{a}_N)^2 / \sum_1^N (a(j) - \bar{a}_N)^2 = (N-1)/(12(N+1))$$

stays bounded. Hence, provided $\max_j (z_j - \bar{z}_N)^2 / \sum_1^N (z_j - \bar{z}_N)^2 \to 0$, condition (9) is satisfied and by Theorem 11, $(S_N - ES_N)/\sqrt{\text{var}(S_N)} \xrightarrow{\mathscr{L}} \mathscr{N}(0,1)$.

4. Using $z_j = j$ in Exercise 3, we easily find that $(S_N - ES_N)/\sqrt{\text{var}(S_N)} \xrightarrow{\mathscr{L}} \mathscr{N}(0,1)$, since we have

$$\max_j (z_j - \bar{z}_N)^2 / \sum_1^N (z_j - \bar{z}_N)^2 = (N-1)/(12N(N+1)) \to 0.$$

The mean of S_N is $N\bar{z}_N \bar{a}_N = N(N+1)^2/4$, and the variance is $N^2(N-1)^2(N+1)^2/(12^2(N-1)) \simeq N^5/12^2$. We may conclude that

$$12\sqrt{N}\left(\frac{1}{N}\sum_{j=1}^{N} \frac{j}{N}\frac{R_j}{N} - \frac{1}{4}\right) \xrightarrow{\mathscr{L}} \mathscr{N}(0,1).$$

Spearman's rank correlation coefficient, ρ_N, is the correlation coefficient between the true ranks j, and the observed ranks, R_j, namely,

$$\rho_N = \frac{12}{N^2 - 1}\left[\frac{1}{N}\sum_1^N jR_j - \frac{(N+1)^2}{4}\right].$$

This result shows that $\sqrt{N}\rho_N \xrightarrow{\mathscr{L}} \mathscr{N}(0,1)$, under the hypothesis of a random ranking.

5. (a) $0 \le \Sigma_1^N \log j - \int_1^N \log(x)\,dx \le \log N$ and $\int_1^N \log(x)\,dx = N(\log N) - N - 1$ shows that $\Sigma_1^N \log j = N(\log N) - N + O(\log N)$. Similarly,

$$\sum_1^N (\log j)^2 = \int_1^N \log(x)^2\,dx + O\big((\log N)^2\big)N(\log n)^2$$

$$- 2N(\log N) + 2N + O\big((\log N)^2\big).$$

Combining these gives

$$\sum_1^N a(j)^2 - \frac{1}{N}\left(\sum_1^N a(j)\right)^2 = N + O\big((\log N)^2\big)$$

It is easy to see that $\max(a(j) - \bar{a}_N)^2 \sim (\log N)^2$. Hence,

$$\frac{\max_j\big(a(j) - \bar{a}_N\big)^2}{\Sigma_1^N\big(a(j) - \bar{a}_N\big)^2} \sim \frac{(\log N)^2}{N}.$$

Condition (9) reduces to

$$\frac{\max_j\big(z_j - \bar{z}_N\big)^2}{\Sigma_1^N\big(z_j - \bar{z}_N\big)^2}\cdot(\log N)^2 \to 0.$$

(b) For $a(j) = 1/\sqrt{j}$, we have $\Sigma_1^N a(j) \sim 2\sqrt{N}$ and $\Sigma_1^N a(j)^2 = \Sigma_1^N 1/j \sim \log N$. So $\Sigma_1^N(a(j - \bar{a}_N)^2 \sim \log N$ and $\max(a(j) - \bar{a}_N)^2 \sim 1$. This gives

$$\frac{\max_j\big(a(j) - \bar{a}_N\big)^2}{\Sigma_1^N\big(a(j) - \bar{a}_N\big)^2} \sim \frac{1}{\log N}.$$

Condition (9) reduces to

$$\frac{N}{\log N}\,\frac{\max_j\big(z_j - \bar{z}_N\big)^2}{\Sigma_1^N\big(z_j - \bar{z}_N\big)^2} \to 0.$$

(c) For $a(j) = 1/j$, we have $\Sigma_1^N a(j) \sim \log N$. So $\Sigma_1^N(a(j) - \bar{a}_N)^2 \sim \Sigma_1^N a(j)^2 = \pi^2/6$ and $\max(a(j) - \bar{a}_N)^2 \sim 1$. Thus,

$$\frac{\max_j\big(a(j) - \bar{a}_N\big)^2}{\Sigma_1^N\big(a(j) - \bar{a}_N\big)^2} \sim \frac{6}{\pi^2}.$$

Condition (9) cannot be satisfied.

6. (a) Each term of the sum

$$S'_N = \sum_1^N (z_{Nj} - \bar{z}_N)(\varphi(U_j) - \bar{\varphi})$$

has mean zero and the $\varphi(U_j)$ are i.i.d., so the asymptotic normality of $S'_N/\sqrt{\mathrm{var}(S'_N)}$ follows immediately from Exercise 6 of Section 5 with z_{nj} replaced by $z_{Nj} - \bar{z}_N$.

(b) The variance of S_N is given in Lemma 1, and $\mathrm{var}(S'_N) = \Sigma_1^N(z_{Nj} - \bar{z}_N)^2\sigma^2$. The covariance is found, as in Lemma 2, to be

$$\mathrm{cov}(S_N, S'_N) = (N/(N-1))\sum_1^N (z_{Nj} - \bar{z}_N)^2 \mathrm{cov}(a(R_{N1}), \varphi(U_1)).$$

From this, the correlation is found as

$$\begin{aligned}\mathrm{corr}(S_N, S'_N) &= \sqrt{N/(N-1)}\,\mathrm{cov}(a(R_{N1}), \varphi(U_1))/ \\ &\qquad \left(\sigma\sqrt{\mathrm{var}(a(R_{N1}))}\right) \\ &= \sqrt{N/(N-1)}\,\mathrm{corr}(a(R_{N1}), \varphi(U_1)).\end{aligned}$$

(c) Given $U_1 = u$, $R_{N1}/N \to u$ with probability 1. As in the Glivenko–Cantelli Theorem, the set of probability 1 on which convergence takes place may be chosen independent of u. Thus, $R_{N1}/N \xrightarrow{\text{a.s.}} U_1$. The function φ, being nondecreasing, has only a countable number of discontinuities. Hence, we have $\varphi(R_{N1}/(N+1)) \xrightarrow{\text{a.s.}} \varphi(U_1)$.

(d) $E\varphi(R_{N1}/(N+1))^2 = (1/N)\Sigma_1^N\varphi(j/(N+1))^2$. If φ were bounded this would be a Riemann approximation to $\int_0^1\varphi(u)^2\,du = E\varphi(U_1)^2$ and we would be done. However, because $(\varphi(u)^+)^2$ is nondecreasing,

$$\begin{aligned}\int_0^{1-(1/(N+1))}(\varphi(u)^+)^2\,du &\le \frac{1}{N+1}\sum_1^N\left(\varphi\left(\frac{j}{N+1}\right)^+\right)^2 \\ &\le \int_{1/(N+1)}^1(\varphi(u)^+)^2\,du,\end{aligned}$$

which shows

$$(1/N)\sum_1^N\left(\varphi\left(\frac{j}{N+1}\right)^+\right)^2 \to \int_0^1(\varphi(u)^+)^2\,du.$$

By symmetry, we have

$$(1/N)\sum_{1}^{N}\left(\varphi\left(\frac{j}{N+1}\right)^{-}\right)^{2} \to \int_0^1 \left(\varphi(u)^{-}\right)^{2} du.$$

This gives $E\varphi(R_{N1}/(N+1))^2 \to E\varphi(U_1)^2$.

(e) By Exercise 8 of Section 2, (c) and (d) together imply that $\varphi(a(R_1)) \xrightarrow{\text{q.m}} \varphi(U_1)$, which is the result to be proved.

(f) By (b) and Exercise 5 of Section 6, it is sufficient to show that $E(a(R_{N1}) - \varphi(U_1))^2/\text{var}(\varphi(U_1)) \to 0$. For this it is sufficient to show that $E(a(R_{N1}) - \varphi(U_1))^2 \to 0$. This follows from (e), and the proof is complete.

7. (a) By Exercise 2 of Section 3, it is sufficient to show that

$$\sqrt{3N}\,\mathbf{b}^T\left(\frac{2}{N(N+1)}\mathbf{S} - \mathbf{p}^*\right) \xrightarrow{\mathscr{L}} \mathscr{N}(\mathbf{0}, \mathbf{b}^T(\mathbf{P} - \mathbf{p}\mathbf{p}^T)\mathbf{b}) \qquad (1)$$

for all k vectors $\mathbf{b}$. If $\mathbf{b}$ is the constant vector $c\mathbf{1}$, where $\mathbf{1}$ is the vector of all 1's, then $\mathbf{b}^T\mathbf{S} = c\sum_1^N j = cN(N+1)/2$ and $\mathbf{b}^T\mathbf{p}^* = c\sum n_j/N = c$, so the left side of (1) is zero. But the right side is the distribution degenerate at zero ($\mathbf{b}^T(\mathbf{P} - \mathbf{p}\mathbf{p}^T)\mathbf{b} = 0$) so the result is true for $\mathbf{b} = c\mathbf{1}$. We now assume that $\mathbf{b}$ is not a constant vector.

Let $N_i = \sum_{h=1}^{i} n_h$ and write S_i in the form $S_i = \sum_{j=1}^{N} z_j^{(i)} a(R_j)$ with

$$a(j) = j \quad \text{and} \quad z_j^{(i)} = \begin{cases} 1, & \text{if } N_{i-1} < j \le N_i, \\ 0, & \text{otherwise}. \end{cases}$$

Thus we have $\mathbf{b}^T\mathbf{S} = \sum_{i=1}^{k} b_i S_i = \sum_{j=1}^{N} z_j R_j$, where $z_j = \sum_{i=1}^{k} b_i z_j^{(i)}$. We use Theorem 12 to show that $\sum_1^N z_j R_j$ is asymptotically normal. From the solution to Exercise 3(d), we see

$$N \max_j \left(a(j) - \bar{a}_N\right)^2 / \sum_1^N \left(a(j) - \bar{a}_N\right)^2 = (N-1)/(12(N+1))$$

stays bounded. So condition (9) holds if and only if $\max_j(z_j - \bar{z}_N)^2/\sum_1^N(z_j - \bar{z}_N)^2 \to 0$. Since $k \le \max_j(z_j - \bar{z}_N) \le 1$, (9) holds if and only if $\sum_1^N(z_j - \bar{z}_N)^2 \to \infty$. We have $\sum_1^N z_j = \sum_1^k b_i n_i$ and $\sum_1^N z_j^2 = \sum_1^k b_i^2 n_i$, so

$$\frac{1}{N}\sum_1^N (z_j - \bar{z})^2 = \sum_1^k \frac{n_i}{N} b_i^2 - \left(\sum_1^k \frac{n_i}{N} b_i\right)^2.$$

Since $n_i/N \to p_i$ as $N \to \infty$,

$$(1/N)\sum_1^N (z_j - \bar{z})^2 \to \sum_1^k p_i b_i^2 - \left(\sum_1^k p_i b_i\right)^2.$$

This is strictly positive from the assumption that $\mathbf{b}$ is not a constant vector. Thus, $\Sigma_1^N (z_j - \bar{z}_N)^2 \to \infty$, which implies that $(\mathbf{b}^T\mathbf{S} - E\mathbf{b}^T\mathbf{S})/\sqrt{\operatorname{var}\mathbf{b}^T\mathbf{S}} \xrightarrow{\mathscr{L}} \mathscr{N}(0, 1)$. We compute the mean and variance of $\mathbf{b}^T\mathbf{S}$.

$$E\mathbf{b}^T\mathbf{S} = \sum_1^N z_j E R_j = ((N+1)/2)\sum_1^N z_j$$

$$= (N(N+1)/2)\sum_1^k b_i n_i / N,$$

and from Lemma 1, $\operatorname{var}\mathbf{b}^T\mathbf{S} = \operatorname{var}\Sigma_1^N z_j R_j = (N/(N-1))\Sigma_1^N (z_j - \bar{z}_N)^2 \operatorname{var}(R_1) = (N/(N-1))\Sigma_1^k n_i (b_i - \bar{b})^2((N^2 - 1)/12$. Using Slutsky's Theorem, we conclude

$$\sqrt{3(N+1)}\left(\frac{2}{N(N+1)}\mathbf{b}^T\mathbf{S} - \mathbf{b}^T\mathbf{p}^*\right) \xrightarrow{\mathscr{L}} \mathscr{N}\left(0, \sum_1^k p_i (b_i - \bar{b})^2\right).$$

The result now follows from

$$\sum_1^k p_i (b_i - \bar{b})^2 = \sum_1^k p_i b_i^2 - \left(\sum_1^k p_i b_i\right)^2 = \mathbf{b}^T\mathbf{P}\mathbf{b} - \mathbf{b}^T\mathbf{p}\mathbf{p}^T\mathbf{b}.$$

(b) From Slutsky's Theorem and part (a),

$$3(N+1)\left(\frac{2}{N(N+1)}\mathbf{S} - \mathbf{p}^*\right)^T \mathbf{P}^{-1}\left(\frac{2}{N(N+1)}\mathbf{S} - \mathbf{p}^*\right)$$

$$\xrightarrow{\mathscr{L}} \mathbf{Y}^T\mathbf{P}^{-1}\mathbf{Y}, \tag{2}$$

where $\mathbf{Y} \in \mathscr{N}(\mathbf{0}, \mathbf{P} - \mathbf{p}\mathbf{p}^T)$. As in the proof of Theorem 9, $\mathbf{Y}^T\mathbf{P}^{-1}\mathbf{Y} \in \chi^2_{k-1}$. Another application of Slutsky's Theorem shows that $\mathbf{P}$ in the left side of (2) can be replaced by $\mathbf{P}^*$.

SOLUTIONS TO THE EXERCISES OF SECTION 13

1. The density of a sample, $Y_1, \dots, Y_{n+1}$, from $\mathscr{G}(1,1)$ is
$$f_{\mathbf{Y}}(y_1, \dots, y_{n+1}) = \exp\{-\textstyle\sum y_j\} I(y_j > 0 \text{ for all } j).$$
The density of $S_k = \Sigma_1^k Y_j$, $k = 1, \dots, n+1$ (Jacobian $= 1$) is
$$f_{\mathbf{S}}(s_1, \dots, s_{n+1}) = \exp\{-s_{n+1}\} I(0 < s_1 < s_2 < \cdots < s_{n+1}).$$
$\{Z_k = S_k / S_{n+1},\ 1 \le k \le n\}$ and $W = S_{n+1}$ (Jacobian $= w^n$) have density
$$g(z_1, \dots, z_n, w) = w^n \exp\{-w\} I\,(0 < z_1 < \cdots < z_n < 1, w > 0).$$
Hence, $(Z_1, \dots, Z_n)$ and S_{n+1} are independent, with $S_{n+1} \in \mathscr{G}(n+1, 1)$ and
$$f_{\mathbf{Z}}(z_1, \dots, z_n) = n! I(z_1, \dots, z_n),$$
exactly the density of the order statistics of a sample of size n from a uniform distribution on [0, 1].
2. Since μ is the median and $f(\mu) = \frac{1}{2}$,
$$\sqrt{n}\,(m_n - \mu) \to \mathscr{N}\left(0, \tfrac{1}{4}/\left(\tfrac{1}{2}\right)^2\right) = \mathscr{N}(0,1).$$
3. Since the first and third quartiles are $\mu - \sigma$ and $\mu + \sigma$ and $f(\mu - \sigma) = f(\mu + \sigma) = 1/(2\pi\sigma)$, we have
$$\sqrt{n}\begin{pmatrix} X_{(n/4)} - (\mu - \sigma) \\ X_{(3n/4)} - (\mu + \sigma) \end{pmatrix} \to \mathscr{N}\left(\begin{pmatrix} 0 \\ 0 \end{pmatrix}, \frac{\pi^2\sigma^2}{4}\begin{pmatrix} 3 & 1 \\ 1 & 3 \end{pmatrix}\right).$$
Now, using Cramér's Theorem with $g(x, y) = (x+y)/2$, $\dot{g}(x, y) = \left(\frac{1}{2}, \frac{1}{2}\right)$
$$\sqrt{n}\left((X_{(n/4)} + X_{(3n/4)})/2 - \mu\right) \to \mathscr{N}(0, \pi^2\sigma^2/2).$$
If $m_n =$ sample median, then $\sqrt{n}\,(m_n - \mu) \to \mathscr{N}(0, \pi^2\sigma^2/4)$ so the midquartile range has efficiency only 50% relative to the sample median.
4. (a) $\sqrt{n}\,(m_n - \mu) \to \mathscr{N}(0, \mu^2)$.
(b)
$$\sqrt{n}\begin{pmatrix} X_{(n/4)} - \mu/2 \\ X_{(3n/4)} - 3\mu/2 \end{pmatrix} \to \mathscr{N}\left(\begin{pmatrix} 0 \\ 0 \end{pmatrix}, \frac{\mu^2}{4}\begin{pmatrix} 3 & 1 \\ 1 & 3 \end{pmatrix}\right)$$
so $\sqrt{n}\,((X_{(n/4)} + X_{(3n/4)})/2 - \mu) \to \mathscr{N}(0, \mu^2/2)$.

(c)

$$\sqrt{n}\,(X_{(3n/4)} - 3\mu/2) \to \mathcal{N}(0, 3\mu^2/4).$$

So,

$$\sqrt{n}\left(\tfrac{2}{3}X_{(3n/4)} - \mu\right) \to \mathcal{N}(0, \mu^2/3).$$

(d) Asymptotically, the midquartile range is twice as efficient as the median. But $2X_{(3n/4)}/3$ is still more efficient. This is not surprising, because the maximum is sufficient for μ, and the closer we get to the maximum/2 the better we shall be.

5. (a) The median of $\mathcal{G}(1, \theta)$ is $\mu = \theta \log(2)$, and $f(\mu|\theta) = 1/(2\theta)$. Hence, $\sqrt{n}\,(m_n - \theta\log(2)) \to \mathcal{N}(0, \theta^2)$ and $\sqrt{n}\,(m_n/\log(2) - \theta) \to \mathcal{N}(0, \theta^2/(\log(2))^2)$.

(b) Similarly,

$$\sqrt{n}\left(X_{(np)} - \theta \log(1/(1-p))\right) \to \mathcal{N}(0, p\theta^2/(1-p)),$$

so that

$$\sqrt{n}\,(X_{(np)}/\log(1/(1-p)) - \theta) \to \mathcal{N}(0, p\theta^2/((1-p)(\log(1-p))^2)).$$

We are to find p to minimize $p/((1-p)(\log(1-p))^2)$. Set the derivative equal to zero, and solve for a root of $2p + \log(1-p) = 0$. Numerical methods give as a solution $p = 0.79681213\cdots$.

6. (a) The median of the distribution, $f(x|\theta)$, is $m(\theta) = (\frac{1}{2})^{1/\theta}$. From $f(m(\theta)|\theta) = \theta 2^{1/\theta}/2$, we find that

$$\sqrt{n}\,(M_n - m(\theta)) \xrightarrow{\mathcal{L}} \mathcal{N}\left(0, 1/\left(4f(m(\theta)|\theta)^2\right)\right) = \mathcal{N}(0, 1/(\theta^2 2^{2/\theta})).$$

(b) Since $M_n \xrightarrow{P} m(\theta)$, we have $\log(M_n) \xrightarrow{P} \log\frac{1}{2}/\theta$ and $\log\frac{1}{2}/\log(M_n) \xrightarrow{P} \theta$.

(c) Let $g(M) = \log\frac{1}{2}/\log M$. Then $g'(M) = -\log\frac{1}{2}/(M(\log M)^2)$, so $g'(m(\theta)) = -\theta^2 2^{1/\theta}/\log\frac{1}{2})$. Hence

$$\sqrt{n}\left(\hat{\theta}_n - \theta\right) = \sqrt{n}\,(g(M_n) - g(m(\theta))) \xrightarrow{\mathcal{L}} \mathcal{N}\left(0, \frac{g'(m(\theta))^2}{\theta^2 2^{2/\theta}}\right)$$

$$= \mathcal{N}\left(0, \frac{\theta^2}{(\log(\frac{1}{2}))^2}\right).$$

SOLUTIONS TO THE EXERCISES OF SECTION 14

1. (a) Since $1 - F(x) = 1 - e^x$ for $x < 0$, we have $x_0 = 0$ and $1 - F(x) = (-x)c(1/(-x))$ where $c(1/(-x)) = (1 - e^x)/(-x) \to 1$ as $x \to 0$. Thus we are in case (b) with $\gamma = 1$ so that $F(b_n x)^n \to G_{2,1}$ as $N \to \infty$, where b_n satisfies $1 - \exp\{-b_n\} = 1/n$. Hence, $b_n = -\log(1 - 1/n) \sim 1/n$ and we may conclude that

$$nM_n \xrightarrow{\mathscr{L}} G_{2,1} = -\mathscr{G}(1,1).$$

Note: In fact, the exact distribution of nM_n is $-\mathscr{G}(1,1)$ for all n, since $F(x/n)^n = (e^{x/n})^n = e^x$.

(b) We have $x_0 = \infty$ and $1 - F(x) = 1/x^2$ for $x > 1$. Thus we are in case (a) with $\gamma = 2$ and $c(x) \equiv 1$, so that $M_n/b_n \to G_{1,2}$ where b_n satisfies $(b_n)^{-2} = 1/N$; that is, $b_n = \sqrt{n}$:

$$M_n/\sqrt{n} \xrightarrow{\mathscr{L}} G_{1,2}.$$

(c) Since $1 - F(x) = \exp\{-x/(1-x)\}$ for $0 < x < 1$, we have $x_0 = 1$ and

$$\begin{aligned}\frac{1 - F(t + xR(t))}{1 - F(t)} &= \exp\left\{-\frac{t + xR(t)}{1 - t - xR(t)} + \frac{t}{1-t}\right\}\\ &= \exp\left\{\frac{-xR(t)}{(1-t)^2 - (1-t)xR(t)}\right\}\\ &\to \exp\{-x\}, \qquad \text{as } t \to 1 \text{ for every } x,\end{aligned}$$

provided $R(t) = (1-t)^2$. Therefore we are in case (c) and $F(a_n + b_n x)^n \to G_3(x)$, where $\exp\{-a_n/(1-a_n)\} = 1/n$, so that

$$a_n = \log(n)/(1 + \log(n))$$

and

$$b_n = (1 - a_n)^2 = 1/(1 + \log(n))^2 \sim 1/(\log(n))^2:$$

$$(\log(n))^2[M_n - \log(n)/(1 + \log(n))] \xrightarrow{\mathscr{L}} G_3.$$

(d) By l'Hospital's rule, $1 - F(x) \sim f(x)$:

$$\frac{1 - F(x)}{f(x)} = \frac{\int_x^\infty t^{\alpha-1}e^{-t}\,dt}{x^{\alpha-1}e^{-x}} \sim \frac{-x^{\alpha-1}e^{-x}}{((\alpha-1) - x)x^{\alpha-2}e^{-x}} \to 1.$$

Therefore, $x_0 = \infty$, and as $t \to \infty$,

$$\frac{1 - F(t + xR(t))}{1 - F(t)} \sim \frac{(t + xR(t))^{\alpha - 1} e^{-t - x R(t)}}{t^{\alpha - 1} e^{-t}} \to e^{-x},$$

if $R(t) \equiv 1$. Therefore by part (c) of Theorem 14, $F(a_n + x)^n \to G_3(x)$, where a_n satisfies $1/n \sim 1 - F(a_n) \sim f(a_n)$. To find an asymptotic expression for a_n, solve as a first approximation, $\exp\{-a_n\}/\Gamma(\alpha) = 1/n$ or $a_n = \log(n/\Gamma(\alpha))$. Replacing a_n by $\log(n/\Gamma(\alpha)) + a'_n$ in $nf(a_n) \to 1$, we find

$$\exp\{-a'_n\}(\log(n/\Gamma(\alpha)) + a'_n)^{\alpha - 1} \to 1.$$

This implies that a'_n must tend to ∞ at a slower rate than a_n, so that $\log(n/\Gamma(\alpha)) + a'_n \sim \log(n/\Gamma(\alpha))$. Hence,

$$\exp\{-a'_n\}(\log(n/\Gamma(\alpha)))^{\alpha - 1} \sim 1$$

or

$$a'_n \sim (\alpha - 1)\log(\log(n/\Gamma(\alpha))).$$

This gives

$$a_n = \log(n/\Gamma(\alpha)) + (\alpha - 1)\log\log(n/\Gamma(\alpha)).$$

Simplifying,

$$M_n - \log(n) - (\alpha - 1)\log\log(n) + \log\Gamma(\alpha) \xrightarrow{\mathscr{L}} G_3.$$

2. Since $P(X < j) = 1 - 2^{-j}$, we have $P(M_n < j) = (1 - 2^{-j})^n$. Hence, if $n(m)/2^m \to \theta$ as $m \to \infty$, we have

$$\begin{aligned} P(M_{n(m)} < m + k) &= (1 - 2^{-(m+k)})^{n(m)} \\ &\to \exp\{-\lim n(m)2^{-(m+k)}\} \\ &= \exp\{-\theta 2^{-k}\}. \end{aligned}$$

3. We have $1 - F(t) = 1 - \exp\{-e^{-t}\}$. As $t \to \infty$, this converges to zero at rate e^{-t}. To see this, apply L'Hospital's rule

$$\frac{1 - F(t)}{e^{-t}} = \frac{1 - \exp\{-e^{-t}\}}{e^{-t}} \sim \frac{-\exp\{-e^{-t}\}e^{-t}}{-e^{-t}} \to 1.$$

Therefore,

$$\frac{1 - F(t + xR(t))}{1 - F(t)} = \frac{e^{-t - x R(t)}}{e^{-t}} = e^{-xR(t)} \to e^{-x},$$

provided $R(t) \equiv 1$. Thus we are in case (c) with $b_n = 1$ and with a_n defined by $1/n = 1 - \exp\{-e^{-a_n}\} \sim e^{-a_n}$. We find that $a_n \sim \log(n)$ and conclude $M_n - \log(n) \xrightarrow{\mathscr{L}} G_3$.

This exercise is somewhat of a joke, since the distribution of $M_n - \log(n)$ is exactly G_3 for all n. In fact, the limiting distributions found in Theorem 14 are all closed up to change of location and scale under the operation of taking the distribution of the maximum. Moreover, these are the only distributions so closed. Take, for example, the distribution G_3. If M_n denotes the maximum of a sample of size n from G_3, the distribution function of $M_n - a$ is $G_3(x + a)^n = \exp\{-ne^{-x-a}\} = \exp\{-ne^{-a}e^{-x}\} = G_3(x)$, provided $ne^{-a} = 1$, or equivalently, $a = \log(n)$.

SOLUTIONS TO THE EXERCISES OF SECTION 15

1. From the result of Example 6 of Section 14

$$(2\log(n))^{1/2}(X_{(n:n)} - \mu) - 2\log(n) + \tfrac{1}{2}\log\log(4\pi n) \to Y$$

where $Y \in G_3$. By symmetry,

$$(2\log(n))^{1/2}(X_{(n:1)} + \mu) + 2\log(n) - \tfrac{1}{2}\log\log(4\pi n) \to -Z,$$

where $Z \in G_3$. By Theorem 15, these two expressions converge jointly with Y and Z independent. Therefore, for the midrange, $M = (X_{(n:n)} + X_{(n:n)})/2$,

$$(2\log(n))^{1/2}(M - \mu) \xrightarrow{\mathscr{L}} (Y - Z)/2.$$

To find the density of $W = (Y - Z)/2$, first write the joint density of Y and Z, $f_{Y,Z}(y, z) = \exp\{-e^{-y} - y - e^{-z} - z\}$, then make the change of variable $W = (Y - Z)/2$ for $Y(dy = 2\,dw)$ and integrate z from $-\infty$ to ∞:

$$f_{W,Z}(w, z) = 2\exp\{-e^{-2w-z} - 2w - z - e^{-z} - z\}$$

$$f_W(w) = 2\exp\{-2w\}\int_{-\infty}^{\infty} \exp\{e^{-z}(e^{2w+1}) - 2z\}\,dz$$

$$= 2\exp\{-2w\}\int_0^{\infty} \exp\{-u(e^{-2w} + 1)\}u\,du$$

$$= 2\exp\{-2w\}/(\exp\{-2w\} + 1)^2,$$

exactly the density of the logistic distribution $\mathscr{L}(0, 1/2)$. Since the sample mean converges to μ at a faster rate [$1/\sqrt{n}$ rather than $1/\sqrt{\log(n)}$], the asymptotic efficiency of the midrange relative to the mean is zero.

2. (a) From Theorem 15(a) applied to the upper two order statistics of a sample of size n from a uniform distribution on (0, 1), we have

$$n\left(1 - U_{(n:n)}, 1 - U_{(n:n-1)}\right) \xrightarrow{\mathscr{L}} (S_1, S_2), \tag{1}$$

where $S_1 = Y_1$ and $S_2 = Y_1 + Y_2$ and Y_1, Y_2 are i.i.d. exponential $\mathscr{G}(1,1)$. If $F(z)$ is the distribution function of $\mathscr{G}(1,1)$, $F(z) = 1 - \exp\{-z\}$, so $Z_1 = F^{-1}(U_{(n:n)})$ and $Z_2 = F^{-1}(U_{(n:n-1)})$ are the upper two order statistics of a sample of size n from $\mathscr{G}(1,1)$. Since $F^{-1}(u) = -\log(1-u)$, we apply Slutsky's Theorem using the transformation $-\log(\cdot)$ on both components of (1) to find

$$(Z_1 - \log(n), Z_2 - \log(n)) \xrightarrow{\mathscr{L}} (W_1, W_2),$$

where $W_1 = -\log(Y_1)$ and $W_2 = -\log(Y_1 + Y_2)$. To find the joint density of W_1, W_2, we take the joint density of Y_1, Y_2, $f(y_1, y_2) = \exp\{-y_1 - y_2\}I(y_1 > 0, y_2 > 0)$, and transform to W_1, W_2. The inverse transformation is $Y_1 = \exp\{-W_1\}$ and $Y_2 = \exp\{-W_2\} - \exp\{-W_1\}$. The Jacobian is $\exp\{-W_1 - W_2\}$. Hence

$$f(w_1, w_2) = \exp\{-e^{-w_2} - w_1 - w_2\}I(w_2 < w_1).$$

(b) Let $V = W_1 - W_2$ be a change of variable for W_1 so that $W_1 = V + W_2$ and the Jacobian is 1. The joint density of V and W_2 is

$$f(v, w_2) = \exp\{-e^{-w_2} - v - 2w_2\}I(v > 0).$$

Thus, V and W_2 are independent, and V is $\mathscr{G}(1,1)$, whereas $-\log(W_2)$ is $\mathscr{G}(2,1)$.

3. From Theorem 14, we have

$$\sqrt{n}\left(\hat{\theta}_1 - \theta\right) \xrightarrow{\mathscr{L}} \mathscr{N}(0, \tfrac{1}{4}).$$

From Example 2, we have

$$n\left(\hat{\theta}_2 - \theta\right) \xrightarrow{\mathscr{L}} Z,$$

where Z has the double exponential distribution with density $f(z) = \exp\{-2|z|\}$. When $n = 100$, the standard deviation of $\hat{\theta}_1$ is about $\frac{1}{20}$ and

$$P\left(|\hat{\theta}_1 - \theta| < \tfrac{2}{20}\right) = 0.95,$$

so the 95% confidence interval for θ is $(\hat{\theta}_1 - 0.1, \hat{\theta}_1 + 0.1)$. To find c

such that $P(|Z| < c) = 0.95$, we solve

$$0.95 = \int_{-c}^{c} e^{-2|z|}\, dz = 1 - e^{-2c}$$

for c and find that $c = \frac{1}{2}\log(20) = 1.50\cdots$. So

$$0.95 = P\big(100|\hat{\theta}_2 - \theta| < 1.50\big) = P\big(|\hat{\theta}_2 - \theta| < 0.015\big),$$

and the 95% confidence interval is $(\hat{\theta}_2 - 0.015, \hat{\theta}_2 + 0.015)$, a big improvement. In fact, the median converges to θ at rate $1/\sqrt{n}$, and the midrange converges to θ at rate $1/n$.

4. From Theorem 15,

$$n(1 - \Phi(Z_{1n}), 1 - \Phi(Z_{2n})) \xrightarrow{\mathscr{L}} (S_1, S_2).$$

But from the definition of a_n and the lemma of Section 14, $n(1 - \Phi(Z_{in})) = (1 - \Phi(Z_{in}))/(1 - \Phi(a_n)) \sim (a_n/Z_{in})\exp\{(a_n^2 - Z_{in}^2)/2\}$. Let $W_{in} = a_n(Z_{in} - a_n)$. Then from Exercise 6 of Section 6,

$$\left(\frac{a_n}{a_n + (W_{1n}/a_n)}\exp\left\{-W_{1n} - \frac{1}{2}(W_{in}^2/a_n^2)\right\},\right.$$

$$\left.\frac{a_n}{a_n + (W_{2n}/a_n)}\exp\left\{-W_{2n} - \frac{1}{2}(W_{2n}^2/a_n^2)\right\}\right) \xrightarrow{\mathscr{L}} (S_1, S_2).$$

This implies that $W_{in}/a_n \xrightarrow{\text{P}} 0$, because otherwise there would be a subsequence n_j such that $W_{in_j} \to \pm\infty$ on a set of positive probability, and any limit of this sequence would have a positive mass at zero or ∞. Thus,

$$(e^{-W_{1n}}, e^{-W_{2n}}) \xrightarrow{\mathscr{L}} (S_1, S_2),$$

and, consequently $(W_{1n}, W_{2n}) \xrightarrow{\mathscr{L}} (-\log S_1, -\log S_2)$, as was to be shown. We may conclude that

$$U_n = \exp\{W_{2n} - W_{1n}\} \xrightarrow{\mathscr{L}} S_1/S_2 \in \mathscr{U}(0,1),$$

and that U_n and W_{2n} are asymptotically independent, since S_1/S_2 and S_2 are independent.

SOLUTIONS TO THE EXERCISES OF SECTION 17

1. There are five conditions to be checked.
   (1) Θ is bounded and closed, hence compact.
   (2) For fixed $x \le 1$, $f(x|\theta) = 1/\theta$, continuous. For $1 < x \le 2$, $f(x|\theta) = 0$ for $\theta < x$, and $= 1/\theta$ for $\theta \ge x$, upper semicontinous. For $x > 2$, $f(x|\theta) = 0$, continuous.
   (3) Let $\theta_0 \in \Theta$. Then $K(x) = \max_{\theta \in \Theta}[f(x|\theta)/f(x|\theta_0)] = \theta_0$ if $x \le 1$, $= \theta_0/x$ if $1 < x \le \theta_0$, and $= \infty$ if $x > \theta_0$. The expectation of $K(X)$, when θ_0 is the true value, is clearly finite.
   (4) If $\varphi(x, \theta, X) = \sup_{|\theta' - \theta| < \rho} f(x|\theta')$, then

$$\begin{aligned}\varphi(x, \theta, \rho) &= 1/(\theta - \rho), && \text{for } x < \theta - \rho\\ &= 1/x, && \text{for } |x - \theta| \le \rho\\ &= 0, && \text{for } x > \theta + \rho,\end{aligned}$$

   clearly measurable.
   (5) $\theta \in \Theta$ is clearly identifiable; for example, different θ have different supports.
2. (a) For $X_{(k)} \le \theta \le X_{(k+1)}$, the likelihood function is

$$L(\theta) = \left(\frac{2}{\theta}\right)^k \left(\prod_{i \le k} X_{(i)}\right) + \left(\frac{2}{1-\theta}\right)^{n-k} \left(\prod_{i > k} X_{(i)}\right).$$

   Since $(\partial/\partial\theta)\log L(\theta) = -(k/\theta) + ((n-k)/(1-\theta))$, $L(\theta)$ is decreasing if $\theta < k/n$ and increasing if $\theta > k/n$.
   (b) Since $L(\theta)$ is continuous and cannot have maxima between the $X_{(k)}$, the maximum-likelihood estimate must be equal to one of the $X(k)$. Moreover, if $(k-1)/n < X_{(k)} < k/n$, then L has a local maximum at $X_{(k)}$.
3. The likelihood function is

$$\begin{aligned}L(\mu_1, \ldots, \mu_n, \sigma) &= \prod_{i=1}^{n} \prod_{j=1}^{d} \frac{1}{\sqrt{2\pi}\,\sigma} \exp\left\{-\frac{1}{2\sigma^2}(X_{ij} - \mu_i)^2\right\}\\ &= \left(\frac{1}{\sqrt{2\pi}\,\sigma}\right)^{nd} \exp\left\{-\frac{1}{2\sigma^2}\sum_{i=1}^{n}\sum_{j=1}^{d}(X_{ij} - \mu_i)^2\right\}.\end{aligned}$$

   The maximum-likelihood estimates of this are found by setting the derivatives of this with respect to the parameters equal to zero and solving:

$$\frac{\partial}{\partial \mu_i} \log L = \frac{1}{\sigma^2} \sum_{j=1}^{d} (X_{ij} - \mu_i) = 0 \Rightarrow \hat{\mu}_i = \overline{X}_i, \qquad \text{for } i = 1, \ldots, n$$

$$\frac{\partial}{\partial \sigma} \log L = -\frac{nd}{\sigma} + \frac{1}{\sigma^3} \sum_{i=1}^{n} \sum_{j=1}^{d} (X_{ij} - \mu_i)^2 = 0$$

$$\Rightarrow \hat{\sigma}^2 = \frac{1}{nd} \sum_{i=1}^{n} \sum_{j=1}^{d} (X_{ij} - \hat{\mu}_i)^2 = \frac{1}{n} \sum_{i=1}^{n} s_i^2,$$

where $s_i^2 = (1/d)\Sigma_{j=1}^d (X_{ij} - \overline{X}_i)^2$.

(b) The s_i^2 and iid with mean $Es_i^2 = ((d-1)/d)\sigma^2$. Hence, from the law of large numbers $\hat{\sigma}^2 \to ((d-1)/d)\sigma^2$ almost surely, so that $\hat{\sigma}^2$ is not consistent.

(c) Here the number of parameters grows to infinity as $n \to \infty$, so the structure of the problem differs from that of Theorem 17.

SOLUTIONS TO THE EXERCISES OF SECTION 18

1. (a) The log-likelihood function is $l_n(\theta) = \log L(\theta) = n \log \theta + (\theta - 1)\Sigma \log X_j$. The likelihood equation is $\dot{l}_n(\theta) = n/\theta + \Sigma \log X_j = 0$, which gives as the MLE,

$$\hat{\theta}_n = \left[(1/n) \sum \log(1/X_j)\right]^{-1}.$$

$\psi(X, \theta) = 1/\theta + \log(X)$, and $\dot{\psi}(X, \theta) = -1/\theta^2$, so that $\mathfrak{I}(\theta) = 1/\theta^2$. This gives

$$\sqrt{n}\left(\hat{\theta}_n - \theta\right) \to \mathcal{N}(0, \theta^2).$$

(b) $l_n(\theta) = n \log(1 - \theta) + \log(\theta) \Sigma X_j$, so

$$\dot{l}_n(\theta) = -n/(1-\theta) + (1/\theta) \Sigma X_j = 0$$

is the likelihood equation; its unique root is

$$\hat{\theta}_n = \overline{X}_n/\left(\overline{X}_n + 1\right).$$

$\psi(X, \theta) = -1/(1-\theta) + X/\theta$, so that $EX = \theta/(1-\theta)$ (because $E\{\psi(X,\theta)\} = 0$), $\dot{\psi}(X,\theta) = -1/(1-\theta)^2 - X/\theta^2$, so that

$$\Im(\theta) = 1/(1-\theta)^2 + 1/\theta(1-\theta) = 1/\theta(1-\theta)^2.$$

This gives

$$\sqrt{n}\left(\hat{\theta}_n - \theta\right) \to \mathcal{N}\left(0, \theta(1-\theta)^2\right).$$

2. Let $D_1 = \partial/\partial\alpha$ and $D_2 = \partial/\partial\beta$. The log-likelihood function is

$$\psi(\alpha, \beta) = -n \log \Gamma(\alpha) - n\alpha \log \beta - (1/\beta)\sum X_j + (\alpha - 1)\sum \log X_j.$$

The likelihood equations are

$$D_1 l_n(\alpha, \beta) = -n\digamma(\alpha) - n \log \beta + \sum \log X_j = 0,$$

$$D_2 l_n(\alpha, \beta) = -n\alpha/\beta + (1/\beta^2)\sum X_j = 0.$$

$D_1^2 \log f = -\digamma'(\alpha)$, $D_1 D_2 \log f = -1/\beta$, and $D_2^2 \log f = \alpha/\beta^2 - 2X/\beta^3$ whose expectation is $\alpha/\beta^2 - 2\alpha\beta/\beta^3 = -\alpha/\beta^2$. Hence,

$$\Im(\alpha, \beta) = \begin{pmatrix} \digamma'(\alpha) & 1/\beta \\ 1/\beta & \alpha/\beta^2 \end{pmatrix},$$

$$\Im(\alpha, \beta)^{-1} = \frac{1}{\alpha\digamma'(\alpha) - 1}\begin{pmatrix} \alpha & -\beta \\ -\beta & \beta^2\digamma'(\alpha) \end{pmatrix}.$$

The asymptotic distribution of the MLEs is

$$\sqrt{n}\left(\hat{\alpha}_n - \alpha, \hat{\beta}_n - \beta\right) \to \mathcal{N}\left((0,0), \Im(\alpha, \beta)^{-1}\right).$$

3. $l_n(\theta_1, \theta_2) = -\theta_2 \sum \cosh(X_j - \theta_1) - n\varphi(\theta_2)$. The likelihood equations are

$$\sum \sinh(X_j - \theta_1) = 0,$$

$$\sum \cosh(X_j - \theta_1) = -n\varphi'(\theta_2).$$

Let $D_1 = \partial/\partial\theta_1$ and $D_2 = \partial/\partial\theta_2$. From $E(D_1 \log f) = E(D_2 \log f) \equiv 0$, it follows that $E \sinh(X - \theta_1) = 0$ and $E \cosh(X - \theta_1) = -\varphi'(\theta_2)$. Hence, since $D_1^2 \log f = -\theta_2 \cosh(X - \theta_2)$, $D_1 D_2 \log f = \sinh(X - \theta_1)$, and $D_2^2 \log f = -\varphi''(\theta_2) = -\mathrm{var}(\cosh(X - \theta_1))$, we find

Fisher information to be

$$\mathfrak{I}(\theta_1, \theta_2) = \begin{pmatrix} -\theta_2\varphi'(\theta_2) & 0 \\ 0 & \varphi''(\theta_2) \end{pmatrix}.$$

The distributions in all of these exercises are exponential families.

4. Let $f(x|\theta)$ and $g(y|\theta)$ be the densities of X and Y given θ, respectively. Then since X and Y are independent, the joint density is $f(x|\theta)g(y|\theta)$ and

$$\psi((x,y),\theta) = \frac{\partial}{\partial\theta}\log f(x|\theta)g(y|\theta)$$

$$= \frac{\partial}{\partial\theta}\log f(x|\theta) + \frac{\partial}{\partial\theta}\log g(y|\theta) = \psi(x,\theta) + \psi(y,\theta).$$

Hence,

$$\mathfrak{I}_{(X,Y)}(\theta) = \mathrm{var}_\theta(\psi((X,Y),\theta))$$

$$= \mathrm{var}_\theta(\psi(X,\theta)) + \mathrm{var}_\theta(\psi(Y,\theta)) = \mathfrak{I}_X(\theta) + \mathfrak{I}_Y(\theta).$$

5. (a) The likelihood equation is

$$\dot{l}_n(\theta) = 2\sum_{i=1}^{n}\frac{(X_i - \theta)}{1 + (X_i - \theta)^2} = 0.$$

For $\theta > X_{(n)}$, each term is negative, so $\dot{l}_n(\theta) < 0$. At $\theta = X_{(n)} - 1$, we have

$$\dot{l}_n(X_{(n)} - 1) = 1 - 2\sum_{i=1}^{n-1}\frac{(X_{(n)} - 1 - X_{(i)})}{1 + (X_{(n)} - 1 - X_{(i)})^2}.$$

If $X_{(n)} - X_{(n-1)} > 2n$, then $X_{(n)} - X_{(i)} > 2n$ for all $i < n$, and

$$\dot{l}_n(X_{(n)} - 1) = 1 - 2\sum_{i=1}^{n-1}\frac{(2n-1)}{1 + (2n-1)^2}$$

$$= 1 - \frac{2(n-1)(2n-1)}{1 + (2n-1)^2} = 1 - \frac{2n^2 - 3n + 1}{2n^2 - 2n + 1} > 0,$$

so there is a root of the likelihood equation in $(X_{(n-1)} - 1, X_{(n)})$.

(b) Suppose without loss of generality that $\theta = 0$. Then from Example 3 of Section 15,

$$\left(\frac{X_{(n-1)}}{n}, \frac{X_{(n)}}{n}\right) \xrightarrow{\mathscr{L}} \left(\frac{1}{X+Y}, \frac{1}{X}\right),$$

where X and Y are independent exponential random variables. Hence,

$$P\big(X_{(n)} > X(n-1) + 2n\big)$$

$$= P\left(\frac{X_{(n)}}{n} > \frac{X_{(n-1)}}{n} + 2\right) \to P\left(\frac{1}{X} > \frac{1}{X+Y} + 2\right) > 0.$$

6. (a) The log-likelihood function is

$$\log L = -2\lambda_1 - 2\lambda_2 + x\log(\lambda_1 + \lambda_2)$$
$$+ y_1 \log(\lambda_1) + y_2 \log(\lambda_2) - \log(x!y_1!y_2!).$$

Setting the partial derivatives to zero gives the equations

$$-2 + \frac{x}{\lambda_1 + \lambda_2} + \frac{y_1}{\lambda_1} = 0 \quad \text{and} \quad -2 + \frac{x}{\lambda_1 + \lambda_2} + \frac{y_2}{\lambda_2} = 0,$$

and solving for λ_1 and λ_2 gives the maximum-likelihood estimates

$$\hat{\lambda}_1 = \frac{Y_1}{2}\left(\frac{X}{Y_1 + Y_2} + 1\right) \quad \text{and} \quad \hat{\lambda}_2 = \frac{Y_2}{2}\left(\frac{X}{Y_1 + Y_2} + 1\right).$$

(b) Let $g(x, y_1, y_2) = (y_1/2)((x/(y_1 + y_2)) + 1)$. Then

$$\dot{g}(x, y_1, y_2) = \left(\frac{y_1}{2(y_1 + y_2)}, \frac{1}{2}\left(\frac{x}{y_1 + y_2} + 1\right)\right.$$
$$\left. - \frac{y_1}{2}\frac{x}{(y_1 + y_2)^2}, -\frac{y_1}{2}\frac{x}{(y_1 + y_2)^2}\right),$$

and we find

$$\dot{g}(\lambda, \lambda_1, \lambda_2) = \left(\frac{\lambda_1}{2\lambda}, 1 - \frac{\lambda_1}{2\lambda}, -\frac{\lambda_1}{2\lambda}\right).$$

The covariance matrix of X, Y_1, Y_2 is diagonal with λ, λ_1, λ_2 along the diagonal, so the asymptotic variance of $\hat{\lambda}_1$ is

$$\dot{g}(\lambda, \lambda_1, \lambda_2)\begin{pmatrix} \lambda & 0 & 0 \\ 0 & \lambda_1 & 0 \\ 0 & 0 & \lambda_2 \end{pmatrix}\dot{g}(\lambda, \lambda_1, \lambda_2)^T = \lambda_1 - \frac{\lambda_1^2}{2\lambda}.$$

7. (a) This is a two-parameter exponential family with

$$L(\theta_1, \theta_2) = \prod_{i=1}^{n} f(x_i | \theta_1, \theta_2) = \frac{1}{(\theta_1 + \theta_2)^n} \exp\{-S_1/\theta_1 - S_2/\theta_2\}.$$

(b) Setting the partial derivatives to zero gives the equations

$$-\frac{n}{\theta_1 + \theta_2} + \frac{S_1}{\theta_1^2} = 0 \quad \text{and} \quad -\frac{n}{\theta_1 + \theta_2} + \frac{S_2}{\theta_2^2} = 0,$$

and solving for θ_1 and θ_2 gives

$$\hat{\theta}_1 = \frac{\sqrt{S_1}}{n}\left(\sqrt{S_1} + \sqrt{S_2}\right) \quad \text{and} \quad \hat{\theta}_2 = \frac{\sqrt{S_2}}{n}\left(\sqrt{S_1} + \sqrt{S_2}\right).$$

It should be checked that this holds if $S_1 = 0$ or $S_2 = 0$. They cannot both be zero.

(c) Taking $n = 1$ and writing $\log f(x|\theta_1, \theta_2) = -\log(\theta_1 + \theta_2) - S_1/\theta_1 - S_2/\theta_2$, we find

$$D_1 \log f = -1/(\theta_1 + \theta_2) + S_1/\theta_1^2$$

and

$$D_2 \log f = -1/(\theta_1 + \theta_2) + S_2/\theta_2^2.$$

This implies $ES_1 = \theta_1^2/(\theta_1 + \theta_2)$,

$$-ED_1^2 \log f = -1/(\theta_1 + \theta_2)^2 + 2ES_1/\theta_1^3 = (\theta_1 + 2\theta_2)/\left[\theta_1(\theta_1 + \theta_2)^2\right]$$

and $-D_1 D_2 \log f = -1/(\theta_1 + \theta_2)^2$. Thus,

$$\mathfrak{I}(\theta_1, \theta_2) = \frac{1}{(\theta_1 + \theta_2)^2}\begin{pmatrix} (\theta_1 + 2\theta_2)/\theta_1 & -1 \\ -1 & (2\theta_1 + \theta_2)/\theta_2 \end{pmatrix}.$$

From this, $\sqrt{n}(\hat{\theta}_n - \theta) \xrightarrow{\mathscr{L}} \mathscr{N}(0, \mathfrak{I}(\theta_1, \theta_2)^{-1})$, where

$$\mathfrak{I}(\theta_1, \theta_2)^{-1} = \frac{(\theta_1 + \theta_2)^2 \theta_1 \theta_2}{4 + 2\theta_1 + 2\theta_2}\begin{pmatrix} (2\theta_1 + \theta_2)/\theta_2 & 1 \\ 1 & (\theta_1 + 2\theta_2/\theta_1) \end{pmatrix}.$$

8. Since

$$\log\left(f_{\theta_0}(x)/f_\theta(x)\right) = (\theta_0 - \theta)T(x) - \left(c(\theta_0) - c(\theta)\right),$$

we have

$$K\left(f_{\theta_0}, f_\theta\right) = (\theta_0 - \theta)E_{\theta_0}T(X) - \left(c(\theta_0) - c(\theta)\right).$$

Using

$$0 = E_\theta(\partial/\partial\theta)\log f_\theta(X) = E_\theta[T(X) - c'(\theta)],$$

we find $E_\theta T(X) = c'(\theta)$, so

$$K\left(f_{\theta_0}, f_\theta\right) = (\theta_0 - \theta)c'(\theta_0) - \left(c(\theta_0) - c(\theta)\right).$$

Fisher Information can be found as

$$\Im(\theta) = -E_\theta(\partial^2/\partial\theta^2)\log f_\theta(X) = c''(\theta).$$

The expansion of $c(\theta)$ to two terms in a Taylor series is $c(\theta) = c(\theta_0) + (\theta - \theta_0)c'(\theta_0) + (\theta - \theta_0)^2 c''(\theta_0)/2 + O(\theta - \theta_0)^3$. From this we may conclude

$$\begin{aligned} K\left(f_{\theta_0}, f_\theta\right) &= -(\theta - \theta_0)^2 c''(\theta_0)/2 - O(\theta - \theta_0)^3 \\ &\sim -(\theta - \theta_0)^2 c''(\theta_0)/2 \\ &= (\theta - \theta_0)^2 \Im(\theta_0)/2. \end{aligned}$$

SOLUTIONS TO THE EXERCISES OF SECTION 19

1. (a) Let $Y_j = -\log(X_j)$. From Exercise 1(a) of Section 18, the MLE of θ is $\hat{\theta}_n = 1/\overline{Y}_n$. Hence the MLE of $1/\theta$ is $\overline{Y}_n$. Because $X_j \in \mathscr{B}(\theta, 1)$, we have $Y_j \in \mathscr{G}(1, 1/\theta)$, so that $E\overline{Y}_n = 1/\theta$ and $\text{var}(\overline{Y}_n) = 1/(n\theta^2)$. From Exercise 1(a) of Section 18, $\Im(\theta) = 1/\theta^2$. The information inequality with $g(\theta) = 1/\theta$ [and $g'(\theta) = -1/\theta^2$] and sample size n then gives $g'(\theta)^2/(n\Im(\theta)) = 1/n\theta^2$ as the lower bound, attained by the MLE.

   (b) Since $X_j \in \mathscr{B}(\theta, 1)$, we have $E\overline{X}_n = \theta/(\theta + 1)$ (unbiased) and $\text{var}(\overline{X}_n) = \theta/n(\theta + 1)^2(\theta + 2)$. The information inequality with $g(\theta) = \theta/(\theta + 1)$ [and $g'(\theta) = 1/(\theta + 1)^2$] and $\Im(\theta) = 1/\theta^2$ gives

$$g'(\theta)^2/(n\Im(\theta)) = \theta^2/n(\theta + 1)^4.$$

   So $\overline{X}_n$ does not achieve the lower bound. In fact, we can do better asymptotically using the MLE, $\hat{\theta}_n/(\hat{\theta}_n + 1)$.

2. Selected components of the 5×5 matrix, $(1-\rho^2)\dot{\psi}$:

$$(1-\rho^2)\dot{\psi}_{11} = -1/\sigma_1^2;$$

$$(1-\rho^2)\dot{\psi}_{12} = \rho/\sigma_1\sigma_2;$$

$$(1-\rho^2)\dot{\psi}_{13} = -2(X-\mu_1)/\sigma_1^3 - \rho(Y-\mu_2)/\sigma_1^2\sigma_2,$$

the expectation of which is 0;

$$(1-\rho^2)\dot{\psi}_{33} = (1-\rho^2)/\sigma_1^2 - 3(X-\mu_1)^2/\sigma_1^4$$
$$- 2\rho(X-\mu_1)(Y-\mu_2)/\sigma_1^3\sigma_1,$$

the expectation of which is $-(2-\rho^2)/\sigma_1^2$;

$$(1-\rho^2)\dot{\psi}_{34} = \rho(X-\mu_1)(Y-\mu_2)/\sigma_1^2\sigma_2^2,$$

the expectation of which is $\rho^2/\sigma_1\sigma_2$;

$$(1-\rho^2)\dot{\psi}_{35} = \big[2\rho(X-\mu_1)^2/\sigma_1^3$$
$$-(1+\rho^2)(X-\mu_1)(Y-\mu_2)/\sigma_1^2\sigma_2\big]/(1-\rho^2),$$

the expectation of which is ρ/σ_1.

3. (a) If $E\hat{\theta} = \mu_1 - \mu_2 = g(\theta)$, then $\dot{g}(\theta) = (1, -1, 0, 0, 0)$ and

$$\operatorname{var}(\hat{\theta}) \geq \dot{g}(\theta)\Im(\theta)^{-1}\dot{g}(\theta)'/n = \left(\sigma_1^2 + \sigma_2^2 - 2\rho\sigma_1\sigma_2\right)/n.$$

   (b) If $E\hat{\theta} = \mu_1/\sigma_1 = g(\theta)$, then $\dot{g}(\theta) = (1/\sigma_1, 0, -\mu_1/\sigma_1^2, 0, 0)$ and $\operatorname{var}(\hat{\theta}) \geq (1 + \mu_1^2/2\sigma_1^2)/n$.

   (c) If $E\hat{\theta} = \rho\sigma_1\sigma_2 = g(\theta)$, then $\dot{g}(\theta) = (0, 0, \rho\sigma_1, \rho\sigma_1, \sigma_1\sigma_2)$ and $\operatorname{var}(\hat{\theta}) \geq \sigma_1^2\sigma_2^2(1+\rho^2)/n$.

4. We think of the X in (1) as a vector of observations, $\mathbf{X} = (X_1, \ldots, X_n)$, and find the Fisher Information for θ based on $\mathbf{X}$. Since the X_i are independent, the Fisher Information based on $\mathbf{X}$ is the sum of the individual informations. The information in X_i is

$$\operatorname{var}\left(\frac{\partial}{\partial\theta}\log f(X_i\theta)\right) = \operatorname{var}(-z_i\exp\{\theta z_i\} + z_i X_i)$$
$$= z_i^2 \operatorname{var}(X_i) = z_i^2\exp\{\theta z_i\}.$$

Hence, the Fisher Information in the whole sample is $\Im(\theta) = \sum_1^n z_i^2\exp\{\theta z_i\}$. When dealing with unbiased estimates, we have $g'(\theta) = 1$ in (1), so we have as a lower bound to the variance of an unbiased estimate, $\hat{\theta}(\mathbf{X})$,

$$\operatorname{var}_\theta \hat{\theta}\ (\mathbf{X}) \geq \frac{1}{\sum_{i=1}^n z_i^2 \exp\{\theta z_i\}}.$$

5. (a) The density of X is $f(x|\theta) = (1/\theta)I_{(0,\theta)}(x)$ and its derivative is $(\partial/\partial\theta) f(x|\theta) = -(1/\theta^2)I_{(0,\theta)}(x)$. If the derivative with respect to θ may be passed under the integral sign in $1 = \int f(x|\theta)\,dx$, we would have $0 = \int(\partial/\partial\theta) f(x|\theta)\,dx = -\int_0^\theta(1/\theta^2)\,dx = -1/\theta$. Thus one of the regularity conditions of the information inequality is not satisfied.
   (b) We have $(\partial/\partial\theta)\log f(x|\theta) = -1/\theta$ for $0 < x < \theta$. This gives $\operatorname{var}((\partial/\partial\theta)\log f(x|\theta)) = 0$ for all $\theta > 0$. So the information inequality would give infinity as a lower bound to a variance.
   (c) We have $E_\theta(2X) = \theta$ and $\operatorname{var}_\theta(2X) = \theta^2/3$. Thus, the information inequality is not valid here.

SOLUTIONS TO THE EXERCISES OF SECTION 20

1. (a) We have

$$\log f(X|\theta) = -(X-\theta) - 2\log(1 + e^{-(X-\theta)}),$$

$$\psi(X,\theta) = \partial \log f(X|\theta)/\partial\theta = 1 - 2e^{-(X-\theta)}/(1 + e^{-(X-\theta)}),$$

and

$$\partial\psi(X,\theta)/\partial\theta = -2\left[e^{-(X-\theta)}/(1 + e^{-(X-\theta)})^2\right].$$

To find $\Im(\theta) = -E_\theta\, \partial\psi(X,\theta)/\partial\theta$, make the change of variable $U = 1 + e^{-(X-\theta)}$ $(dU = -e^{-(x-\theta)}\,dX)$ and find

$$\Im(\theta) = 2E\left[e^{-(X-\theta)}/(1 + e^{-(X-\theta)})^2\right] = 2\int_1^\infty \left[(u-1)/u^2\right]/u^2\,du$$

$$= 2\int_1^\infty \{u^{-3} - u^{-4}\}\,du = 2\{\tfrac{1}{2} - \tfrac{1}{3}\} = \tfrac{1}{3}.$$

   (b) We have

$$\log f(X|\theta) = -\log(\pi) - \log\left(1 + (X-\theta)^2\right),$$

$$\psi(X,\theta) = 2(X-\theta)/\left(1 + (X-\theta)^2\right),$$

and

$$\partial\psi(X,\theta)/\partial\theta = -2\left(1-(X-\theta)^2\right)/\left(1+(X-\theta)^2\right)^2.$$

We change variables, $Y = (X-\theta)$ $(dY = dX)$ to find

$$\mathfrak{I}(\theta) = 2E(1-Y^2)/(1+Y^2)^2 = (2/\pi)\int_{-\infty}^{\infty}(1-y^2)/(1+y^2)^3\,dy$$

$$= (2/\pi)\left[2\int_{-\infty}^{\infty}(1+y^2)^{-3}\,dy - \int_{-\infty}^{\infty}\left(1+y^2\right)^{-2}\right)dy\right].$$

To find $\int_{-\infty}^{\infty}(1+y^2)^{-m}\,dy$, we integrate by parts:

$$\int_{-\infty}^{\infty}(1+y^2)^{-m}\,dy = y(1+y^2)^{-m}\big|_{-\infty}^{\infty} + m\int_{-\infty}^{\infty}y(1+y^2)^{-(m+1)}2y\,dy$$

$$= 0 + 2m\int_{-\infty}^{\infty}(1+y^2)^{-m}\,dy$$

$$- 2m\int_{-\infty}^{\infty}(1+y^2)^{-(m+1)}\,dy,$$

giving the recursion for $m \geq 1$,

$$\int_{-\infty}^{\infty}(1+y^2)^{-(m+1)}\,dy = [(2m-1)/2m]\int_{-\infty}^{\infty}(1+y^2)^{-m}\,dy.$$

Now using the fact that $(1/\pi)\int_{-\infty}^{\infty}(1+y^2)^{-1}\,dy = 1$, we find $\int_{-\infty}^{\infty}(1+y^2)^{-2}\,dy = \pi/2$, and $\int_{-\infty}^{\infty}(1+y^2)^{-3}\,dy = 3\pi/8$. Hence, $\mathfrak{I}(\theta) = (2/\pi)[6\pi/8 - \pi/2] = \frac{1}{2}$.

2. Since $\log L(\theta) = -n\log\pi - \Sigma_1^n \log(1+(X_j-\theta)^2)$, the likelihood equations are

$$\partial \log L(\theta)/\partial\theta = 2\sum_1^n (X_j-\theta)/\left(1+(X_j-\theta)^2\right) = 0.$$

(There may be many roots.) Since $\mathfrak{I}(\theta) = \frac{1}{2}$, the scores are

$$\mathfrak{I}(\theta)^{-1}(\partial \log L(\theta)/\partial\theta)/n = (4/n)\sum(X_j-\theta)/\left(1+(X_j-\theta)^2\right).$$

From Example 2 of Section 10 the asymptotic distribution of the median m_n is given by $\sqrt{n}\,(m_n-\theta) \to \mathscr{N}(0,\pi^2/4)$. This may be improved by adding the scores

$$m_n^* = m_n + (4/n)\sum(X_j-m_n)/\left(1+(X_j-m_n)^2\right)$$

to obtain an asymptotically efficient estimate: $\sqrt{n}\,(m_n^*-\theta) \to \mathscr{N}(0,2)$.

3. Since $EX_j = (1 - \theta) + 2\theta = 1 + \theta$, the method of moments equates $\overline{X}_n$ and $1 + \theta$ to give the estimate $\theta_n^* = \overline{X}_n - 1$. This estimate cannot be admissible, since it may estimate θ to be negative or to be greater than one. Since $EX_j^2 = 2(1 - \theta) + 6\theta = 2 + 4\theta$, we have that

$$\operatorname{var}(X_j) = (2 + 4\theta) - (1 + \theta)^2 = 1 + 2\theta - \theta^2.$$

Therefore by the Central Limit Theorem, $\sqrt{n}\,(\theta_n^* - \theta) \to \mathcal{N}(0, 1 + 2\theta - \theta^2)$. The asymptotically efficient estimate given by one iteration of Newton's method is

$$\hat{\theta}_n = \theta_n^* + \frac{\Sigma_1^n (X_j - 1)/(1 + \theta_n^*(X_j - 1))}{\Sigma_1^n (X_j - 1)^2/(1 + \theta_n^*(X_j - 1))^2}.$$

4. (a) The mean and variance of this exponential distribution are $1/\theta$ and $1/\theta^2$. The method-of-moments estimator of θ is $\tilde{\theta}_n = 1/\overline{X}_n$. Its asymptotic distribution is $\sqrt{n}\,(\tilde{\theta}_n - \theta) \xrightarrow{\mathcal{L}} \mathcal{N}(0, \theta^2)$. Fisher information is $\mathcal{I}(\theta) = 1/\theta^2$, so the estimator $\tilde{\theta}_n$ is fully efficient.
   (b) In the information inequality, let $\hat{\theta}(X) = X$. Then $g(\theta) = 1/\theta$, and the information inequality becomes $\operatorname{var}_\theta(X) \geq (-1/\theta^2)^2/\mathfrak{I}(\theta)$. Using $\operatorname{var}_\theta(X) = 1/\theta^2$, this inequality becomes $\mathfrak{I}(\theta) \geq 1/\theta^2$. This lower bound to Fisher information is achieved by the given exponential distribution.

SOLUTIONS TO THE EXERCISES OF SECTION 21

1. Fisher Information for the Poisson distribution is $\mathfrak{I}(\theta) = 1/\theta$, and the maximum-likelihood estimate of θ is $\overline{X}_n$. The posterior density is approximately the normal density centered at $\overline{X}_n$ with variance equal to θ_0, where θ_0 is the true value of θ. Since θ_0 is unknown, it may be useful to approximate this density by the normal density with mean $\overline{X}_n$ and variance $\overline{X}_n$. Mathematically, we may say that if θ_0 is the true value, the posterior density $\sqrt{n}\,(\theta - \overline{X}_n)$ converges to the density of $\mathcal{N}(0, \theta_0)$ in L_1 almost surely.
2. Let $g_n(\theta)$ (resp. $h_n(\zeta)$) represent the conditional density of θ (resp. ζ) given $X_1, \ldots, X_n$. We are to show that for all ζ, $h_n(\zeta) \to (1/\theta_0)\exp\{-\zeta/\theta_0\}I(\zeta > 0)$ almost surely as $n \to \infty$. We have

$$g_n(\theta) = g(\theta)\theta^{-n}I(M_n < \theta)/C_n,$$

where C_n is the normalizing constant,

$$C_n = \int_{M_n}^{\infty} g(\theta)\theta^{-n}\, d\theta.$$

Changing variables to $\zeta = n(\theta - M_n)$ with $d\theta = d\zeta/n$, we have

$$h_n(\zeta) = g(M_n + \zeta/n)(1 + \zeta/(nM_n))^{-n} I(0 < \zeta)/D_n,$$

where

$$D_n = \int_0^{\infty} g(M_n + \zeta/n)(1 + \zeta/(nM_n))^{-n}\, d\zeta.$$

Since M_n converges to θ_0 almost surely, the numerator of $h_n(\zeta)$ converges to $g(\theta_0)\exp\{-\zeta/\theta_0\}I(0 < \zeta)$ almost surely. To complete the proof, we must show that D_n converges to $g(\theta_0)\theta_0$ almost surely. Using the assumption that $g(\theta)$ is bounded, and using the fact that the convergence of $(1 + \zeta/(nM))^{-n}$ to $\exp\{-\zeta/M\}$, for fixed positive ζ and M, is monotone decreasing in n, we can bound the integrand in D_n above by a function of the form const. times $(1 + \zeta/M')^{-2}$, which is integrable. Then the Lebesgue Bounded Convergence Theorem gives the result.

SOLUTIONS TO THE EXERCISES OF SECTION 22

1.

$$L(\theta) = (2\pi\sigma_x\sigma_y)^{-n} \exp\left\{-\left[\sum (X_j - \mu_x)^2/\sigma_x^2 + \sum (Y_j - \mu_y)^2/\sigma_y^2\right]/2\right\}.$$

The general MLEs are $\hat{\mu}_x = \overline{X}$, $\hat{\mu}_y = \overline{Y}$, $\hat{\sigma}_x^2 = (1/n)\Sigma(X_j - \overline{X})^2$, and $\hat{\sigma}_y^2 = (1/n)\Sigma(Y_j - \overline{Y})^2$. Under H_0, the X_j and Y_j together form a sample of size $2n$ from a single normal distribution, so the MLEs are

$$\mu_x^* = \mu_y^* = (\overline{X} + \overline{Y})/2,$$

$$\sigma_x^{*2} = \sigma_y^{*2} = \left[\sum (X_j - \mu_x^*)^2 + \sum (Y_j - \mu_y^*)^2\right]/2n.$$

From this, we find

$$L(\theta^*) = (2\pi\sigma^{*2})^{-n} \exp\{-n\}, \qquad L(\hat{\theta}\ ) = \left(2\pi\hat{\sigma}_x\hat{\sigma}_y\right)^{-n} \exp\{-n\}.$$

There are two restrictions under H_0, so that

$$-2\log\lambda = n\left[2\log\sigma^{*2} - \log\hat{\sigma}_x^2 - \log\hat{\sigma}_y^2\right] \to \chi_2^2.$$

2. $L(\theta, \mu) = \theta^n \mu^n \exp\{-\theta \sum X_j - \mu \sum Y_j\}$. The general MLEs are $\hat{\theta} = 1/\bar{X}$ and $\hat{\mu} = 1/\bar{Y}$. Under H_0, the likelihood function is $L(\theta) = 2^n \theta^{2n} \exp\{-\theta(\sum X_j + 2\sum Y_j)\}$, which leads to the MLEs $\theta^* = 2/(\bar{X} + 2\bar{Y})$, $\mu^* = 2\theta^*$. Hence, $L(\hat{\theta}, \hat{\mu}) = \bar{X}^{-n}\bar{Y}^{-n} \exp\{-2n\}$ and $L(\theta^*, \mu^*) = 2^n(\theta^*)^{2n} \exp\{-2n\}$. Since there is a single restriction under H_0, we have

$$-2\log\lambda = 2n\left[2\log\left((\bar{X} + 2\bar{Y})/2\right) - \log\bar{X} - \log 2\bar{Y}\right] \to \chi_1^2$$

3. As is well known, the MLEs for the θ's are $\hat{\theta}_i = \bar{X}_{i\cdot}$. If all the θ's are the same, then the X_{ij} form a sample of size nk from the Poisson, so that the MLE is $\theta^* = \bar{X}_{\cdot\cdot}$. Since the log likelihood is

$$\log L(\theta) = \sum_i \sum_j \left[-\theta_i + X_{ij}\log\theta_i - \log X_{ij}!\right],$$

$$= -n\sum\theta_i + n\sum \bar{X}_{i\cdot}\log\theta_i - \sum_i\sum_j \log X_{ij}!$$

and since there are $k - 1$ restrictions under H_0,

$$-2\log\lambda = 2\left[\log L(\hat{\theta}\ ) - \log L(\theta^*)\right]$$

$$= 2n\left[\sum \bar{X}_{i\cdot}\log\bar{X}_{i\cdot} - k\bar{X}_{\cdot\cdot}\log\bar{X}_{\cdot\cdot}\right] \to \chi_{k-1}^2.$$

4. Find an orthogonal matrix $\mathbf{Q}$ such that $\mathbf{QPQ}^T = \begin{pmatrix} \mathbf{I}_r & \mathbf{0} \\ \mathbf{0} & \mathbf{0} \end{pmatrix}$; call it $\mathbf{D}$. Let $\mathbf{W} = \mathbf{QZ}$. Then $\mathbf{W} \in \mathcal{N}(\mathbf{Q}\boldsymbol{\delta}, \mathbf{I}_k)$ and $\mathbf{Z}^T\mathbf{PZ} = \mathbf{W}^T\mathbf{QPQ}^T\mathbf{W} = \mathbf{W}^T\mathbf{DW} = \sum_{i=1}^r W_j^2$. This has a noncentral χ^2 distribution with r degrees of freedom and noncentrality parameter φ equal to the sum of the squares of the first r coordinates of $\mathbf{Q}\boldsymbol{\delta}$, namely, the square of the length of the vector $\mathbf{DQ}\boldsymbol{\delta}$. Thus, $\mathbf{Z}^T\mathbf{PZ} \in \chi_r^2(\varphi)$, where $\varphi = \boldsymbol{\delta}^T\mathbf{Q}^T\mathbf{DDQ}\boldsymbol{\delta} = \boldsymbol{\delta}^T\mathbf{P}\boldsymbol{\delta}$.
5. (a) The distribution of $-2\log\lambda_n$ is approximately noncentral chi-square, $\chi_1^2(\varphi)$, where the noncentrality parameter φ has the form, $\varphi = \delta_1^2(G_1 - G_2^2/G_3)$, since all of these matrices reduce to scalars. Using $\delta_1 = \sqrt{1000}\,(0.1)$ and

$$\Im(\mu, \sigma) = \begin{pmatrix} 1/\sigma^2 & 0 \\ 0 & 2/\sigma^2 \end{pmatrix},$$

we find that $\varphi = 10/\sigma_0^2$.

(b) Again the asymptotic distribution is noncentral chi-square, $\chi_1^2(\varphi)$, with the same formula for φ and the same value of δ_1, but this time

$$\mathfrak{I}(\mu, \sigma) = \begin{pmatrix} \digamma(\alpha) & 1/\beta \\ 1/\beta & \alpha/\beta^2 \end{pmatrix},$$

so that $\varphi = 10(\digamma(1) - 1)$ independent of β. Replacing $\digamma(1)$ by its value, $\pi^2/6$, we find that $\varphi = 6.449$.

6. From Eq. (4), $-2\log\lambda_n \sim n(\hat{\boldsymbol{\theta}}_n - \boldsymbol{\theta}_0)^T \mathscr{I}(\theta_0)(\hat{\boldsymbol{\theta}}_n - \boldsymbol{\theta}_0)$, where $\hat{\boldsymbol{\theta}}_n$ is the unrestricted maximum-likelihood estimate, which from Theorem 16 has an asymptotic normal distribution,

$$\sqrt{n}\left(\hat{\boldsymbol{\theta}}_n - \boldsymbol{\theta}_0\right) \xrightarrow{\mathscr{L}} \mathscr{N}\left(\mathbf{0}, \mathscr{I}(\boldsymbol{\theta}_0)^{-1}\right).$$

Therefore, the asymptotic problems may be reduced to the following fixed sample problems for the normal distribution.

Suppose $\mathbf{X} \in \mathscr{N}(\boldsymbol{\theta}, \boldsymbol{\Sigma})$, where $\boldsymbol{\Sigma} = \mathscr{I}(\boldsymbol{\theta}_0)^{-1}$ is known. Find the distribution of $-2\log\lambda$, where λ is the likelihood ratio test statistic for testing H_0: $\theta_1 = 0$, $\theta_2 = 0$ against (a) H_1: $\theta_1 > 0$, θ_2 unrestricted, or (b) H_1: $\theta_1 \geq 0$, $\theta_2 \geq 0$, $\boldsymbol{\theta} \neq 0$. We reformulate this problem by transforming to independent normal variables. Let $Y_1 = X_1/\sigma_1$ and

$$Y_2 = ((X_2/\sigma_2) - \rho(X_1/\sigma_1))/\sqrt{1 - \rho^2}.$$

Then $\mathbf{Y} \in \mathscr{N}(\boldsymbol{\mu}, \mathbf{I})$, where $\mu_1 = \theta_1/\sigma_1$ and $\mu_2 = ((\theta_2/\sigma_2) - \rho(\mu_1/\sigma_1))/\sqrt{1-\rho^2}$. The hypotheses have become H_0: $\mu_1 = 0$, $\mu_2 = 0$ against (a) H_1: $\mu_1 > 0$ μ_2 unrestricted, or (b) H_1: $\mu_1 \geq 0$, $\rho\mu_1 + \sqrt{1-\rho^2}\,\mu_2 \geq 0$, $\boldsymbol{\mu} \neq \mathbf{0}$.

(a) The unrestricted MLE of $\boldsymbol{\mu}$ is $\mathbf{Y}$. The MLE under $H_0 \cup H_1$ is (Y_1^+, Y_2). On the half plane $Y_1 > 0$, $-2\log\lambda$ is the squared distance of $\mathbf{Y}$ to $\mathbf{0}$. This occurs with probability $\frac{1}{2}$ under H_0, which gives χ_2^2 with probability $\frac{1}{2}$. On the half plane $Y_1 < 0$, $\mathbf{Y}$ is projected onto the line $Y_1 = 0$; thus, $-2\log\lambda$ is the squared distance of Y_1 to zero which gives a χ_1^2 with probability $\frac{1}{2}$.

(b) Now the MLE under $H_0 \cup H_1$ is the projection of $\mathbf{Y}$ onto the cone $Y_1 \geq 0$, $\rho Y_1 + \sqrt{1-\rho^2}\,Y_2 \geq 0$. Thus there are four regions. On the cone itself, $\mathbf{Y}$ is unchanged, giving a χ_2^2 distribution with the probability of the cone. On $Y_1 < 0$, $Y_2 \geq 0$, $\mathbf{Y}$ is projected onto the line $Y_1 = 0$, giving a χ_1^2 distribution with probability $\frac{1}{4}$. Similarly, on the set $\rho Y_1 + \sqrt{1-\rho^2}\,Y_2 < 0$, those $\mathbf{Y}$ whose perpendicular projection onto the line $\rho Y_1 + \sqrt{1-\rho^2}\,Y_2 = 0$ ends up with $Y_1 > 0$ are so projected. This occurs also with probability $\frac{1}{4}$ and gives a χ_1^2

distribution. All remaining points are projected into the origin giving a $\delta_0 = \chi_0^2$ distribution with the remaining probability. The probability of the cone under H_0 is the angle ϑ of the cone divided by 2π. ϑ is the angle between the line $\rho Y_1 + \sqrt{1-\rho^2}\, Y_2 = 0$ with $Y_1 > 0$ and the line $Y_1 = 0$ with $Y_2 > 0$. This is easily found to be $\vartheta = \pi - \arccos \rho$.

SOLUTIONS TO THE EXERCISES OF SECTION 23

1. The minimum χ^2 estimate is the value of $\boldsymbol{\theta}$ that minimizes $Q_n(\boldsymbol{\pi}(\boldsymbol{\theta}))$. Its asymptotic variance is

$$V = \left(\dot{A}(\boldsymbol{\theta})'\, \Sigma(\boldsymbol{\pi}(\boldsymbol{\theta}))^{-1} \dot{A}(\boldsymbol{\theta})\right)^{-1}$$

where $\Sigma(\boldsymbol{\pi})$ denotes $(d/d\boldsymbol{\pi})\dot{\varphi}(\boldsymbol{\pi})$. Because $A(\boldsymbol{\theta}) = \varphi(\boldsymbol{\pi}(\boldsymbol{\theta}))$, we have $\dot{A}(\boldsymbol{\theta}) = \Sigma(\boldsymbol{\pi}(\boldsymbol{\theta}))\dot{\boldsymbol{\pi}}(\boldsymbol{\theta})$ and $V = (\dot{\boldsymbol{\pi}}(\boldsymbol{\theta})'\, \Sigma(\boldsymbol{\pi}(\boldsymbol{\theta}))\dot{\boldsymbol{\pi}}(\boldsymbol{\theta}))^{-1}$. For the exponential family,

$$\log f(x|\boldsymbol{\theta}) = \boldsymbol{\pi}(\boldsymbol{\theta})'\mathbf{T}(\mathbf{x}) - \varphi(\boldsymbol{\pi}(\theta)),$$

and Fisher Information is

$$\begin{aligned}\mathfrak{I}(\theta) &= \mathrm{var}_\theta\{\dot{\boldsymbol{\pi}}(\theta)'\mathbf{T}(X) - \dot{\varphi}(\boldsymbol{\pi}(\boldsymbol{\theta}))\dot{\boldsymbol{\pi}}(\boldsymbol{\theta})\} = \dot{\boldsymbol{\pi}}(\boldsymbol{\theta})'\,\mathrm{var}_{\boldsymbol{\theta}}\{\mathbf{T}(X)\}\dot{\boldsymbol{\pi}}(\boldsymbol{\theta}) \\ &= \dot{\boldsymbol{\pi}}(\boldsymbol{\theta})'\,\Sigma(\boldsymbol{\theta})\dot{\boldsymbol{\pi}}(\boldsymbol{\theta}) = V^{-1}.\end{aligned}$$

Thus the MLE and the minimum χ^2 estimates have the same asymptotic variance.

2. (a)

$$\chi^2 = \frac{4}{\frac{1}{3} - \theta} + \frac{25}{\frac{2}{3} - \theta} + \frac{9}{2\theta} - 100.$$

So solving

$$(d/d\theta)\chi^2 = \frac{4}{\left(\frac{1}{3} - \theta\right)^2} + \frac{25}{\left(\frac{2}{3} - \theta\right)^2} - \frac{9}{2\theta^2} = 0$$

gives $\hat{\theta} = 0.1471$.

(b)

$$\begin{aligned}\chi^2_{\mathrm{mod}} &= 20(2/3 - 5\theta)^2 + 50\left(\tfrac{1}{3} - 2\theta\right)^2 + 30(1 - 20\theta/3)^2, \\ (d/d\theta)\chi^2_{\mathrm{mod}} &= -200\left(\tfrac{2}{3} - 5\theta\right) - 200\left(\tfrac{1}{3} - 2\theta\right) - 400(1 - 20\theta/3) \\ &= 0\end{aligned}$$

gives $\hat{\theta} = 0.1475$.

(c) The log likelihood is proportional to $20\log(1/3 - \theta) + 50\log(2/3 - \theta) + 30\log(2\theta)$. The likelihood equation is thus $-20/(\frac{1}{3} - \theta) - 50/(\frac{2}{3} - \theta) + 30/\theta = 0$. The MLE is $\hat{\theta} = 0.1472$.

3. (a) Let $\text{probit}(p) = \Phi^{-1}(p)$. The transformed χ^2 becomes

$$\chi^2_{\text{tr}} = n\sum \frac{\left(\text{probit}(n_j/n) - (\alpha + \beta x_j)\right)^2 \varphi\left((\alpha + \beta x_j)\right)^2}{\Phi(\alpha + \beta x_j)\left(1 - \Phi(\alpha + \beta x_j)\right)},$$

using $d\Phi^{-1}(p)/dp = 1/\Phi'(\Phi^{-1}(p))$. Applying modification:

$$\text{probit } \chi^2 = n\sum \frac{\left(\text{probit}(f_j) - (\alpha + \beta x_j)\right)^2 \varphi\left(\Phi^{-1}(f_j)\right)^2}{f_j(1 - f_j)}.$$

(b) Let $\text{cogit}(p) = \tan(\pi p - \pi/2)$. The transformed modified χ^2 is

$$\text{cogit } \chi^2 = n\sum \frac{\left(\text{cogit}(f_j) - (\alpha + \beta x_j)\right)^2 \cos^4(\pi f_j - \pi/2)}{f_j(1 - f_j)\pi^2}.$$

4. The minimum χ^2 equation of Example 4 is

$$20\left[\frac{-e^{-\theta}}{1 - e^{-\theta}} + \frac{(0.4 - e^{-\theta/2})/2}{1 - e^{-\theta/2}} + \frac{(0.8 - e^{-\theta/4})/4}{1 - e^{-\theta/4}}\right] = 0.$$

We may simplify by replacing the denominators by their estimates

$$-e^{-\theta} + \frac{(0.4 - e^{-\theta/2})/2}{0.6} + \frac{(0.8 - e^{-\theta/4})/4}{0.2} = 0.$$

This reduces to

$$e^{-\theta} + \frac{e^{-\theta/2}}{1.2} + \frac{e^{-\theta/4}}{0.8} = \frac{4}{3}.$$

Solution by numerical methods gives $\theta_n^* = 1.7407\cdots$.

5. $n_1 = 30$, $n_2 = 20$, $n_3 = 50$, $z_1 = \log(0.3)$, $z_2 = \log(0.2)$, $z_3 = \log(0.3)$, $x_1 = 0$, $x_2 = 1$, and $x_3 = -1$. The linearized constraint $\sum n_j a_j = \sum n_j z_j$ gives $\theta_0 = 0.3\theta_1 + c$, where

$$c = 0.3\log 0.3 + 0.2\log 0.2 + 0.5\log 0.5 = -1.0297.$$

$(\partial/\partial\theta_1)Q_n = 0$ leads to the equation

$$\theta_1 = (9\log 0.3 + 26\log 0.2 - 35\log 0.5)/(2.7 + 33.8 + 24.5) = -0.4659,$$

from which we find $\theta_0 = -1.1694$. This results in $p_1 = \exp\{\theta_0\} = 0.3105$, $p_2 = \exp\{\theta_0 + \theta_1\} = 0.1949$, and $p_3 = \exp\{\theta_0 - \theta_1\} = 0.4948$. Because the sum is 1.0002, slightly too large, we modify θ_0 by subtracting $\log(1.0002) = 0.0002$, to make $\theta_0 = -1.1692$.

6. (a) We make the transformation $g(x) = \arcsin(x)$, $g'(x) = (1 - x^2)^{1/2}$, on each coordinate to arrive at the transformed χ^2

$$\chi^2_{\text{tr}} = n \sum (Z_i - \theta_1 x_i - \theta_2)^2,$$

where $Z_i = \arcsin(\bar{Y}_{i\cdot})$ for $i = 1, \ldots, d$. This is now a simple least-squares problem so that

$$\hat{\theta}_1 = \frac{s_{xz}}{s_x^2} \quad \text{and} \quad \hat{\theta}_2 = \bar{Z} - \hat{\theta}_1 \bar{x}.$$

(b) In the transformed χ^2, $\mathbf{A}(\boldsymbol{\theta}) = \theta_1 \mathbf{x} + \theta_2 \mathbf{1}$, so that $\dot{\mathbf{A}}(\boldsymbol{\theta})$ is the $d \times 2$ matrix $(\mathbf{x}\mathbf{1})$. We have

$$\sqrt{n}\left(\hat{\boldsymbol{\theta}}_n - \boldsymbol{\theta}\right) \to \mathscr{N}(\mathbf{0}, \boldsymbol{\Sigma}), \qquad \text{where } \boldsymbol{\Sigma} = \left(\dot{\mathbf{A}}'\mathbf{M}\dot{\mathbf{A}}\right)^{-1}.$$

For the transformed χ^2, $\mathbf{M}$ is the unit matrix, so

$$\boldsymbol{\Sigma} = \left(\dot{\mathbf{A}}'\dot{\mathbf{A}}\right)^{-1} = \begin{pmatrix} \sum X_j^2 & \sum X_j \\ \sum X_j & d \end{pmatrix}^{-1} = \frac{1}{d s_x^2} \begin{pmatrix} 1 & -\bar{X} \\ -\bar{X} & \sum X_j^2 / d \end{pmatrix}.$$

(c) To minimize $\operatorname{var}(\hat{\theta}_1)$, we maximize s_x^2; that is, we put $d/2$ observations at 0 and $d/2$ at 1. The same is true if we try to minimize the determinant. To minimize the asymptotic variance of $\hat{\theta}_2$, we obviously put all the observations at 0, but this gives us no information about $\hat{\theta}_1$. In general, we should put m observations at 0 and $d - m$ at 1, where $m \geq d/2$. A reasonable compromise might be $m = 2d/3$.

SOLUTIONS TO THE EXERCISES OF SECTION 24

1. (a) Under H_0, all expected cell frequencies are equal to 20. So,

$$\chi^2_{H_0} = \frac{(10 - 20)^2}{20} + \frac{(24 - 20)^2}{20} + \cdots + \frac{(16 - 20)^2}{20} = 9.2.$$

This is close to the 10% cutoff point, $\chi^2_5(0.90) = 9.24$, so we accept at the 5% level.

(b) If p_1 and p_6 are known to be equal, then they are estimated as $(n_1 + n_6)/(2n)$, et cetera. The expected cell frequencies become 13, 24, 23, 23, 24, and 13, respectively. We find

$$\chi^2_{H_1} = \frac{(10 - 13)^2}{13} + \cdots = 2.167.$$

Since this χ^2 distribution has 3 degrees of freedom, we obviously accept H_1.

(c) For testing H_0 against H_1, we use $\chi^2_{H_0} - \chi^2_{H_1} = 9.2 - 2.167 = 7.133$. Since this is beyond $\chi^2_2(0.95) = 5.99$ we would reject H_0 if it were known that H_1 were true.

(d) The noncentrality parameters may be computed in the same way as the χ^2's above, but pretending that the observations were 15, 15, 15, 15, 30, and 30, respectively. We find $\phi_{H_0} = (15 - 20)^2/20 + \cdots = 15$. At 5 degrees of freedom at the 5% level, we find the power from the Fix tables (Table 3) to be about $\beta = 0.86$. Similarly, under H_1 we estimate $p_1 = p_6 = (15 + 30)/240$ et cetera and compute $\phi_{H_1} = (15 - 22.5)^2/22.5 + \cdots = 10$. At 3 degrees of freedom, we find the power to be $\beta = 0.86$ again. The noncentrality parameter for the test of H_0 against H_1 is the difference, $\phi = \phi_{H_0} - \phi_{H_1} = 5$. At 2 degrees of freedom, this gives a power of $\beta = 0.50$.

2. (a) Estimate p_{11} by n_{11}/n, $p_{12} = p_{21}$ by $(n_{12} + n_{21})/(2n)$, et cetera, and evaluate the χ^2 as

$$\chi^2_{H_1} = 2\left[\frac{(6 - 8.5)^2}{8.5} + \frac{(10 - 16.5)^2}{16.5} + \frac{(20 - 17.5)^2}{17.5}\right] = 7.306.$$

The χ^2 has 3 degrees of freedom, and since $\chi^2_3(0.95) = 7.81$, we are close to rejecting at the 5% level.

(b) Under hypothesis H_0, the likelihood is proportional to

$$\begin{aligned} L &\sim p_1^{2n_{11}}(p_1 p_2)^{n_{12}+n_{21}}(p_1 p_3)^{n_{13}+n_{31}} p_2^{2n_{22}}(p_2 p_3)^{n_{23}+n_{32}} p_3^{2n_{33}} \\ &= p_1^{n_{1.}+n_{.1}} p_2^{n_{2.}+n_{.2}} p_3^{n_{3.}+n_{.3}}. \end{aligned}$$

We find the maximum-likelihood estimates of p_1, p_2, and p_3 to be $\hat{p}_1 = (n_{1.} + n_{.1})/(2n) = (31 + 49)/400 = 0.20$, $\hat{p}_2 = 0.18$, and $\hat{p}_3 = 0.62$ from which we may compute the table of expected values,

$$\begin{bmatrix} 8 & 7.2 & 24.8 \\ 7.2 & 6.48 & 22.32 \\ 24.8 & 22.32 & 76.88 \end{bmatrix},$$

from which the χ^2 may be computed as $\chi^2_{H_0} = (15 - 8)^2/8 + \cdots = 24.09$. Nine cells and two parameters estimated leaves 6 degrees of freedom. Since $\chi^2_6(0.95) = 12.59$, we reject H_0 strongly.

(c) Our χ^2 is now $\chi^2_{H_0} - \chi^2_{H_1} = 16.78$, again highly significant when compared to $\chi^2_3(0.95) = 7.81$.

3. We find the maximum-likelihood estimates of the p_{ij} under the two hypotheses. The likelihood function, $L(\mathbf{p})$ is proportional to

$$L(\mathbf{p}) \propto \prod_{i=1}^{I} \prod_{j=1}^{J} p_{ij}^{n_{ij}}.$$

(a) Under H, we seek to maximize $L(\mathbf{p})$ under the constraints $\Sigma_{j=1}^{J} p_{ij} = 1/I$. This occurs at $\hat{p}_{ij} = n_{ij}/(In_{i\cdot})$ for all i and j, where $n_{i\cdot} = \Sigma_{j=1}^{J} n_{ij}$. The χ^2 statistic is

$$\chi_a^2 = \sum_{i=1}^{I} \sum_{j=1}^{J} \frac{(n_{ij} - N\hat{p}_{ij})^2}{N\hat{p}_{ij}} = \sum_{i=1}^{I} \frac{(n_{i\cdot} - (N/I))^2}{N/I}.$$

For each i, $J - 1$ parameters were estimated so the χ^2 has $(IJ - 1) - I(J - 1) = I - 1$ degrees of freedom.

(b) Under H_0, we seek to maximize L when p_{ij} is replaced by p_j and we have the constraint $\Sigma_{j=1}^{J} p_j = 1/I$. The maximum-likelihood estimates are $p_j^* = n_{\cdot j}/(IN)$, and the chi-square is

$$\chi_b^2 = \sum_{i=1}^{I} \sum_{j=1}^{J} \frac{(n_{ij} - Np_j^*)^2}{np_j^*}.$$

It has $(IJ - 1) - (J - 1) = IJ - J$ degrees of freedom.

(c) To test H_0 against $H - H_0$, we use $\chi_b^2 - \chi_a^2$. It has $(IJ - J) - (I - 1) = IJ - I - J + 1 = (I - 1)(J - 1)$ degrees of freedom. Under H_0, $\chi_b^2 - \chi_a^2$ is asymptotically equivalent to the χ^2 of Example 1 for testing the homogeneity of a contingency table.

4. All tests are of the form: Reject H_0 if

$$\chi^2 = \sum_{i,j,k} \frac{(n_{ijk} - N\hat{p}_{ijk})^2}{N\hat{p}_{ijk}} \geq \chi^2_{\text{d.f.};\,\alpha}$$

(a) $L \propto \Pi_{ijk}(p_i q_j r_k)^{n_{ijk}} = (\Pi p_i^{n_{i\cdot\cdot}})(\Pi p_j^{n_{\cdot j \cdot}})(\Pi p_k^{n_{\cdot\cdot k}})$, so $\hat{p}_i = n_{i\cdot\cdot}/N$, $\hat{p}_j = n_{\cdot j \cdot}/N$, and $\hat{p}_k = n_{\cdot\cdot k}/N$.

$$\begin{aligned} \text{d.f.} &= (IJK - 1) - (I - 1) - (J - 1) - (K - 1) \\ &= IJK - I - J - K + 2. \end{aligned}$$

(b) $L \propto \prod_{ijk}(p_i q_{jk})^{n_{ijk}} = (\prod p_i^{n_{i\cdot\cdot}})(\prod q_{jk}^{n_{\cdot jk}})$, so $\hat{p}_i = n_{i\cdot\cdot}/N$, $\hat{q}_{jk} = n_{\cdot jk}/N$. d.f. $= (IJK - 1) - (I - 1) - (JK - 1) = (I - 1)(JK - 1)$.

(c) $L \propto \prod_{ijk}(\pi_i q_{jk})^{n_{ijk}} = (\prod \pi_i^{n_{i\cdot\cdot}})(\prod q_{jk}^{n_{\cdot jk}})$, so $\hat{q}_{jk} = n_{\cdot jk}/N$. d.f. $= (IJK - 1) - (JK - 1) = IJK - JK$.

(d) $L \propto \prod_{ijk}(p_{i|k} q_{j|k} r_k)^{n_{ijk}} = (\prod p_{i|k}^{n_{i\cdot k}})(\prod q_{j|k}^{n_{\cdot jk}})(\prod r_k^{n_{\cdot\cdot k}})$, so $\hat{p}_{i|k} = n_{i\cdot k}/n_{\cdot\cdot k}$, $\hat{q}_{j|k} = n_{\cdot jk}/n_{\cdot\cdot k}$, and $\hat{r}_k = n_{\cdot\cdot k}/N$. d.f. $= (IJK - 1) - K(I - 1) - K(J - 1) - (K - 1) = IJK - IK - JK - K$.

(e) $L \propto \prod_{ijk}(p_i q_j r_{k|ij})^{n_{ijk}} = (\prod p_i^{n_{i\cdot\cdot}})(\prod q_j^{n_{\cdot j\cdot}})(\prod r_{k|ij}^{n_{ijk}})$, so $\hat{p}_i = n_{i\cdot\cdot}/N$, $\hat{q}_j = n_{\cdot j\cdot}/N$, and $\hat{r}_{k|ij} = n_{ijk}/n_{ij\cdot}$. $d.f. = (IJK - 1) - (I - 1) - (J - 1) - IJ(K - 1) = (I - 1)(J - 1)$.

5. (a) In this problem, there are 10 independent χ^2's with two cells each. Let n_{ij} and X_{ij} represent the total number of ticks and the number of dead ticks, respectively, of species S_i given treatment T_j. Then, collapsing the two-celled χ^2's into one-celled, we have a χ^2 of the form

$$\chi^2 = \sum_{j=1}^{5} \frac{(X_{1j} - n_{1j}p_j)^2}{n_{1j}p_j(1 - p_j)} + \sum_{j=1}^{5} \frac{(X_{2j} - n_{2j}\pi_j)^2}{n_{2j}\pi_j(1 - \pi_j)},$$

with 10 degrees of freedom. If $p_j = \pi_j$, the common value of p_j and π_j is estimated by the total number of deaths divided by the total number of observations, namely, $\hat{p}_j = \hat{\pi}_j = (X_{1j} + X_{2j})/(n_{1j} + n_{2j})$. Thus, $\hat{p}_1 = \hat{\pi}_1 = (30 + 42)/(50 + 77) = 0.567$, $\hat{p}_2 = 0.728$, $\hat{p}_3 = 0.552$, $\hat{p}_4 = 0.308$, $\hat{p}_5 = 0.400$. Replacing the p_j and the π_j in the χ^2 by their estimates, we find

$$\chi^2 = \frac{1.65^2}{12.28} + \frac{3.42^2}{10.5} + \frac{0.08^2}{28.1} + \frac{1.23^2}{13.0} + \frac{0.2^2}{6.72}$$
$$+ \frac{1.65^2}{18.9} + \frac{3.42^2}{12.08} + \frac{0.08^2}{9.89} + \frac{1.23^2}{9.16} + \frac{0.2^2}{12.48} = 2.73. \quad (1)$$

Since we lost 5 degrees of freedom estimating five parameters, this χ^2 has five degrees of freedom, so the null hypothesis is obviously accepted.

(b) The numerators of the χ^2 in (1) depend on the X_{1j} and X_{2j} only through the differences, $(X_{1j}/n_{1j}) - (X_{2j}/n_{2j})$. In fact,

$$(X_{1j} - \hat{p}_j)^2 = \frac{n_{1j}^2 n_{2j}^2}{(n_{1j} + n_{2j})^2}\left(\frac{X_{1j}}{n_{1j}} - \frac{X_{2j}}{n_{2j}}\right)^2.$$

The noncentrality parameter at any alternative such that $p_j - \pi_j =$

0.1 may be found by replacing the differences $(X_{1j}/n_{1j}) - (X_{2j}/n_{2j})$ by 0.1 in the numerators of the χ^2.

$$\phi = \frac{3.03^2}{12.28} + \frac{2.84^2}{10.5} + \frac{2.96^2}{28.1} + \frac{2.52^2}{13.0} + \frac{1.82^2}{6.72}$$

$$\frac{3.03^2}{18.9} + \frac{2.84^2}{12.08} + \frac{2.96^2}{9.89} + \frac{2.52^2}{9.16} + \frac{1.82^2}{12.48} = 5.81.$$

From the Fix Tables at $\alpha = .05$ and 5 degrees of freedom, we find that the power is only about 0.42.

References

R. R. Bahadur (1958). Examples of inconsistency of maximum likelihood estimates. *Sankhyā 20*, 207–210.

O. E. Barndorff-Nielsen and D. R. Cox (1989). *Asymptotic Techniques for Use in Statistics*. Chapman and Hall, London, New York.

A. C. Berry (1941). The accuracy of the Gaussian approximation to the sum of independent variates. *Trans. Amer. Math. Soc. 49*, 122–136.

R. Bhattacharya (1990). Asymptotic expansions in statistics. In *Asymptotic Statistics. DMV Seminar, Band 14*. Birkhäuser Verlag, 9–66.

J. A. Bucklew (1990). *Large Deviation Techniques in Decision, Simulation, and Estimation*. John Wiley & Sons, New York.

K. L. Chung (1974). *A Course in Probability Theory*, 2/e. Harcourt Brace and World, New York.

H. Cramér (1946). *Mathematical Methods of Statistics*. Princeton University Press, Princeton, NJ.

M. Denker (1985). *Asymptotic Distribution Theory in Nonparametric Statistics*. Friedr. Vieweg & Sohn, Braunschweig.

G. Esseen (1944). Fourier analysis of distribution functions. A mathematical study of the Gauss-Laplacian law. *Acta Math. 77*, 1–125.

W. Feller. *An Introduction to Probability Theory and Its Applications*, Vol. 1 (3/e, 1968); Vol. 2 (1966). John Wiley & Sons, New York.

E. Fix (1949). Tables of the non-central χ^2. *Univ. Calif. Pub. in Statist. 1*, 15–19.

J. Galambos (1978). *Asymptotic Theory of Extreme Order Statistics*. John Wiley & Sons, New York.

J. Hájek (1961). Some extensions of the Wald-Wolfowitz-Noether theorem. *Ann. Math. Statist. 32*, 506–523.

J. Hájek and Z. v. Sidák (1967). *Theory of Rank Tests*. Academic Press, New York.

P. Hall (1992). *The Bootstrap and Edgeworth Expansion*. Springer-Verlag, New York.

W. Hoeffding (1948). A class of statistics with asymptotically normal distribution. *Ann. Math. Statist. 19*, 293.

L. Le Cam (1953). On some asymptotic properties of maximum likelihood estimates and related estimates. *Univ. Calif. Publ. in Statist. 1*, 277–330.

L. Le Cam (1986). *Asymptotic Methods in Statistical Decision Theory*. Springer-Verlag, New York.

L. Le Cam and G. L. Yang (1990). *Asymptotics in Statistics*, Springer-Verlag, New York.

J. Neyman (1949). Contribution to the theory of the χ^2 test. *Proc. (First) Berkeley Symp. on Math. Statist. and Prob.*, 239–273.

J. Neyman and E. L. Scott (1948). Consistent estimates based on partially consistent observations. *Econometrica 16*, 1–32.

G. E. Noether (1949). On a theorem of Wald and Wolfowitz. *Ann. Math. Statist. 20*, 455.

E. H. Oliver (1972). A maximum likelihood oddity. *American Statistician 26*, No. 2, 43–44.

T. Parthasarathy (1972). *Selection Theorems and their Applications*. Lecture Notes in Mathematics 263. Springer-Verlag, New York.

B. L. S. Prakasa Rao (1987). *Asymptotic Theory of Statistical Inference*. John Wiley & Sons, New York.

C. R. Rao (1973). *Linear Statistical Inference and Its Applications*, 2/e. John Wiley & Sons, New York.

H. Scheffé (1947). A useful convergence theorem for probability distributions. *Ann. Math. Statist. 18*, 434–458.

P. K. Sen and J. M. Singer (1993). *Large Sample Methods in Statistics*. Chapman and Hall, London, New York.

J. M. Steele (1994). Le Cam's inequality and Poisson approximation. *Amer. Math. Monthly 101*, 48–54.

P. van Beek (1972). An application of Fourier methods to the problem of sharpening the Berry-Esseen inequality. *Z. Wahrscheinlichkeitstheorie verw. Geb. 23*, 187–196.

J. von Neumann (1949). On rings of operators. Reduction theory. *Ann. Math. 50*, 401–485.

A. Wald (1949). Note on the consistency of the maximum likelihood estimate, *Ann. Math. Statist. 20*, 595–601.

A. Wald and J. Wolfwitz (1944). Statistical tests based on permutations of the observations. *Ann. Math. Statist. 15*, 358–372.

S. S. Wilks (1938). The large-sample distribution of the likelihood ratio for testing composite hypotheses. *Ann. Math. Statist. 9*, 60–62.

Index